Medical Data Processing and Analysis—2nd Edition

Medical Data Processing and Analysis—2nd Edition

Guest Editors

Wan Azani Mustafa
Hiam Alquran

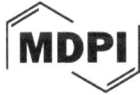

Basel • Beijing • Wuhan • Barcelona • Belgrade • Novi Sad • Cluj • Manchester

Guest Editors

Wan Azani Mustafa
Faculty of Engineering & Technology
Universiti Malaysia Perlis
Perlis
Malaysia

Hiam Alquran
Department of Biomedical Systems and Informatics Engineering
Yarmouk University
Irbid
Jordan

Editorial Office
MDPI AG
Grosspeteranlage 5
4052 Basel, Switzerland

This is a reprint of the Special Issue, published open access by the journal *Diagnostics* (ISSN 2075-4418), freely accessible at: https://www.mdpi.com/journal/diagnostics/special_issues/QQZ4N5NO56.

For citation purposes, cite each article independently as indicated on the article page online and as indicated below:

Lastname, A.A.; Lastname, B.B. Article Title. *Journal Name* **Year**, *Volume Number*, Page Range.

ISBN 978-3-7258-3503-4 (Hbk)
ISBN 978-3-7258-3504-1 (PDF)
https://doi.org/10.3390/books978-3-7258-3504-1

© 2025 by the authors. Articles in this book are Open Access and distributed under the Creative Commons Attribution (CC BY) license. The book as a whole is distributed by MDPI under the terms and conditions of the Creative Commons Attribution-NonCommercial-NoDerivs (CC BY-NC-ND) license (https://creativecommons.org/licenses/by-nc-nd/4.0/).

Contents

About the Editors vii

Preface ix

Wan Azani Mustafa and Hiam Alquran
Editorial for the Special Issue "Medical Data Processing and Analysis—2nd Edition"
Reprinted from: *Diagnostics* **2025**, *15*, 1170, https://doi.org/10.3390/diagnostics15091170 1

Kagan Tur
Multi-Modal Machine Learning Approach for COVID-19 Detection Using Biomarkers and X-Ray Imaging
Reprinted from: *Diagnostics* **2024**, *14*, 2800, https://doi.org/10.3390/diagnostics14242800 6

Jeferson David Gallo-Aristizabal, Daniel Escobar-Grisales, Cristian David Ríos-Urrego, Jesús Francisco Vargas-Bonilla, Adolfo M. García and Juan Rafael Orozco-Arroyave
Towards Parkinson's Disease Detection Through Analysis of Everyday Handwriting
Reprinted from: *Diagnostics* **2025**, *15*, 381, https://doi.org/10.3390/diagnostics15030381 19

Insu Jeon, Minjoong Kim, Dayeong So, Eun Young Kim, Yunyoung Nam, Seungsoo Kim, et al.
Reliable Autism Spectrum Disorder Diagnosis for Pediatrics Using Machine Learning and Explainable AI
Reprinted from: *Diagnostics* **2024**, *14*, 2504, https://doi.org/10.3390/diagnostics14222504 32

Karim Gasmi, Hajer Ayadi, Mouna Torjmen
Enhancing Medical Image Retrieval with UMLS-Integrated CNN-Based Text Indexing
Reprinted from: *Diagnostics* **2024**, *14*, 1204, https://doi.org/10.3390/diagnostics14111204 68

Mohd Anjum, Hong Min and Zubair Ahmed
A Novel Framework for Data Assessment That Uses Edge Technology to Improve the Detection of Communicable Diseases
Reprinted from: *Diagnostics* **2024**, *14*, 1148, https://doi.org/10.3390/diagnostics14111148 86

Ahmed Alsayat, Mahmoud Elmezain, Saad Alanazi, Meshrif Alruily, Ayman Mohamed Mostafa and Wael Said
Multi-Layer Preprocessing and U-Net with Residual Attention Block for Retinal Blood Vessel Segmentation
Reprinted from: *Diagnostics* **2023**, *13*, 3364, https://doi.org/10.3390/diagnostics13213364 106

Ahila Amarnath, Poongodi Manoharan, Buvaneswari Natarajan, Roobaea Alroobaea, Majed Alsafyani, Abdullah M. Baqasah, et al.
Medical Image Despeckling Using the Invertible Sparse Fuzzy Wavelet Transform with Nature-Inspired Minibatch Water Wave Swarm Optimization
Reprinted from: *Diagnostics* **2023**, *13*, 2919, https://doi.org/10.3390/diagnostics13182919 126

Mohammed Alsalatie, Hiam Alquran, Wan Azani Mustafa, Ala'a Zyout, Ali Mohammad Alqudah, Reham Kaifi and Suhair Qudsieh
A New Weighted Deep Learning Feature Using Particle Swarm and Ant Lion Optimization for Cervical Cancer Diagnosis on Pap Smear Images
Reprinted from: *Diagnostics* **2023**, *13*, 2762, https://doi.org/10.3390/diagnostics13172762 142

Muhammad Shahzad, Muhammad Atif Tahir, Musaed Alhussein, Ansharah Mobin, Rauf Ahmed Shams Malick and Muhammad Shahid Anwar
NeuPD—A Neural Network-Based Approach to Predict Antineoplastic Drug Response
Reprinted from: *Diagnostics* **2023**, *13*, 2043, https://doi.org/10.3390/diagnostics13122043 . . . . **161**

Masyitah Abu, Nik Adilah Hanin Zahri, Amiza Amir, Muhammad Izham Ismail, Azhany Yaakub, Fumiyo Fukumoto and Yoshimi Suzuki
Analysis of the Effectiveness of Metaheuristic Methods on Bayesian Optimization in the Classification of Visual Field Defects
Reprinted from: *Diagnostics* **2023**, *13*, 1946, https://doi.org/10.3390/diagnostics13111946 . . . . **178**

Muhammad Amin, Khalil Ullah, Muhammad Asif, Habib Shah, Arshad Mehmood and Muhammad Attique Khan
Real-World Driver Stress Recognition and Diagnosis Based on Multimodal Deep Learning and Fuzzy EDAS Approaches
Reprinted from: *Diagnostics* **2023**, *13*, 1897, https://doi.org/10.3390/diagnostics13111897 . . . . **196**

Abdullah M. Albarrak
Improving the Trustworthiness of Interactive Visualization Tools for Healthcare Data through a Medical Fuzzy Expert System
Reprinted from: *Diagnostics* **2023**, *13*, 1733, https://doi.org/10.3390/diagnostics13101733 . . . . **247**

Ratchakit Phetrittikun, Kerdkiat Suvirat, Kanakorn Horsiritham, Thammasin Ingviya and Sitthichok Chaichulee
Prediction of Acid-Base and Potassium Imbalances in Intensive Care Patients Using Machine Learning Techniques
Reprinted from: *Diagnostics* **2023**, *13*, 1171, https://doi.org/10.3390/diagnostics13061171 . . . . **265**

Bader M. Albahlal
Emerging Technology-Driven Hybrid Models for Preventing and Monitoring Infectious Diseases: A Comprehensive Review and Conceptual Framework
Reprinted from: *Diagnostics* **2023**, *13*, 3047, https://doi.org/10.3390/diagnostics13193047 . . . . **288**

About the Editors

Wan Azani Mustafa

Wan Azani Mustafa received his degree in Biomedical Electronic Engineering (2013) and a PhD in Mechatronic Engineering (2017) from University Malaysia Perlis (UniMAP). He is a member of the Board of Engineers Malaysia (BEM) (2014) and the Malaysia Board of Technologists (MBOT) (2017), and he is a Senior Member of the IEEE. He is currently a Senior Lecturer at University Malaysia Perlis, Malaysia. He has published more than 390 academic articles with Scopus H-Index 21, and his current interests include image processing, biomechanics, intelligence systems, and computer science.

Hiam Alquran

Hiam Alquran, Professor at Department of Biomedical Systems and Informatics Engineering, Yarmouk University, Jordan. Alquran received her PhD (2014) degree in Biomedical and Biotechnology Engineering from Massachusetts Lowell University, USA, her M.Sc. degree (2008) in Automation Engineering from Yarmouk University, and her B.S.c in Biomedical Engineering from JUST -Jordan (2005). Her research interests pertain to medical image processing, digital signal processing, pattern recognition and deep learning.

Preface

This Special Issue, "Medical Data Processing and Analysis", explores cutting-edge advancements in biomedical data processing, modeling, and analysis to address critical challenges in healthcare. Medical data encompass various forms of patient information, such as signals, images, and biochemical components, offering significant insights into a patient's condition and disease progression. The evolution of computer-aided diagnostic (CAD) systems, fueled by advancements in artificial intelligence (AI), machine learning (ML), and deep learning, has transformed how medical data are processed and analyzed. These technologies enable accurate image segmentation, classification, and region-of-interest identification, leading to improved diagnostic and prognostic capabilities.

This Special Issue aims to showcase innovative approaches to healthcare applications, including patient monitoring, disease diagnosis and progression, rehabilitation, and medical image analysis. It highlights how robust signal processing, data modeling, and novel computational tools facilitate a better understanding of patient status, disease stages, and treatment planning. Addressing challenges such as limited datasets and data variability, these works emphasize the critical role of technological innovation in overcoming barriers to accurate, personalized healthcare solutions.

Through this collection, we aim to inspire researchers and practitioners to leverage these advancements, fostering collaborations that push the boundaries of biomedical data processing and accelerate the development of impactful, patient-centered solutions in modern medicine.

Wan Azani Mustafa and Hiam Alquran
Guest Editors

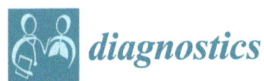

Editorial

Editorial for the Special Issue "Medical Data Processing and Analysis—2nd Edition"

Wan Azani Mustafa [1,2,*] and Hiam Alquran [3]

1. Faculty of Electrical Engineering & Technology, Campus Pauh Putra, Universiti Malaysia Perlis, Arau 02600, Malaysia
2. Advanced Computing (AdvComp), Centre of Excellence (CoE), Universiti Malaysia Perlis, Arau 02600, Malaysia
3. Department of Biomedical Systems and Informatics Engineering, Yarmouk University, Irbid 21163, Jordan; heyam.q@yu.edu.jo
* Correspondence: wanazani@unimap.edu.my

Medical data processing and analysis have become central to advancements in healthcare, driven largely by the need for accurate diagnosis, personalized treatment, and efficient healthcare system management [1–3]. A major trend in this domain is addressing the limitations of insufficient quality data through human-in-the-loop (HITL) approaches [4], explainable AI (XAI) frameworks [5], and blockchain-based security models [6]. Current expansions in machine learning, computer vision, and edge computing have significantly impacted the early detection and diagnosis of various types of diseases [7–11]. Many studies demonstrate innovative applicable approaches to neurological disorders, infectious diseases, developmental conditions, and medical image retrieval.

On the other hand, Tur [12] introduced a multi-modal machine learning framework for identifying COVID-19 utilizing a combination of many biochemical biomarkers and chest X-ray imaging. The proposed hybrid model combines data from both sources, and ensemble learning was employed to enhance its diagnostic accuracy over single-modality approaches. The study emphasized the impact of multimodal data fusion when concentrating on heterogeneous manifestations of infectious diseases. However, Jeon et al. [13] surveyed machine learning and explainable AI (XAI) for the dependable diagnosis of autism spectrum disorder (ASD) in pediatric patients. They developed neurodevelopmental features and behavioral assessments for building a high-performance diagnostic model. Prominently, utilizing XAI modified the interpretation, and the assessments were shown to be appropriate for clinical adoption by enhancing trustable models. In contrast, Gasmi et al. [14] investigated the enhancement of medical image retrieval by incorporating Unified Medical Language System (UMLS) concepts with a convolutional neural network (CNN)-based text indexing method. Their proposed system develops semantics that recognize medical reports and can combine these semantics with related images. Their recommended approach fills the gap between clinical language and image databases, assisting image retrieval precisely in clinical decision support systems.

Mosqueira-Rey et al. [15] emphasized the role of HITL in overcoming data bottlenecks in deep learning models for pancreatic cancer treatment, combining synthetic data augmentation using generative adversarial networks (GANs) and expert feedback through active learning. Together, these works highlight an increasing focus on privacy-preserving models and patient acceptance, though obstacles such as encryption overheads and equitable technology access persist. Singh and Mantri [16] similarly focused on improving preprocessing and feature selection strategies via Rough Set Theory (RST) to optimize data dimensionality, enhancing the performance of clinical decision support systems (CDSS). Hussain and Mishra [17] demonstrated the application of AI and big data in COVID-19 diagnosis, employing deep learning on medical images amid data scarcity challenges. Collectively, these studies underscore that while data augmentation and expert integration help mitigate data limitations, complexities in model integration and data quality assurance remain persistent issues. Parallel to data-centric innovations, patient trust and data security have emerged as critical considerations. Paccoud et al. [18] explored patient perspectives on adopting digital medical devices (DMDs) for Parkinson's disease management, finding a general willingness tempered by demographic differences. Addressing confidentiality concerns, Affum and Enchill [19] introduced a division-free gradient descent multivariate regression approach to encrypted medical data, ensuring secure machine learning without exposing sensitive patient information.

Advancements in electronic medical record (EMR) processing have also demonstrated strong potential but revealed dependencies on robust feature extraction and explainable model structures. Pham et al. [20] developed a validated case definition for rheumatoid arthritis (RA) using a tree-based ensemble, identifying XGBoost as particularly effective for generating interpretable outcomes suitable for primary care. Singh and Mantri [16] achieved improved classification for diseases like breast cancer and thyroid disorders through integrated machine learning models and advanced feature selection. Hussain and Mishra [17] similarly used convolutional neural networks and transfer learning to enhance COVID-19 diagnosis accuracy. Although these techniques produced promising results, their reliance on structured datasets limits their real-world applicability, where data heterogeneity is common. Alongside technical challenges, interpretability and ethical concerns have come to the forefront. Hakkoum et al. [21] conducted a comprehensive evaluation of interpretability techniques for supervised machine learning models, emphasizing the tension between model transparency and performance in medical applications. Hossain et al. echoed this concern, noting healthcare professionals' hesitancy to adopt deep neural networks (DNNs) due to their "black-box" nature, thus advocating for stronger development of XAI methods. Shakhovska et al. [22] proposed a hybrid XAI system combining multiple neural network architectures to improve interpretability and clinical relevance, suggesting a promising avenue toward balancing performance and transparency.

Ethical challenges in AI-driven healthcare also involve the heavy reliance on statistical generalizations rather than individualized patient evidence. Holm [23] argued that AI systems based solely on statistical estimations can lead to ethical dilemmas in resource allocation, resonating with critiques from Hakkoum et al. [21] and Hossain et al. [24] regarding the need for more trustworthy, context-sensitive AI models. While statistical models may provide transparency, they often lack the nuanced sensitivity to handle complex biological variations, highlighting a need for future models that integrate statistical clarity with deep learning capabilities.

From a practical application standpoint, machine learning has been increasingly utilized to predict healthcare outcomes and optimize system behaviors. Park et al. [25] illustrated this by predicting the closure of medical and dental clinics using administrative health insurance data combined with Support Vector Machines (SVMs), Random Forests (RF), and Extreme Gradient Boosting (XGBoost). Similarly, Maheshwari et al. [26] applied machine learning and blockchain technologies to predict transaction types within healthcare systems, advancing decentralized healthcare data management. Security, data integrity, and system optimization have become key priorities in handling decentralized medical data. Khan et al. [27] highlighted the importance of blockchain in facilitating secure communications among heterogeneous medical devices integrated through AI-enabled machine learning models.

Karthiyayini et al. [28] addressed challenges in the secure transmission of medical image data by proposing the Enhanced Model for Medical Image Data Security (EM-MIDS), incorporating machine learning approaches such as K-Means Clustering (KMC) and Random Forest (RF) for classification, supported by Support Vector Machine (SVM) for security evaluation. The integration of chaotic maps and channel-based methodologies added robustness to the encryption–decryption framework. Comparative studies suggested EM-MIDS's superiority over existing models, particularly concerning data accuracy and privacy integrity. Meanwhile, Alyahyan [29] introduced a Transformer-based Attention-Guided CNN (TAGCNN) for disease diagnosis, achieving notable improvements in accuracy compared to conventional models like ResNet50, AlexNet, and DenseNet169. While both studies demonstrated the growing efficacy of machine learning in medical imaging, a potential limitation is the narrow focus on specific datasets, such as benchmark medical images or osteoporosis X-rays, which may limit generalizability across broader clinical applications.

Machine learning's application in triaging outpatient care through heterogeneous data further illustrates the transformative potential of automated systems. Salman et al. [30] developed an early triage prediction model using multiple machine learning algorithms, such as SVM, Random Forest, Decision Tree, Logistic Regression, Naive Bayes, and K-Nearest Neighbor, with Decision Tree algorithms achieving the highest performance of 93.5%. That study emphasized the importance of integrating diverse Internet of Medical Things (IoMT) data, including ECG, blood pressure, and SpO2 measurements, into patient assessment processes. Complementing this, Kural et al. [31] explored the application of supervised and unsupervised learning methods like Sammon mapping and Extreme Gradient Boosting (XGBoost) for identifying anaphylaxis in claims databases. Their findings highlighted the value of automated feature selection pipelines for refining disease identification algorithms, particularly in settings where ground truth data are sparse or varied. However, both research efforts acknowledged the complexity of handling heterogeneous medical datasets, often complicated by inconsistencies in data quality and format, underlining a need for more robust, adaptable models capable of handling real-world clinical variability. The challenge of generalization in artificial intelligence (AI) models for healthcare remains significant, particularly when confronting biases intrinsic to training datasets. Ong Ly et al. [32] systematically investigated shortcut learning, where models inadvertently learn irrelevant patterns from biased data acquisition processes rather than genuine clinical features. Their development of PEst, a bias-corrected external accuracy estimator, significantly improved generalization assessments without requiring external datasets, reducing overestimation of model performance by an average of 20%.

In conclusion, medical data processing and analysis are rapidly advancing through human-in-the-loop approaches, privacy-preserving AI, blockchain-based security, and explainable machine learning frameworks. However, the field must address crucial challenges related to model generalizability, ethical considerations, patient trust, equitable access, and computational efficiency. Future research must prioritize interdisciplinary strategies that integrate technical innovation with patient-centered, transparent, and secure healthcare solutions to ensure AI-driven tools are both accurate and ethically sound.

Author Contributions: Conceptualization, W.A.M. and H.A.; methodology, W.A.M.; software, W.A.M.; validation, W.A.M. and H.A.; formal analysis, H.A.; investigation, H.A.; resources, W.A.M.; data curation, H.A.; writing—original draft preparation, H.A.; writing—review and editing, W.A.M. and H.A.; visualization, H.A.; supervision, W.A.M.; project administration, W.A.M.; funding acquisition, W.A.M. All authors have read and agreed to the published version of the manuscript.

Funding: This research received no external funding.

Conflicts of Interest: The authors declare no conflicts of interest.

References

1. Yean, C.W.; Ahmad, W.K.W.; Mustafa, W.A.; Murugappan, M.; Rajamanickam, Y.; Adom, A.H.; Omar, M.I.; Zheng, B.S.; Junoh, A.K.; Razlan, Z.M.; et al. An emotion assessment of stroke patients by using bispectrum features of EEG signals. *Brain Sci.* **2020**, *10*, 672. [CrossRef]
2. Yin, P.; Yin, T.; Zhao, S.; Yu, S. Construction of a secure storage and sharing model for medical data under computer network technology. *Appl. Math. Nonlinear Sci.* **2024**, *9*, 888. [CrossRef]
3. Alsalatie, M.; Alquran, H.; Mustafa, W.A.; Mohd Yacob, Y.; Ali Alayed, A. Analysis of Cytology Pap Smear Images Based on Ensemble Deep Learning Approach. *Diagnostics* **2022**, *12*, 2756. [CrossRef]
4. Budd, S.; Robinson, E.C.; Kainz, B. A survey on active learning and human-in-the-loop deep learning for medical image analysis. *Med. Image Anal.* **2021**, *71*, 102062. [CrossRef] [PubMed]
5. van der Velden, B.H.M.; Kuijf, H.J.; Gilhuijs, K.G.A.; Viergever, M.A. Explainable artificial intelligence (XAI) in deep learning-based medical image analysis. *Med. Image Anal.* **2022**, *79*, 102470. [CrossRef] [PubMed]
6. Qu, J. Blockchain in medical informatics. *J. Ind. Inf. Integr.* **2022**, *25*, 100258. [CrossRef]
7. Schaefer, J.; Lehne, M.; Schepers, J.; Prasser, F.; Thun, S. The use of machine learning in rare diseases: A scoping review. *Orphanet J. Rare Dis.* **2020**, *15*, 145. [CrossRef]
8. Chittora, P.; Chaurasia, S.; Chakrabarti, P.; Kumawat, G.; Chakrabarti, T.; Leonowicz, Z.; Jasinski, M.; Jasinski, L.; Gono, R.; Jasinska, E.; et al. Prediction of Chronic Kidney Disease—A Machine Learning Perspective. *IEEE Access* **2021**, *9*, 17312–17334. [CrossRef]
9. Kaur, C.; Kumar, M.S.; Anjum, A.; Binda, M.B.; Mallu, M.R.; Ansari, M.S. Al Chronic Kidney Disease Prediction Using Machine Learning. *J. Adv. Inf. Technol.* **2023**, *14*, 384–391. [CrossRef]
10. Mustafa, W.A.; Halim, A.; Jamlos, M.A.; Syed Idrus, Z.S. A Review: Pap Smear Analysis Based on Image Processing Approach. *J. Phys. Conf. Ser.* **2020**, *1529*, 1–13. [CrossRef]
11. Mustafa, W.A.B.W.; Yazid, H.; Yaacob, S.B.; Basah, S.N. Bin Blood vessel extraction using morphological operation for diabetic retinopathy. In Proceedings of the 2014 IEEE Region 10 Symposium, Kuala Lumpur, Malaysia, 14–16 April 2014; pp. 208–212. [CrossRef]
12. Tur, K. Multi-Modal Machine Learning Approach for COVID-19 Detection Using Biomarkers and X-Ray Imaging. *Diagnostics* **2024**, *14*, 2800. [CrossRef]
13. Jeon, I.; Kim, M.; So, D.; Kim, E.Y.; Nam, Y.; Kim, S.; Shim, S.; Kim, J.; Moon, J. Reliable Autism Spectrum Disorder Diagnosis for Pediatrics Using Machine Learning and Explainable AI. *Diagnostics* **2024**, *14*, 2504. [CrossRef]
14. Gasmi, K.; Ayadi, H.; Torjmen, M. Enhancing Medical Image Retrieval with UMLS-Integrated CNN-Based Text Indexing. *Diagnostics* **2024**, *14*, 1204. [CrossRef] [PubMed]
15. Mosqueira-Rey, E.; Hernández-Pereira, E.; Bobes-Bascarán, J.; Alonso-Ríos, D.; Pérez-Sánchez, A.; Fernández-Leal, Á.; Moret-Bonillo, V.; Vidal-Ínsua, Y.; Vázquez-Rivera, F. Addressing the data bottleneck in medical deep learning models using a human-in-the-loop machine learning approach. *Neural Comput. Appl.* **2024**, *36*, 2597–2616. [CrossRef]
16. Singh, K.N.; Mantri, J.K. Clinical decision support system based on RST with machine learning for medical data classification. *Multimed. Tools Appl.* **2024**, *83*, 39707–39730. [CrossRef]
17. Hussain, M.J.; Mishra, A. Transforming Public Health with AI and Big Data Deep Learning for COVID-19 Detection in Medical Imaging. *J. Intell. Syst. Internet Things* **2025**, *16*, 42–59. [CrossRef]
18. Paccoud, I.; Valero, M.M.; Marín, L.C.; Bontridder, N.; Ibrahim, A.; Winkler, J.; Fomo, M.; Sapienza, S.; Khoury, F.; Corvol, J.-C.; et al. Patient perspectives on the use of digital medical devices and health data for AI-driven personalised medicine in Parkinson's Disease. *Front. Neurol.* **2024**, *15*, 1453243. [CrossRef]
19. Affum, E.; Enchill, M. Data Confidentiality in Machine Learning: Exploring Multivariate Regression and Its Application on Encrypted Medical Data. *SN Comput. Sci.* **2024**, *5*, 335. [CrossRef]
20. Pham, A.N.Q.; Barber, C.E.H.; Drummond, N.; Jasper, L.; Klein, D.; Lindeman, C.; Widdifield, J.; Williamson, T.; Jones, C.A. Development and validation of a rheumatoid arthritis case definition: A machine learning approach using data from primary care electronic medical records. *BMC Med. Inform. Decis. Mak.* **2024**, *24*, 360. [CrossRef]
21. Hakkoum, H.; Idri, A.; Abnane, I. Global and local interpretability techniques of supervised machine learning black box models for numerical medical data. *Eng. Appl. Artif. Intell.* **2024**, *131*, 107829. [CrossRef]
22. Shakhovska, N.; Shebeko, A.; Prykarpatskyy, Y. A novel explainable ai model for medical data analysis. *J. Artif. Intell. Soft Comput. Res.* **2024**, *14*, 121–137. [CrossRef]
23. Holm, S. Data-driven decisions about individual patients: The case of medical AI. *J. Eval. Clin. Pract.* **2024**, *30*, 735–740. [CrossRef] [PubMed]

24. Hossain, M.D.I.; Zamzmi, G.; Mouton, P.R.; Salekin, M.D.S.; Sun, Y.; Goldgof, D. Explainable AI for Medical Data: Current Methods, Limitations, and Future Directions. *ACM Comput. Surv.* **2025**, *57*, 148. [CrossRef]
25. Park, Y.-T.; Kim, D.; Jeon, J.S.; Kim, K.G. Predictors of Medical and Dental Clinic Closure by Machine Learning Methods: Cross-Sectional Study Using Empirical Data. *J. Med. Internet Res.* **2024**, *26*, e46608. [CrossRef] [PubMed]
26. Maheshwari, S.; Jain, P.K.; Al-Sharify, N.T.; Ghosh, S.; Dubey, D.; Kaur, G. Medical data analysis and transaction type prediction using machine learning and blockchain technology. *IET Blockchain* **2025**, *5*, e70001. [CrossRef]
27. Khan, A.A.; Laghari, A.A.; Baqasah, A.M.; Bacarra, R.; Alroobaea, R.; Alsafyani, M.; Alsayaydeh, J.A.J. BDLT-IoMT—A novel architecture: SVM machine learning for robust and secure data processing in Internet of Medical Things with blockchain cybersecurity. *J. Supercomput.* **2025**, *81*, 271. [CrossRef]
28. Karthiyayini, S.; John Simon Christopher, J.; Sheik Arafat, I.; Syed Moomin, F.M.H. Enhanced Model for Medical Image Data Security Using Machine Learning. *SN Comput. Sci.* **2024**, *5*, 1103. [CrossRef]
29. Alyahyan, S. Applying machine learning classification techniques for disease diagnosis from medical imaging data using Transformer based Attention Guided CNN (TAGCNN). *Multimed. Tools Appl.* **2024**, *83*, 72861–72887. [CrossRef]
30. Salman, O.S.; Latiff, N.M.A.; Arifin, S.H.S.; Salman, O.H. Early Triage Prediction for Outpatient Care Based on Heterogeneous Medical Data Utilizing Machine Learning. *Pertanika J. Sci. Technol.* **2024**, *32*, 2343–2367. [CrossRef]
31. Kural, K.C.; Mazo, I.; Walderhaug, M.; Santana-Quintero, L.; Karagiannis, K.; Thompson, E.E.; Kelman, J.A.; Goud, R. Using machine learning to improve anaphylaxis case identification in medical claims data. *JAMIA Open* **2024**, *7*, ooae037. [CrossRef]
32. Ong Ly, C.; Unnikrishnan, B.; Tadic, T.; Patel, T.; Duhamel, J.; Kandel, S.; Moayedi, Y.; Brudno, M.; Hope, A.; Ross, H.; et al. Shortcut learning in medical AI hinders generalization: Method for estimating AI model generalization without external data. *NPJ Digit. Med.* **2024**, *7*, 124. [CrossRef] [PubMed]

Disclaimer/Publisher's Note: The statements, opinions and data contained in all publications are solely those of the individual author(s) and contributor(s) and not of MDPI and/or the editor(s). MDPI and/or the editor(s) disclaim responsibility for any injury to people or property resulting from any ideas, methods, instructions or products referred to in the content.

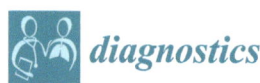

Article

Multi-Modal Machine Learning Approach for COVID-19 Detection Using Biomarkers and X-Ray Imaging

Kagan Tur

Internal Medicine Department, Faculty of Medicine, Ahi Evran University, Kirsehir 40200, Turkey; kagan.tur@ahievran.edu.tr; Tel.: +90-50-577-339-27

Abstract: *Background*: Accurate and rapid detection of COVID-19 remains critical for clinical management, especially in resource-limited settings. Current diagnostic methods face challenges in terms of speed and reliability, creating a need for complementary AI-based models that integrate diverse data sources. *Objectives*: This study aimed to develop and evaluate a multi-modal machine learning model that combines clinical biomarkers and chest X-ray images to enhance diagnostic accuracy and provide interpretable insights. *Methods*: We used a dataset of 250 patients (180 COVID-19 positive and 70 negative cases) collected from clinical settings. Biomarkers such as CRP, ferritin, NLR, and albumin were included alongside chest X-ray images. Random Forest and Gradient Boosting models were used for biomarkers, and ResNet and VGG CNN architectures were applied to imaging data. A late-fusion strategy integrated predictions from these modalities. Stratified k-fold cross-validation ensured robust evaluation while preventing data leakage. Model performance was assessed using AUC-ROC, F1-score, Specificity, Negative Predictive Value (NPV), and Matthews Correlation Coefficient (MCC), with confidence intervals calculated via bootstrap resampling. *Results*: The Gradient Boosting + VGG fusion model achieved the highest performance, with an AUC-ROC of 0.94, F1-score of 0.93, Specificity of 93%, NPV of 96%, and MCC of 0.91. SHAP and LIME interpretability analyses identified CRP, ferritin, and specific lung regions as key contributors to predictions. *Discussion*: The proposed multi-modal approach significantly enhances diagnostic accuracy compared to single-modality models. Its interpretability aligns with clinical understanding, supporting its potential for real-world application.

Keywords: multi-modal machine learning; COVID-19 diagnostics; biomarkers and imaging; SHAP and LIME analysis

Citation: Tur, K. Multi-Modal Machine Learning Approach for COVID-19 Detection Using Biomarkers and X-Ray Imaging. *Diagnostics* **2024**, *14*, 2800. https://doi.org/10.3390/diagnostics14242800

Academic Editors: Wan Azani Mustafa and Hiam Alquran

Received: 5 November 2024
Revised: 11 December 2024
Accepted: 12 December 2024
Published: 13 December 2024

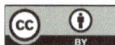

Copyright: © 2024 by the author. Licensee MDPI, Basel, Switzerland. This article is an open access article distributed under the terms and conditions of the Creative Commons Attribution (CC BY) license (https://creativecommons.org/licenses/by/4.0/).

1. Introduction

COVID-19 continues to challenge global healthcare systems, underscoring the need for rapid, accurate, and scalable diagnostic methods. While RT-PCR remains the gold standard for COVID-19 detection, it is often hampered by high false-negative rates, slow processing times, and limited accessibility in resource-constrained environments [1–3]. These limitations have prompted growing interest in complementary diagnostic approaches that integrate advanced technologies, such as machine learning and artificial intelligence (AI), to analyze clinical and imaging data [4,5].

Clinical biomarkers such as C-reactive protein (CRP), ferritin, and Neutrophil-to-Lymphocyte Ratio (NLR) provide systemic insights into inflammation and immune responses, while chest X-ray images visualize respiratory pathology, including ground-glass opacities and consolidations commonly observed in COVID-19 patients [6–8]. Integrating these data sources has the potential to significantly enhance diagnostic accuracy. Recent studies have shown that chest X-rays are particularly valuable for identifying COVID-19-related pneumonia and distinguishing it from other respiratory conditions, yet these approaches often lack the systemic context provided by biomarkers [9,10].

Machine learning has been widely applied to COVID-19 diagnostics, but most studies focus on a single data modality—either imaging or biomarkers—leaving a gap in utilizing their combined diagnostic potential. For example, deep learning architectures like ResNet and VGG have demonstrated high AUC-ROC scores (>0.9) in analysing chest X-ray data, making them effective tools for detecting COVID-19-related lung abnormalities. However, these models often lack insights into systemic inflammation and immune responses that can be captured through biomarkers [11,12]. Similarly, biomarker-based models excel in identifying systemic features of COVID-19 but lack the detailed imaging insights critical for understanding localized lung pathology [13]. Recent research, such as COVID-Net, has explored interpretability in imaging but focuses exclusively on X-ray data, neglecting the systemic context that biomarkers could provide [14]. This represents a significant gap in leveraging the complementary strengths of multi-modal data.

Transparency and interpretability are essential for the adoption of machine learning models in clinical settings. However, most existing studies lack robust interpretability frameworks, limiting their clinical applicability. While some imaging-focused studies use Grad-CAM or saliency maps to highlight regions of interest, these approaches are largely confined to single-modality datasets, failing to generalize across multi-modal data combinations [15,16]. Few studies incorporate advanced interpretable techniques like SHAP or LIME to provide a detailed understanding of how models arrive at predictions, leaving a critical gap in aligning machine learning outputs with clinical reasoning [17].

This study addresses these critical gaps by developing a multi-modal machine learning framework that integrates systemic biomarkers with imaging data for COVID-19 detection. The novelty of this approach lies in three main contributions.

First, the study leverages synergistic integration, combining systemic biomarkers such as CRP, ferritin, and NLR with imaging features extracted from chest X-rays. This integration enhances diagnostic accuracy by combining localized and systemic disease information, bridging the gap left by single-modality models. Second, it employs state-of-the-art interpretability techniques, including SHAP and LIME, to ensure that the model predictions align with clinical reasoning and physiological mechanisms. This interpretability adds a critical layer of transparency and trust, enabling clinicians to better understand and utilize the model predictions. Finally, this study addresses dataset imbalance by utilizing stratified k-fold cross-validation, ensuring fair and unbiased performance evaluation across COVID-19-positive and negative cases.

The proposed multi-modal framework represents a significant advancement over traditional approaches, offering a robust, interpretable, and clinically applicable tool for improving COVID-19 diagnostics.

2. Materials and Methods

The dataset used in this study included a diverse sample of 250 cases, comprising 180 COVID-19 positive cases and 70 COVID-19 negative cases, providing a robust basis for evaluating model performance. Patient data comprised demographic information, blood biomarkers, and chest X-ray images, enabling a comprehensive multi-modal analysis. The dataset included patients from Middle and Greater Anatolia, ensuring demographic diversity in terms of age, gender, and geographic distribution. This inclusion enhances the generalizability of the findings and aligns the study with the clinical demographics encountered in regional healthcare settings.

Key biomarkers analyzed included C-reactive protein (CRP), ferritin, the Neutrophil-to-Lymphocyte Ratio (NLR), the Monocyte-to-Lymphocyte Ratio (MLR) and albumin [18]. These biomarkers were selected for their established associations with COVID-19 severity and inflammatory response. Elevated CRP and ferritin levels, for instance, are indicative of heightened inflammatory processes and cellular damage, while NLR reflects immune dysregulation commonly observed in COVID-19 patients [19,20]. Conversely, albumin levels often decrease in severe cases, serving as a marker for poor prognosis [21]. This biomarker selection allowed for a multi-faceted approach to COVID-19 detection, reflecting both immune response and systemic disease progression.

Data preprocessing involved several critical steps to ensure uniformity and enhance model performance. Missing values in biomarker data were imputed using mean values, a standard technique to manage incomplete clinical datasets effectively while maintaining data integrity [22]. Continuous biomarker variables were normalized to standardize value ranges, addressing the sensitivity of machine learning algorithms to feature scale [23]. For chest X-ray images, preprocessing included resizing the images to a consistent resolution of 224 × 224 pixels and converting them to grayscale. This reduced computational complexity while preserving key diagnostic features. To further improve the robustness of the imaging models, data augmentation techniques such as rotation, horizontal flipping, and contrast adjustment were employed. These techniques artificially expanded the training dataset and mitigated overfitting, a frequent issue in medical imaging models due to limited sample sizes [24,25].

Machine learning models were tailored to the distinct characteristics of each data modality. For tabular biomarker data, both Random Forest and Gradient Boosting models were implemented, as these ensemble methods are robust against overfitting and can effectively capture complex relationships within clinical variables [26,27]. Hyperparameter tuning was performed to optimize these models specifically for AUC-ROC, ensuring they maximally leveraged the information within the biomarker data. For imaging data, convolutional neural network (CNN) architectures, specifically ResNet and VGG, were selected due to their demonstrated effectiveness in medical image classification tasks. Transfer learning was employed with these CNNs, initializing the models with pretrained weights from large datasets and then fine-tuning them on the COVID-19 X-ray images. This approach enhanced model accuracy by leveraging generalized visual features [28,29]. To create a unified multi-modal model, a late fusion approach was applied, whereby predictions from the biomarker and imaging models were combined post-training. The Gradient Boosting and VGG combination achieved the highest accuracy, indicating that integrating diverse data types enhances diagnostic power in COVID-19 detection [27,30].

To evaluate model performance, AUC-ROC was used as the primary metric for assessing each model's ability to distinguish between COVID-19 positive and negative cases. Secondary metrics, including F1-score, precision, recall, specificity, Negative Predictive Value (NPV), and Matthews Correlation Coefficient (MCC), were calculated to provide a comprehensive understanding of each model's predictive performance. Confidence intervals (CI 95%) were calculated using bootstrap resampling, ensuring the statistical reliability of the reported metrics [1,31]. This multi-metric evaluation approach is critical for understanding the clinical applicability of the model, as high recall is particularly important in COVID-19 detection to minimize missed cases.

To enhance the interpretability of the multi-modal model, SHAP (SHapley Additive exPlanations) and LIME (Local Interpretable Model-Agnostic Explanations) analyses were conducted. SHAP identified influential biomarkers, particularly CRP, ferritin, NLR, and albumin, providing transparency into the biomarker-based predictions and aligning the model's features with known clinical insights. Elevated CRP, ferritin, and NLR levels were found to increase the likelihood of COVID-19 positivity, while lower albumin levels were associated with worse outcomes, consistent with prior findings on the inflammatory response in COVID-19 [19,29]. Meanwhile, LIME was applied to the imaging component, enabling the identification of key lung regions that significantly influenced predictions. LIME highlighted areas commonly associated with COVID-19 pathology, such as ground-glass opacities and consolidations in lower lung regions, providing a visual overlay that supports clinician understanding of the model's decisions [24,26].

To validate the performance differences between the proposed multi-modal models and single-modality models, several statistical tests were employed. For paired continuous metrics, such as AUC-ROC, the Wilcoxon Signed-Rank Test was used to evaluate the statistical significance of performance differences between models across cross-validation folds. This nonparametric test considers the rank differences between paired observations, providing robust comparisons for small sample sizes.

To assess overall differences among all evaluated models, the Friedman test was employed as a nonparametric equivalent to repeated-measures ANOVA. Post-hoc comparisons were conducted using the Nemenyi test to identify pairwise differences.

Additionally, bootstrap resampling was performed to calculate 95% confidence intervals (CIs) for key metrics, such as AUC-ROC, precision, recall, and F1-score. Bootstrap methods ensure robust estimation of variability and statistical reliability. All preprocessing steps and statistical analyses adhered to the methodology described by Japkowicz and Shah [32].

This study adhered to ethical guidelines approved by the Ethics Committee of Ahi Evran University, in accordance with the Declaration of Helsinki (Decision no: 2022-23/200, Date: 20 December 2022). All patient data were fully de-identified to ensure confidentiality and comply with relevant data protection regulations, maintaining ethical integrity throughout the study.

3. Results

3.1. Sample Characteristics and Clinical Features

The dataset consisted of 250 cases, with 180 COVID-19 positive cases (72%) and 70 COVID-19 negative cases (28%). Patients were drawn from Middle and Greater Anatolia, representing a demographically diverse cohort. The mean age of the participants was 55.4 years (SD $\pm$ 15.2), with a nearly equal gender distribution (52% male, 48% female). Clinical characteristics included comorbidities such as hypertension (42%), diabetes (34%), and chronic obstructive pulmonary disease (19%). Key biomarkers, including CRP, ferritin, NLR, and albumin, were collected to represent systemic inflammation, immune dysregulation, and disease severity.

In COVID-19 positive cases, CRP and ferritin levels were significantly elevated compared to negative cases (CRP: 120 mg/L vs. 10 mg/L; ferritin: 600 ng/mL vs. 150 ng/mL). Conversely, albumin levels were lower in positive cases (3.2 g/dL vs. 4.2 g/dL). These differences were consistent with known clinical markers of severe COVID-19 and informed the selection of features for the machine learning models.

3.2. Missing Data Comparison

To address missing values, mean imputation was applied across the dataset. A sensitivity analysis was conducted to evaluate the impact of this method. The analysis compared model performance before and after mean imputation, revealing negligible differences in key performance metrics. For instance, the AUC-ROC for the Gradient Boosting + VGG model was 0.94 (95% CI: 0.91–0.96) with imputation and 0.93 (95% CI: 0.90–0.95) without imputation. Similar trends were observed for F1-score, precision, and recall, with variations remaining within the confidence intervals.

The findings indicate that mean imputation preserved the integrity of the dataset without introducing significant bias. Alternative imputation strategies, such as median imputation or advanced methods like multiple imputation, were not explored in this study due to the minimal impact of missing data (missingness rate < 5%).

3.3. Model Development and Input Variables

The multi-modal machine learning framework integrated complementary diagnostic information from biomarkers and imaging data. Biomarkers such as CRP, ferritin, NLR, and albumin were chosen for their strong associations with COVID-19 pathophysiology. In parallel, chest X-ray images captured radiological features indicative of COVID-19-related pneumonia, including ground-glass opacities and consolidations.

Two distinct machine learning pipelines were established. For tabular biomarker data, ensemble models like Random Forest and Gradient Boosting were employed for their ability to handle non-linear feature interactions. For imaging data, convolutional neural networks (CNNs) such as ResNet and VGG were selected due to their robust performance in medical imaging tasks. Transfer learning was utilized to initialize the CNNs with pretrained weights, followed by fine-tuning on the COVID-19 dataset. Hyperparameter tuning through grid search ensured model optimization for AUC-ROC, the primary evaluation metric.

3.4. Validation Strategy

Robust evaluation of the models was ensured using stratified k-fold cross-validation, which preserved the original class distribution of 180 positive and 70 negative cases across all folds. Preprocessing steps, including data augmentation for imaging and normalization for biomarkers, were applied exclusively to the training data, preventing data leakage during validation.

An independent test set, entirely separate from the training and validation data, was used to assess generalizability. Key performance metrics included AUC-ROC, precision, recall, F1-score, specificity, Matthews Correlation Coefficient (MCC), and Negative Predictive Value (NPV). Confidence intervals (CI 95%) were calculated for all metrics using bootstrap resampling, ensuring statistical reliability and robustness.

3.5. Model Performance, Statistical Analysis and Diagnostic Accuracy

The performance of single-modality and multi-modal models, along with their respective confidence intervals (CI 95%), is summarized in Table 1. Confidence intervals were computed for all metrics, including AUC-ROC, F1-score, precision, and recall, to ensure the statistical reliability of the results and are presented in Table 1. Single-modality models trained solely on biomarkers or imaging data achieved reasonable accuracy. For example, Random Forest (biomarkers) attained an AUC-ROC of 0.85 (95% CI: 0.82–0.88), while VGG (X-ray) achieved an AUC-ROC of 0.83 (95% CI: 0.80–0.86). However, integrating these modalities through multi-modal models significantly improved diagnostic accuracy and robustness. AUC-ROC curves for all models are given in Figure 1.

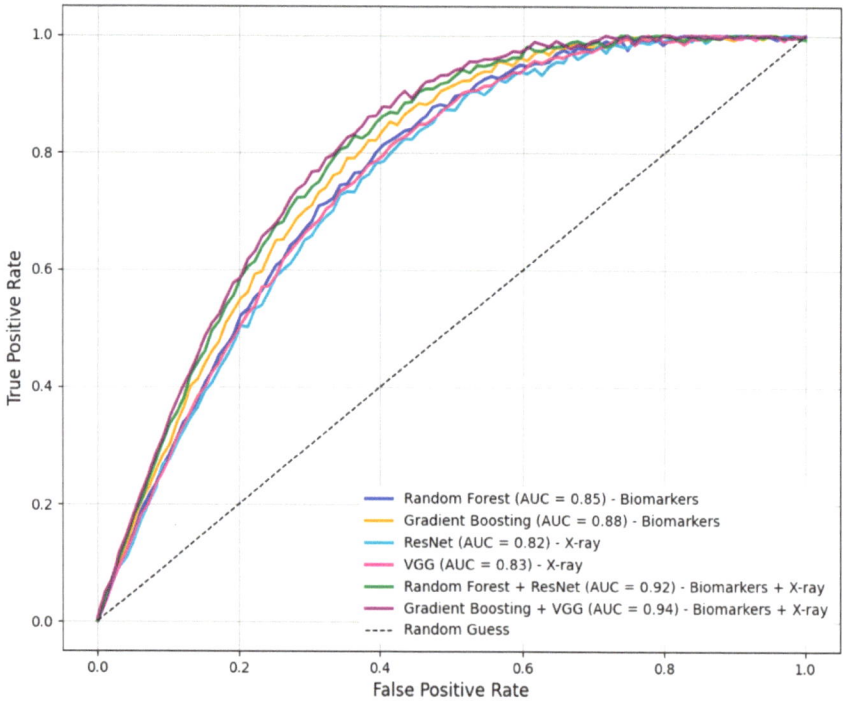

Figure 1. AUC-ROC curves for models.

Table 1. Model performance metrics.

Model	Modality	AUC-ROC (95% CI)	F1-Score (95% CI)	Precision (95% CI)	Recall (95% CI)
Random Forest	Biomarkers Only	0.85 (0.82–0.88)	0.83 (0.80–0.85)	0.85 (0.83–0.87)	0.86 (0.83–0.88)
Gradient Boosting	Biomarkers Only	0.88 (0.85–0.91)	0.85 (0.82–0.87)	0.88 (0.85–0.90)	0.87 (0.84–0.89)
ResNet	X-ray Only	0.82 (0.79–0.85)	0.80 (0.77–0.83)	0.79 (0.77–0.81)	0.81 (0.78–0.84)
VGG	X-ray Only	0.83 (0.80–0.86)	0.81 (0.78–0.83)	0.80 (0.78–0.82)	0.82 (0.79–0.84)
Random Forest + ResNet	Biomarkers + X-ray	0.92 (0.89–0.94)	0.91 (0.89–0.93)	0.93 (0.91–0.95)	0.92 (0.90–0.94)
Gradient Boosting + VGG	Biomarkers + X-ray	0.94 (0.91–0.96)	0.93 (0.91–0.95)	0.97 (0.95–0.98)	0.96 (0.94–0.98)

The Gradient Boosting + VGG combination achieved the best overall performance, with an AUC-ROC of 0.94 (95% CI: 0.91–0.96), F1-score of 0.93 (95% CI: 0.91–0.95), precision of 0.97 (95% CI: 0.95–0.98), and recall of 0.96 (95% CI: 0.94–0.98). These results highlight the advantage of combining biomarkers with imaging data to leverage their synergistic diagnostic potential.

The performance of single-modality and multi-modal models is summarized in Table 2, with the addition of specificity, NPV, and MCC for the Gradient Boosting + VGG model. Specificity was calculated as 0.93, indicating strong identification of true negatives. The NPV was 0.87, reflecting the probability of correctly identifying negative cases. The MCC score of 0.86, a robust metric accounting for class imbalance, underscores the model's balanced performance across both classes.

Table 2. Comprehensive metrics for Gradient Boosting + VGG Model.

Metric	Value
AUC-ROC	0.94
F1-Score	0.93
Precision	0.97
Recall (Sensitivity)	0.96
Specificity (Sp)	0.93
Negative Prediction Value (NPV)	0.87
Matthews Corellation Coefficient (MCC)	0.86

To determine the superiority of the Gradient Boosting + VGG multi-modal model, several statistical analyses were conducted. The Wilcoxon Signed-Rank Test compared AUC-ROC values across cross-validation folds for Gradient Boosting + VGG versus Random Forest. The test resulted in a statistic of 10.00 and a p-value of 0.0313, indicating significant improvements in performance by the multi-modal model.

For overall comparisons across all models, the Friedman test demonstrated statistically significant differences (test statistic = 27.89, p = 0.0001). Post-hoc analyses identified the Gradient Boosting + VGG model as significantly superior to other models.

Bootstrap resampling provided 95% confidence intervals for AUC-ROC values, with the Gradient Boosting + VGG model achieving a CI of 0.93–0.96. These findings, summarized in Table 3, validate the robustness and statistical reliability of the proposed multi-modal framework.

Table 3. Statistical test results for model performance comparisons.

Test	Value
Wilcoxon Signed-Rank Test Statistic	10.00
Wilcoxon p-value	0.0313
Friedman Test Statistic	27.89
Friedman p-value	0.0001
Bootstrap CI (Gradient Boosting + VGG)	0.93–0.96

3.6. Confusion Matrix and Biomarker Distribution

The confusion matrix for the Gradient Boosting + VGG model (Figure 2) demonstrated high accuracy, correctly identifying 170 of 180 COVID-19 positive cases and 65 of 70 negative cases. This resulted in a recall (sensitivity) of 0.96, precision of 0.97, and specificity of 0.93. The balance between sensitivity and specificity highlights the model's robustness in minimizing both false negatives and false positives.

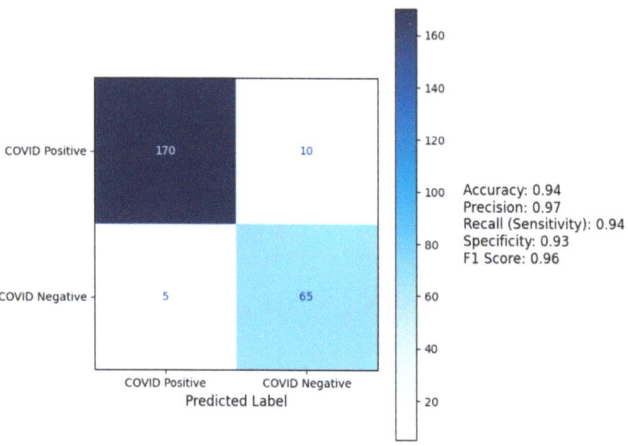

Figure 2. Confusion matrix for Gradient Boosting + VGG Model.

Key biomarkers (CRP, ferritin, NLR, and albumin) exhibited distinct distributions across COVID-19 positive and negative cases (Figure 3). Elevated CRP, ferritin, and NLR levels were consistently observed in positive cases, while albumin levels were lower, aligning with known clinical characteristics of COVID-19.

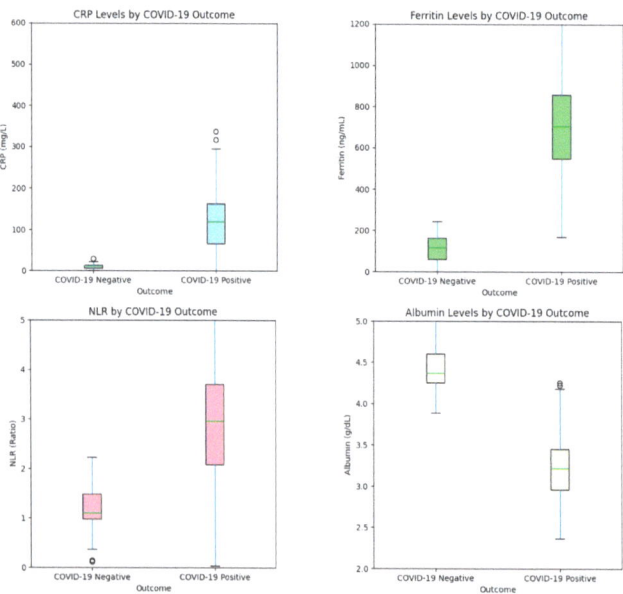

Figure 3. Distribution of key biomarkers by COVID-19 outcome (**top left**: CRP, **top right**: Ferritin, **bottom left**: NLR, **bottom right**: Albumin).

3.7. Interpretability Analysis

SHAP and LIME analyses provided interpretability to the multi-modal model. SHAP identified CRP, ferritin, NLR, and albumin as the most influential biomarkers (Figure 4), while LIME highlighted radiological features in lung regions, such as ground-glass opacities and consolidations, reinforcing clinical relevance (Figure 5).

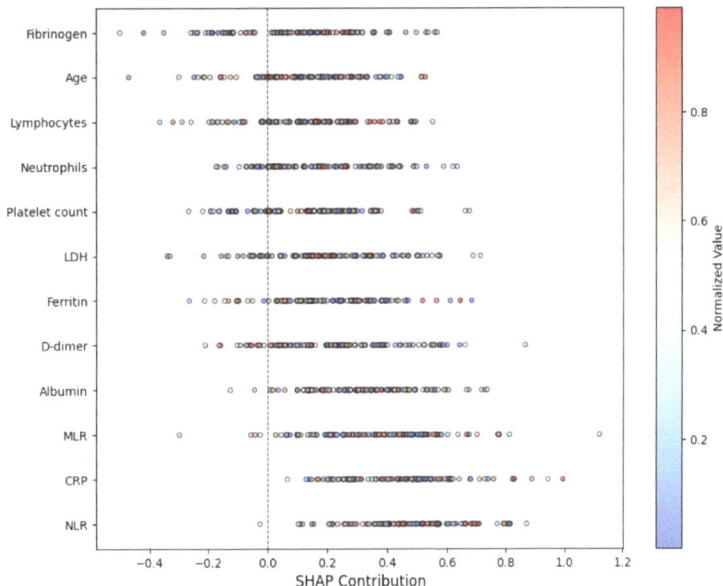

Figure 4. SHAP summary for key biomarkers.

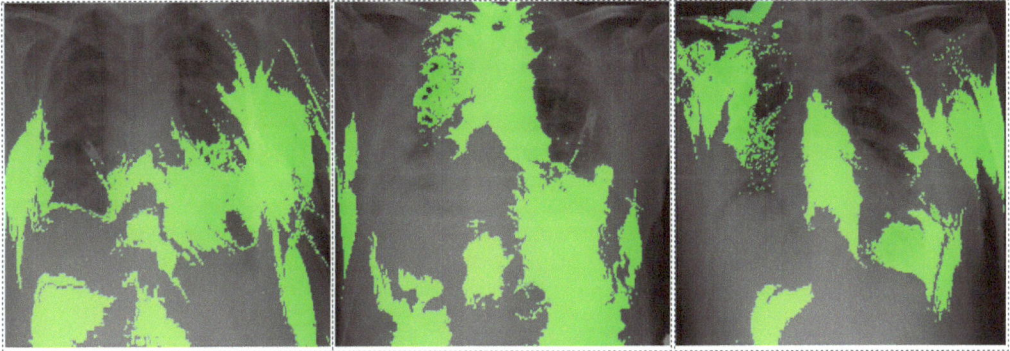

Figure 5. LIME explanation of key X-ray regions.

4. Discussion

4.1. Implications for Clinical Practice

This study demonstrates the diagnostic superiority of multi-modal models integrating biomarkers and X-ray imaging over single-modality approaches. The Gradient Boosting + VGG model achieved the highest AUC-ROC (0.94, 95% CI: 0.91–0.96), F1-score (0.93, 95% CI: 0.91–0.95), precision (0.97, 95% CI: 0.95–0.98), and recall (0.96, 95% CI: 0.94–0.98). These metrics confirm the model's ability to minimize both false positives and false negatives, crucial for clinical scenarios.

The confusion matrix (Figure 2) highlights the practical relevance of this multi-modal model, with 170 of 180 COVID-19 positive cases correctly identified (recall: 0.94) and 65 of 70 negative cases accurately classified (specificity: 0.93). High recall minimizes missed diagnoses, reducing the risk of uncontained transmission and worsening patient outcomes [33]. Simultaneously, high precision (0.97) minimizes false positives, reducing unnecessary treatments and psychological stress for patients [34].

The biomarker distribution analysis further underscores the clinical significance of CRP, ferritin, NLR, and albumin. Elevated CRP and ferritin levels in COVID-19 positive cases highlight systemic inflammatory responses triggered by the virus. Studies consistently show that CRP correlates with COVID-19 severity, serving as a predictive marker for adverse outcomes [34–38]. Similarly, high ferritin levels are associated with cytokine storm syndrome, a severe immune response causing multi-organ damage [39,40]. Elevated NLR reflects immune dysregulation and a pro-inflammatory state linked to poor outcomes, corroborating previous findings [18,41]. Low albumin levels observed in positive cases align with literature identifying hypoalbuminemia as a marker of poor prognosis in COVID-19, likely due to its role in immune modulation and vascular integrity maintenance [21,42]. The statistical analyses demonstrated the superiority of the Gradient Boosting + VGG multi-modal model, with significant improvements in AUC-ROC confirmed by the Wilcoxon Signed-Rank Test ($p < 0.05$) and overall differences validated by the Friedman test ($p = 0.0001$). Bootstrap resampling further established the model's robustness, with AUC-ROC confidence intervals of 0.93–0.96. These results underscore the diagnostic advantage of integrating biomarker and imaging data, providing a reliable and interpretable framework for COVID-19 detection.

Integrating these biomarkers with imaging data captures both systemic immune responses and localized lung pathology, providing a robust diagnostic framework. X-ray imaging reveals radiological patterns such as ground-glass opacities and consolidations, commonly associated with COVID-19 pneumonia. Combining these modalities addresses the limitations of each; biomarkers lack spatial information, while imaging data alone may overlook systemic responses [43,44].

4.2. Comparison with Previous Studies

The results align with prior research on single-modality approaches but demonstrate significant improvements in diagnostic accuracy through multi-modal integration. Previous imaging-only studies, such as those using ResNet or VGG, report AUC-ROC scores ranging from 0.85 to 0.90, reflecting their capacity to capture radiological features [21,26]. Similarly, biomarker-only models, which often focus on CRP and NLR, have shown promise but typically achieve lower AUC-ROC scores (e.g., 0.80–0.88) [44,45].

Few studies have explored multi-modal frameworks for COVID-19 diagnosis. While frameworks like COVID-Net leverage imaging data effectively, they often lack systemic insights provided by biomarkers, limiting their ability to capture the full disease spectrum [46]. This study advances the field by demonstrating how multi-modal integration enhances diagnostic accuracy while incorporating interpretability tools such as SHAP and LIME, which align AI predictions with established clinical markers and radiological signs [34].

4.3. Study Limitations

This study demonstrates the feasibility and clinical relevance of combining biomarkers and X-ray imaging for COVID-19 diagnosis. The use of SHAP and LIME tools ensures transparency and trust in model predictions, aligning outputs with clinical reasoning and making the model practical for real-world use. Additionally, the inclusion of confidence intervals for all metrics reinforces statistical reliability.

However, limitations must be acknowledged. First, the dataset size ($n = 250$ cases) remains modest compared to larger public datasets. The inclusion of 70 negative cases improved class balance but may still introduce bias in performance metrics, particularly precision and specificity. Additionally, the dataset derives from patients in university medical hospitals in Central and Greater Anatolia, limiting the generalizability of findings to similar populations and healthcare settings. Expanding the dataset with diverse and representative populations is essential for broader applicability.

The reliance on mean imputation for missing data, though validated through sensitivity analysis, could be refined further. Advanced techniques like multiple imputation or deep learning-based imputation may provide more robust handling of missingness. Finally, the study focused on X-ray imaging and systemic biomarkers. Incorporating additional modalities, such as CT imaging or genomic data, could further enhance diagnostic accuracy.

4.4. Interpretability and Clinical Relevance

SHAP and LIME analyses enhance the model's interpretability, ensuring alignment with clinical observations. SHAP identified CRP, ferritin, NLR, and albumin as critical predictors, consistent with their roles in systemic inflammation, immune dysregulation, and poor prognosis. Elevated CRP and ferritin levels correlate with adverse outcomes, while high NLR reflects pro-inflammatory states, and low albumin levels signal systemic severity [35–39,41,47–50]. LIME further validated the focus on radiological features such as ground-glass opacities and consolidations, aligning with established COVID-19 pathology [40,51].

These tools provide actionable insights, making AI-driven diagnostics more accessible and trustworthy. By elucidating the rationale behind predictions, SHAP and LIME enable clinicians to better understand and validate the model's outputs, fostering confidence in its integration into diagnostic workflows.

4.5. Future Research Directions

Future research should prioritize the expansion and validation of datasets to enhance the model's generalizability. Larger and more diverse datasets with balanced class distributions are essential for ensuring robust performance across different populations and healthcare settings. Collaborations with multi-center hospitals and public health organizations can facilitate the collection of such datasets, providing a broader representation of patient demographics and clinical conditions.

Another important direction is the integration of additional diagnostic modalities. Incorporating advanced imaging techniques, such as CT scans, alongside genomic data or outputs from wearable devices, could enrich the diagnostic framework. These modalities would provide complementary insights, offering a more comprehensive understanding of COVID-19 and other diseases, further enhancing the multi-modal approach [52].

Improvements in data handling techniques should also be explored. Advanced imputation methods, such as multiple imputation, could address issues arising from missing data more effectively, while refined feature selection algorithms can bolster preprocessing robustness. These enhancements would strengthen the reliability and accuracy of the models, particularly in scenarios with incomplete or complex datasets.

Finally, evaluating the real-world implementation of multi-modal models in clinical workflows is critical. Such studies would provide insights into the utility, scalability, and operational constraints of the models in practical settings. Federated learning and privacy-preserving approaches could enable broader data access while safeguarding patient confidentiality, promoting the secure and ethical use of AI-driven diagnostics [53,54].

By addressing these areas, multi-modal models have the potential to evolve into robust, scalable, and clinically impactful tools, capable of revolutionizing diagnostic processes across various healthcare contexts.

5. Conclusions

This study introduces a novel multi-modal machine learning framework for the early detection of COVID-19, integrating blood biomarkers and chest X-ray imaging data. By leveraging systemic inflammation markers such as CRP, ferritin, NLR, and albumin alongside imaging insights, the framework achieves superior diagnostic accuracy compared to single-modality approaches. The Gradient Boosting + VGG model demonstrated the highest performance, achieving an AUC-ROC of 0.94, precision of 0.97, and recall of 0.96. These results highlight the diagnostic power of combining systemic and localized data to provide a comprehensive understanding of COVID-19 pathology.

What sets this approach apart is its focus on interpretability. By incorporating SHAP and LIME analyses, the model ensures that predictions align with known clinical markers and imaging features associated with COVID-19. This transparency not only enhances clinical trust but also facilitates practical adoption in healthcare settings, bridging the gap between traditional diagnostics and AI-driven solutions. The interpretability tools provide clinicians with actionable insights, fostering confidence in the model's outputs and supporting its integration into diagnostic workflows.

This framework is particularly valuable in resource-limited settings where access to advanced diagnostic tools, such as CT imaging or genomic sequencing, may be restricted. By utilizing commonly available data sources—blood tests and X-rays—this approach offers a scalable and cost-effective solution for rapid and accurate COVID-19 detection. The robustness of the model in identifying critical COVID-19 markers positions it as a significant asset for improving diagnostic outcomes, reducing diagnostic delays, and supporting timely clinical interventions.

Future research should focus on validating this framework with larger and more diverse datasets, encompassing a broader range of patient demographics and healthcare settings. Expanding the scope to include additional modalities, such as CT imaging or genomic data, could further enhance the diagnostic accuracy and applicability of the model. By addressing these areas, this multi-modal approach could evolve into a cornerstone of infectious disease diagnostics, proposing a novel way for more comprehensive and interpretable AI solutions in healthcare.

Funding: This research received no external funding.

Institutional Review Board Statement: This study was conducted in accordance with the Declaration of Helsinki and approved by the Ethics Committee of Ahi Evran University Faculty of Medicine Ethics Committee (Decision no: 2022-23/200, Date: 20 December 2022).

Informed Consent Statement: Informed consent was obtained from all subjects involved in the study.

Data Availability Statement: The original contributions presented in this study are included in the article. Further inquiries can be directed to the corresponding author.

Acknowledgments: The author would like to express their gratitude to Erkan Tur for his invaluable assistance with data analysis, visualization, and support with machine learning models. His expertise and insights were instrumental in enhancing the quality and accuracy of this research.

Conflicts of Interest: The author declares no conflicts of interest.

References

1. Shenoy, V.; Malik, S.B. CovXr: Automated detection of COVID-19 pneumonia in chest X-rays through machine learning. In Proceedings of the 2021 IEEE Symposium Series on Computational Intelligence (SSCI), Virtual Conference, 5–7 December 2021; pp. 1–6.
2. Das, N.N.; Kumar, N.; Kaur, M.; Kumar, V.; Singh, D. Automated deep transfer learning-based approach for detection of COVID-19 infection in chest X-rays. *Ing. Rech. Biomed.* **2020**, *43*, 114–119.
3. Altan, A.; Karasu, S. Recognition of COVID-19 disease from X-ray images by hybrid model consisting of 2D curvelet transform, chaotic salp swarm algorithm, and deep learning technique. *Chaos Solitons Fractals* **2020**, *140*, 110071. [CrossRef] [PubMed]
4. Panday, A.; Kabir, M.A.; Chowdhury, N.K. A survey of machine learning techniques for detecting and diagnosing COVID-19 from imaging. *Quant. Biol.* **2021**, *10*, 188–207. [CrossRef]
5. Rehouma, R.; Buchert, M.; Chen, Y.P. Machine learning for medical imaging-based COVID-19 detection and diagnosis. *Int. J. Intell. Syst.* **2021**, *36*, 5085–5115. [CrossRef]
6. Mathesul, S.; Swain, D.; Satapathy, S.K.; Rambhad, A.; Acharya, B.; Gerogiannis, V.C.; Kanavos, A. COVID-19 detection from chest X-ray images based on deep learning techniques. *Algorithms* **2023**, *16*, 494. [CrossRef]
7. Tamal, M.; Alshammari, M.; Alabdullah, M.; Hourani, R.; Abu Alola, H.; Hegazi, T.M. An integrated framework with machine learning and radiomics for accurate and rapid early diagnosis of COVID-19 from chest X-ray. *Expert Syst. Appl.* **2020**, *180*, 115152. [CrossRef]

8. Bardhan, S.; Roga, S. Feature-based automated detection of COVID-19 from chest X-ray images. In *Emerging Technologies During the Era of COVID-19 Pandemic*; Springer: Cham, Switzerland, 2021; pp. 115–131.
9. Rasheed, J.; Hameed, A.A.; Djeddi, C.; Jamil, A.; Al-Turjman, F. A machine learning-based framework for diagnosis of COVID-19 from chest X-ray images. *Interdiscip. Sci. Comput. Life Sci.* **2021**, *13*, 103–117. [CrossRef]
10. Rafique, Q.; Rehman, A.; Afghan, M.S.; Ahmad, H.M.; Zafar, I.; Fayyaz, K.; Ain, Q.; Rayan, R.A.; Al-Aidarous, K.M.; Rashid, S.; et al. Reviewing methods of deep learning for diagnosing COVID-19, its variants and synergistic medicine combinations. *Comput. Biol. Med.* **2023**, *163*, 107191. [CrossRef]
11. Jain, G.; Mittal, D.; Thakur, D.; Mittal, M.K. A deep learning approach to detect COVID-19 coronavirus with X-Ray images. *Biocybern. Biomed. Eng.* **2020**, *40*, 1391–1405. [CrossRef]
12. Apostolopoulos, I.D.; Mpesiana, T.A. COVID-19: Automatic detection from X-ray images utilizing transfer learning with convolutional neural networks. *Phys. Eng. Sci. Med.* **2020**, *43*, 635–640. [CrossRef]
13. Khan, A.I.; Shah, J.L.; Bhat, M.M. CoroNet: A deep neural network for detection and diagnosis of COVID-19 from chest X-ray images. *Comput. Methods Programs Biomed.* **2020**, *196*, 105581. [CrossRef]
14. Wang, L.; Lin, Z.Q.; Wong, A. COVID-Net: A tailored deep convolutional neural network design for detection of COVID-19 cases from chest X-ray images. *Sci. Rep.* **2020**, *10*, 19549. [CrossRef] [PubMed]
15. Oh, Y.; Park, S.; Ye, J.C. Deep Learning COVID-19 Features on CXR Using Limited Training Data Sets. *IEEE Trans. Med. Imaging* **2020**, *39*, 2688–2700. [CrossRef] [PubMed]
16. Waheed, A.; Goyal, M.; Gupta, D.; Khanna, A.; Al-Turjman, F.; Pinheiro, P.R. Covidgan: Data augmentation using auxiliary classifier gan for improved COVID-19 detection. *IEEE Access* **2020**, *8*, 91916–91923. [CrossRef] [PubMed]
17. Hussain, E.; Hasan, M.; Rahman, A.; Lee, I.; Tamanna, T.; Parvez, M.Z. CoroDet: A deep learning-based classification for COVID-19 detection using chest X-ray images. *Chaos Solitons Fractals* **2020**, *142*, 110495. [CrossRef]
18. Citu, C.; Gorun, F.; Motoc, A.; Sas, I.; Gorun, O.M.; Burlea, B.; Tuta-Sas, I.; Tomescu, L.; Neamtu, R.; Malita, D.; et al. The predictive role of NLR, d-NLR, MLR, and SIRI in COVID-19 mortality. *Diagnostics* **2022**, *12*, 122. [CrossRef]
19. Ali, E.T.; Jabbar, A.S.; Al Ali, H.S.; Hamadi, S.S.; Jabir, M.S.; Albukhaty, S. Extensive Study on Hematological, Immunological, Inflammatory Markers, and Biochemical Profile to Identify the Risk Factors in COVID-19 Patients. *Int. J. Inflamm.* **2022**, *2022*, 5735546. [CrossRef]
20. Jamal, M.; Bangash, H.I.; Habiba, M.; Lei, Y.; Xie, T.; Sun, J.; Wei, Z.; Hong, Z.; Shao, L.; Zhang, Q. Immune dysregulation and system pathology in COVID-19. *Virulence* **2021**, *12*, 918–936. [CrossRef]
21. Aziz, M.; Fatima, R.; Lee-Smith, W.; Assaly, R. The association of low serum albumin level with severe COVID-19: A systematic review and meta-analysis. *Crit. Care* **2020**, *24*, 255. [CrossRef]
22. Ismael, A.M.; Şengür, A. The investigation of multiresolution approaches for chest X-ray image based COVID-19 detection. *Health Inf. Sci. Syst.* **2020**, *8*, 29. [CrossRef]
23. Gouda, W.; Almurafeh, M.; Humayun, M.; Jhanjhi, N.Z. Detection of COVID-19 based on chest X-rays using deep learning. *Healthcare* **2022**, *10*, 343. [CrossRef] [PubMed]
24. Ibrahim, D.M.; Elshennawy, N.M.; Sarhan, A.M. Deep-chest: Multi-classification deep learning model for diagnosing COVID-19, pneumonia, and lung cancer chest diseases. *Comput. Biol. Med.* **2021**, *132*, 104348. [CrossRef] [PubMed]
25. Oraibi, Z.A.; Albasri, S. Prediction of COVID-19 from chest X-ray images using multiresolution texture classification with robust local features. In Proceedings of the 2021 IEEE 45th Annual Computers, Software, and Applications Conference (COMPSAC), Madrid, Spain, 12–16 July 2021; pp. 663–668.
26. Dong, S.; Yang, Q.; Fu, Y.; Tian, M.; Zhuo, C. RCoNet: Deformable mutual information maximization and high-order uncertainty-aware learning for robust COVID-19 detection. *IEEE Trans. Neural Netw. Learn. Syst.* **2021**, *32*, 3401–3411. [CrossRef] [PubMed]
27. Chauhan, A.; Jagadish, D.N.; Harish, M.; Mahto, L. Multimodality data fusion for COVID-19 diagnosis. In Proceedings of the 2021 IEEE International Conference on Big Data (Big Data), Orlando, FL, USA, 15–18 December 2021.
28. Rajpal, S.; Agarwal, M.; Rajpal, A.; Lakhyani, N.; Saggar, A.; Kumar, N. Cov-elm classifier: An extreme learning machine based identification of COVID-19 using chest X-ray images. *Intell. Decis. Technol.* **2022**, *16*, 193–203. [CrossRef]
29. Abbas, Q.; Mahmood, K.; Rehman, S.U.; Imran, M. COVID-19 image classification using hybrid averaging transfer learning model. *Mehran Univ. Res. J. Eng. Technol.* **2023**, *42*, 72–83. [CrossRef]
30. Mondal, M.R.H.; Bharati, S.; Podder, P. CO-IRv2: Optimized InceptionResNetV2 for COVID-19 detection from chest CT images. *PLoS ONE* **2021**, *16*, e0259179. [CrossRef]
31. Ogunpola, A.; Saeed, F.; Basurra, S.; Albarrak, A.M.; Qasem, S.N. Machine learning-based predictive models for detection of cardiovascular diseases. *Diagnostics* **2024**, *14*, 144. [CrossRef]
32. Japkowicz, N.; Shah, M. Performance evaluation in machine learning. In *Machine Learning in Radiation Oncology: Theory and Applications*; Springer: Cham, Switzerland, 2015; pp. 41–56.
33. Hussain, S.; Xu, S.; Aslam, M.; Hussain, F. Clinical predictions of COVID-19 patients using deep stacking neural networks. *J. Investig. Med.* **2023**, *72*, 112–127. [CrossRef]
34. Afifi, A.; Hafsa, N.E.; Ali MA, S.; Alhumam, A.; Alsalman, S. An ensemble of global and local-attention-based convolutional neural networks for COVID-19 diagnosis on chest X-ray images. *Symmetry* **2021**, *13*, 113. [CrossRef]
35. Tjendra, Y.; Al Mana, A.F.; Espejo, A.P.; Akgun, Y.; Millan, N.C.; Gomez-Fernandez, C.; Cray, C. Predicting Disease Severity and Outcome in COVID-19 Patients: A Review of Multiple Biomarkers. *Arch. Pathol. Lab. Med.* **2020**, *144*, 1465–1474. [CrossRef]

36. Romiti, G.F.; Corica, B. Assessing inflammatory status in COVID-19: A role in the pandemic? *Intern. Emerg. Med.* **2021**, *16*, 1423–1425.
37. Alam, J.M.; Asghar, S.S.; Ali, H.; Mahmood, S.R.; Ansari, M.A. Profiling of inflammatory biomarkers in mild to critically ill severe acute respiratory syndrome corona virus-19 (SARS COVID-19) patients from Karachi, Pakistan. *Pak. J. Pharm. Sci.* **2021**, *34*, 429–433. [PubMed]
38. Smail, S.W.; Babaei, E.; Amin, K. Hematological, inflammatory, coagulation, and oxidative/antioxidant biomarkers as predictors for severity and mortality in COVID-19: A prospective cohort-study. *Int. J. Gen. Med.* **2023**, *16*, 565–580. [CrossRef] [PubMed]
39. Patil, S.; Toshniwal, S.; Acharya, A.G.; Narwade, G. Role of Ferritin in COVID-19 Pneumonia: Sensitive Marker of Inflammation, Predictor of Mechanical Ventilation, and Early Marker of Post-COVID Lung Fibrosis. *Muller J. Med. Sci. Res.* **2022**, *13*, 28–34. [CrossRef]
40. Carubbi, F.; Salvati, L.; Alunno, A.; Maggi, F.; Borghi, E.; Mariani, R.; Mai, F.; Paoloni, M.; Ferri, C.; Desideri, G.; et al. Ferritin is associated with the severity of lung involvement but not with worse prognosis in patients with COVID-19: Data from two Italian COVID-19 units. *Sci. Rep.* **2021**, *11*, 4863. [CrossRef]
41. Gurusamy, E.; Mahalakshmi, S.; Kaarthikeyan, G.; Ramadevi, K.; Arumugam, P.; Gayathri, M. Biochemical predictors for SARS-CoV-2 severity. *Bioinformation* **2021**, *17*, 834–839. [CrossRef]
42. Zerbato, V.; Sanson, G.; De Luca, M.; Di Bella, S.; di Masi, A.; Caironi, P.; Marini, B.; Ippodrino, R.; Luzzati, R. The impact of serum albumin levels on COVID-19 mortality. *Infect. Dis. Rep.* **2022**, *14*, 278–286. [CrossRef]
43. Wang, W.; Liu, S.; Yu, C.; Li, Y. A mixture of machine learning models for COVID-19 diagnosis using chest X-ray images. *IEEE Access* **2020**, *8*, 110386–110393.
44. Khan, I.U.; Aslam, N.; Anwar, T.; Alsaif, H.S.; Chrouf, S.M.B.; Alzahrani, N.A.; Alamoudi, F.A.; Kamaleldin, M.M.A.; Awary, K.B. Using a deep learning model to explore the impact of clinical data on COVID-19 diagnosis using chest X-ray. *Sensors* **2022**, *22*, 669. [CrossRef]
45. Prinzi, F.; Militello, C.; Scichilone, N.; Gaglio, G.; Vitabile, S. Explainable machine-learning models for COVID-19 prognosis prediction using clinical, laboratory, and radiomic features. *IEEE Access* **2023**, *11*, 121492–121510. [CrossRef]
46. El-bana, S.; Abdeltawab, H.; Eltahan, E. A pipeline for specialized COVID-19 detection using medical imaging. *Comput. Biol. Med.* **2020**, *131*, 104256.
47. Singh, A.; Bhadani, P.P.; Surabhi; Sinha, R.; Bharti, S.; Kumar, T.; Nigam, J.S. Significance of immune-inflammatory markers in predicting clinical outcome of COVID-19 patients. *Indian J. Pathol. Microbiol.* **2023**, *66*, 111–117. [CrossRef] [PubMed]
48. Oktavia, N.; Efrida, E.; Rofinda, Z. Comparison in Levels of Interleukin 6, Ferritine and Neutrophil-Lymphocyte Ratio in COVID-19 Patients Treated in ICU and Non-ICU. *J. Profesi Med. J. Kedokt. Dan Kesehat.* **2022**, *16*, 120–127. [CrossRef]
49. Zali, F.; Mardani, R.; Farahmand, M.; Ahmadi, N.; Shahali, M.; Salehi-Vaziri, M.; Doroud, D.; Aghasadeghi, M.; Sadeghi, S.; Mousavi-Nasab, S. Predictive Value Alteration of Laboratory Routine and Ferritin/Transferrin Ratio in Monitoring of COVID-19 Patients. *Clin. Lab.* **2022**, *68*, 10. [CrossRef]
50. Agha, N.; Rezaei, S.A.; Abdulrahman, B.K.; Al-khayat, Z. Study of D-dimer, CRP & ferritin status as independent risk factors for severity of the clinical aspects in patients with COVID-19 in Erbil, Iraq. *Afr. J. Health Sci.* **2023**, *35*, 709–720.
51. Cervantes, E.G.; Chan, W.Y. Lime-enabled investigation of convolutional neural network performances in COVID-19 chest X-ray detection. In Proceedings of the 2021 IEEE Canadian Conference on Electrical and Computer Engineering (CCECE), Virtual Conference, 2–17 September 2021; pp. 1–6.
52. Sáez, C.; Romero, N.; Conejero, J.A.; García-Gómez, J.M. Potential limitations in COVID-19 machine learning due to data source variability: A case study in the nCov2019 dataset. *J. Am. Med. Inform. Assoc.* **2020**, *28*, 360–364. [CrossRef]
53. Nguyen, D.; Kay, F.; Tan, J.; Yan, Y.; Ng, Y.S.; Iyengar, P.; Peshock, R.; Jiang, S. Deep Learning–Based COVID-19 Pneumonia Classification Using Chest CT Images: Model Generalizability. *Front. Artif. Intell.* **2021**, *4*, 694875. [CrossRef]
54. Yang, D.; Xu, Z.; Li, W.; Myronenko, A.; Roth, H.R.; Harmon, S.; Xu, S.; Turkbey, B.; Turkbey, E.; Wang, X.; et al. Federated semi-supervised learning for COVID region segmentation in chest CT using multi-national data from China, Italy, Japan. *Med. Image Anal.* **2020**, *70*, 101992. [CrossRef]

Disclaimer/Publisher's Note: The statements, opinions and data contained in all publications are solely those of the individual author(s) and contributor(s) and not of MDPI and/or the editor(s). MDPI and/or the editor(s) disclaim responsibility for any injury to people or property resulting from any ideas, methods, instructions or products referred to in the content.

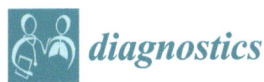

Article

Towards Parkinson's Disease Detection Through Analysis of Everyday Handwriting

Jeferson David Gallo-Aristizabal [1], Daniel Escobar-Grisales [1], Cristian David Ríos-Urrego [1], Jesús Francisco Vargas-Bonilla [1], Adolfo M. García [2,3,4,5] and Juan Rafael Orozco-Arroyave [1,6,*]

[1] GITA Lab., Faculty of Engineering, University of Antioquia, Medellín 510010, Colombia; jeferson.gallo@udea.edu.co (J.D.G.-A.); daniel.esobar@udea.edu.co (D.E.-G.); cdavid.rios@udea.edu.co (C.D.R.-U.); jesus.vargas@udea.edu.co (J.F.V.-B.)
[2] Cognitive Neuroscience Center, Universidad de San Andrés, Buenos Aires B1644BID, Argentina; adolfomartingarcia@gmail.com
[3] Global Brain Health Institute (GBHI), University of California San Francisco, San Francisco, CA 94143, USA
[4] Trinity College Dublin, D02 R590 Dublin, Ireland
[5] Departamento de Lingüística y Literatura, Facultad de Humanidades, Universidad de Santiago de Chile, Santiago 9170020, Chile
[6] LME Lab., University of Erlangen, 91054 Erlangen, Germany
* Correspondence: rafael.orozco@udea.edu.co

Abstract: Background: Parkinson's disease (PD) is the second most prevalent neurodegenerative disorder worldwide. People suffering from PD exhibit motor symptoms that affect the control of upper and lower limb movement. Among daily activities that depend on proper upper limb control is the handwriting process, which has been studied in state-of-the-art research, mainly considering non-semantic drawings like spirals, geometric figures, cursive lines, and others. **Objectives:** This paper analyzes the suitability of modeling the handwriting process of digits from 0 to 9 to automatically discriminate between PD patients and healthy control subjects. The main hypothesis is that modeling these numbers allows a more natural evaluation of upper limb control. **Methods:** Two approaches are considered: modeling of the images resulting from the strokes collected by the digital tablet and modeling of the time series yielded by the digital tablet while performing the strokes, i.e., time-dependent signals. The first approach is implemented by fine-tuning a CNN-based architecture, while the second approach is based on hand-crafted features measured upon the time series, namely pressure and kinematic measurements. Features extracted from time-dependent signals are represented following two strategies, one based on statistical functionals and the other one based on creating Gaussian Mixture Models (GMMs). **Results:** The experiments indicate that pressure-based features modeled with functionals are the ones that yield the highest accuracy, indicating that PD-related symptoms are better modeled with dynamic approaches than those based on images. **Conclusions:** The dynamic approach outperformed the image-based model, indicating that the writing process, modeled with signals collected over time, reveals motor symptoms more clearly than images resulting from handwriting. This finding is in line with previous results in the state-of-the-art research and constitutes a step forward to create more accurate and informative methods to detect and monitor PD symptoms.

Keywords: Parkinson's disease; handwriting; convolutional neural networks; dynamic analysis; natural handwriting tasks

1. Introduction

Parkinson's disease (PD) is a neurodegenerative disorder that affects the central nervous system, and it is characterized by the progressive loss of dopaminergic neurons in the midbrain [1]. These neurons are mainly responsible for the production of dopamine, which is a neurotransmitter in charge of keeping operational neural pathways associated with mood, motor control, and other functions [2]. Among motor symptoms derived from PD are muscular rigidity, resting tremor, postural instability, and bradykinesia [3]. Motor symptoms negatively impact activities that require highly coordinated movements like handwriting [4]. Anomalies in handwriting include micrographia (abnormal reduction in writing size) and dysgraphia (deficits in graphomotor production) [5]. Other neurodegenerative disorders also affect the handwriting process, for instance, Alzheimer's disease patients are known for producing abnormal strokes in different handwriting tasks [6,7] Handwriting analyses are carried out via online data or offline data. Online data refer to handwriting signals acquired using digital devices, such as tablets or smart pens; offline data consist of traditional methods like writing with an ink pen on paper. Handwriting using conventional methods could be more natural for elderly patients; however, online data allow dynamic analyses of the handwriting process and enable sensing-relevant bio-signals such as pressure, in-air movements, dynamic horizontal and vertical positions, pen inclinations, and other relevant information [8,9]. For a comprehensive review of methods used to evaluate neurodegenerative disorders considering handwriting biosignals, please see [10].

Online and offline handwriting studies typically consider geometric-based tasks, namely, drawings that involve figures like spirals, meanders, geometric figures, and others [11]. Studies have explored the use of different features including kinematic [12–14], geometric, and pressure [15]. One of the main advantages of online handwriting is that it provides the sensor-based signals and also the resulting image, i.e., the drawing. This characteristic has motivated researchers to use image processing methods, mainly based on Convolutional Neural Networks (CNNs), to model those images. For instance, in [16], the authors used time series-based images from drawing tasks. Raw signals collected from the tablet were transformed into matrices to form images which were further processed by a CNN architecture pre-trained on the ImageNet dataset. In another study presented in [17], the authors created spectral representations from tablet signals to model tremor and other symptoms. These signal representations were stacked to form an image and then feed a CNN model with kernel sizes of 1×5 and 1×3. In [18], authors analyzed drawings from three datasets (PaHaW [19], HandPD [20], and NewHandPD [11]) to increase sample-size. They used an AlexNet model pre-trained on ImageNet and data augmentation techniques. Finally, in [21], authors implemented a CNN with two blocks containing three convolutional layers and one pooling layer. Similarly, in [22], the authors used pre-trained models based on ImageNet to improve the model's generalization capability. Other datasets like MNIST and UJIpenchars2, which are semantically similar to writing tasks, have also been used to pre-train models [23].

Regarding modeling dynamic information from raw tablet signals, previous studies suggest that dynamic analysis of online handwriting provides suitable information to detect PD motor symptoms such as tremor and bradykinesia [9]. Regarding the offline approach, deep learning architectures mainly based on CNNs have been used to analyze handwritten drawings. On the one hand, the majority of handwriting-related studies consider drawings of geometric figures and spirals. On the other hand, writing tasks that request the patient to write numbers, letters, words, or sentences [19] are more natural and closer to activities of daily living, which is what expert neurologists usually focus on during clinical check-ups. Models focused on these kinds of tasks eventually produce better systems to perform accurate monitoring of patients. Additionally, these semantic writing tasks may have a higher cognitive load to patients, therefore providing information about motor planning (e.g., between-letter or word transitions), which is affected due to lack of coordination in PD [10]. Dynamic signals extracted from writing tasks have been modeled using different dimensions such as kinematic [24,25], spectro-temporal [26], and non-linear [27].

State-of-the-art research shows that deep learning architectures (mainly based on CNN architectures) have been used to model images resulting either from offline handwriting images or from images created by considering online signals. Most studies with promising results are based on drawing tasks [22,28,29]. However, these approaches are not as natural as those based on regular writing tasks, i.e., writing of letters, numbers, words, or sentences, making those models not suitable for performing non-intrusive monitoring of the neurological state of patients.

This paper introduces and compares two different approaches based on online handwriting signals collected from PD patients and healthy controls (HCs). One approach considers resulting images of the tablet handwriting to feed a CNN architecture pre-trained with adapted samples of the MNIST corpus and fine-tuned with Parkinson's data. The second approach consists of considering online signals and extracting different features, including those related to the pressure and movements of the pen (namely, kinematic). The resulting features are compressed and represented with two statistical approaches: statistical functionals and Gaussian Mixture Models (GMMs). Statistical representations are used as input to a Support Vector Machine (SVM) classifier, the parameters of which are optimized following a k-fold cross-validation strategy. Results show that image-based features are outperformed by dynamic analyses with the pressure feature set using statistical functionals. This likely indicates that vertical control of hand movement is more challenging for PD patients.

The rest of the paper is organized as follows. Section 2 introduces the data considered for this study, Section 3 explains the methodology followed in the paper, Section 4 shows experiments and results, Section 5 elaborates a discussion about findings reported in the study, and finally, Section 6 presents the conclusions derived from this work.

2. Data Acquisition and Participants

Our handwriting database (Hw-DB) consists of 104 participants, including 51 PD patients and 53 HC subjects. Forty-seven of the patients were evaluated by an expert neurologist according to the MDS-UPDRS-III scale. The remaining four patients could not come to the clinic for their neurological evaluation because they live in the countryside and were not available for these clinical screenings. Subjects were asked to write the numbers from 0 to 9 using a Wacom Cintiq 13 HD tablet, with a sampling frequency of 180 Hz. This tablet provides six signals: x and y position, z (distance from the tablet surface to the pen tip), azimuth and altitude angles, and pen pressure. Additional details about the participants are shown in Table 1.

Table 1. Demographic and clinical information of the participants.

	PD Patients		HC	
	Male	Female	Male	Female
Number of subjects	24	27	32	21
Age ($\mu \pm \sigma$) ⋆	69.2 ± 10.0	62.1 ± 12.0	67.1 ± 10.6	58.8 ± 10.8
Age range	50–90	29–84	49–85	43–83
MDS-UPDRS-III ($\mu \pm \sigma$)	39.2 ± 17.0	32.3 ± 15.9		
Range of MDS-UPDRS-III	16–82	14–77		

⋆ Indicates that there is no statistical difference between the two groups according to a t-test with p-value = 0.45. Gender bias was discarded through a Chi-squared test with p-value = 0.2439.

3. Methodology

Figure 1 summarizes the methodology addressed in this paper. The information from the sequence of numbers is analyzed following two approaches: image-based and dynamic. The first approach only uses the data of the image generated by the position information of the tablet, making this task similar to offline handwriting. This approach considers a Convolutional Neural Network (CNN) pre-trained using sequences created with numbers from the MNIST database. Sizes of digits in the MNIST corpus are changed to artificially create the effect of micrographia. Then, the CNN model is fine-tuned using the handwriting digits of PD and HC subjects. The second approach constitutes a dynamic analysis where we use all information available when data are captured using a digital tablet. Two sets of classical handwriting features are computed from the 6 time-series signals available in online handwriting (x and y position, z (distance from the tablet surface to the pen tip), azimuth and altitude angles, and pen pressure). Finally, feature vectors obtained from the image-based and dynamic analyses are used independently to train two Support Vector Machine (SVM) classifiers to discriminate between PD patients and HC subjects.

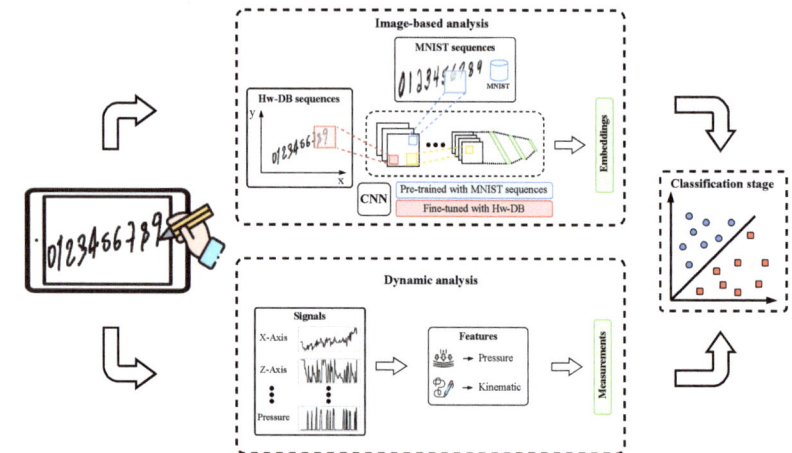

Figure 1. General methodology proposed in this study.

3.1. Feature Extraction

3.1.1. Image-Based Analysis

This model is based on a CNN architecture, a widely used modeling strategy in image processing [30]. In each layer, different filters are trained to detect patterns while the spatial dimensions of the image are reduced to obtain a compressed image representation. The CNN model training requires many samples to generalize patterns and avoid model overfitting; this represents a limitation in the study of medical data, where only a few samples are available. Transfer Learning (TL) and Data Augmentation (DA) techniques have emerged to address the problem of data scarcity [28,31–33].

In this study, we created 7000 synthetic sequences of numbers from 0 to 9 using the digits of the MNIST database [34]. Half of the sequences contain concatenated digits, while the rest are modified to model micrographia, which is a distinct symptom of handwriting in PD patients. The idea behind this approach is to pre-train the architecture to recognize non-modified sequences (synthetic samples of HC subjects, i.e., without micrographia) vs. modified sequences (synthetic samples of PD patients, i.e., with micrographia), which implicitly means having an architecture properly trained to detect micrographia. The starting digit for the modified sequence is randomly chosen from 0 to 5. Once the first modified digit is chosen, the rest of the sequence, until 9, is progressively reduced until the last digit (9) results in half of its original size. Examples of the modified and non-modified sequences of digits from MNIST are shown in Figure 2. In addition, given the fact that several sequences in the Hw-DB exhibited slight rotations resulting from the writing process of participants, all the synthetic sequences (modified and non-modified) were randomly rotated at angles of $-15°, -5°, 0°, 5°, 15°$. From the set of generated sequences, a subset of 6000 synthetic sequences was used to train a CNN architecture to classify between modified and non-modified sequences. The remaining synthetic sequences were used as a test set. The CNN model employed in this experiment is based on a LeNet architecture because it constitutes a simple model appropriate for the size of the corpus that we could access to develop this study. Additionally, this architecture showed as good results as in a previous work where we modeled digits [35]. This network consists of 3 convolutional layers with 16, 8, and 4 filters, employing a (5×5) kernel. Max-pooling layers were used to reduce the size of each feature map by half. The output feature map was flattened to feed three fully connected layers with 512, 64, and 2 neurons, respectively. The first two fully connected layers employed a rectified linear unit (ReLU) activation function, and the last one made the final decision using a Softmax activation function. The shape of input images is 144 in height and 216 in width.

The pre-trained architecture and its weights are used as the starting point to fine-tune a specific architecture for the automatic discrimination between PD and HC subjects. The fine-tuning process is performed with data from the Hw-DB corpus. Once the architecture is fine-tuned, we take the embedding of the flattened feature map as a feature vector to feed the SVM classifier.

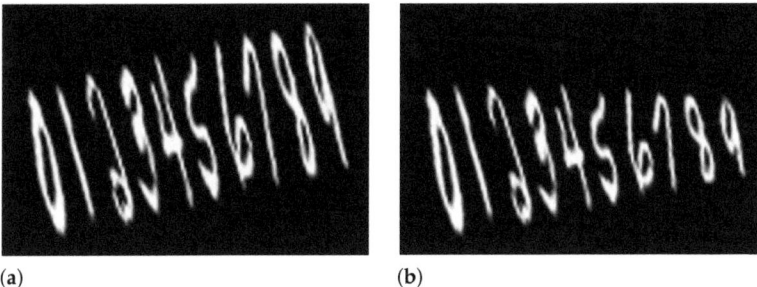

(a)   (b)

Figure 2. Sequences created by MNIST database. (a) Non-modified sequence. (b) Modified sequence.

3.1.2. Dynamic Analysis

Although the image-based representation method has the advantage of being suitable for online and offline handwriting, it does not allow modeling motor problems such as rigidity, bradykinesia, or freezing of the upper limbs. These motor problems affect the dynamics of handwriting, leading to changes in velocity, acceleration, and fluency, which cannot be captured from the resulting image. In contrast, the dynamic approach leverages all the available data from online handwriting, where different feature sets are computed using the time series signals provided by the digital tablet. Table 2 shows a summary of all computed features, the details of which are described below.

Pressure-based features: Pressure features describe the mechanical force exerted on the pen tip during on-surface movements produced along the writing process. Common pressure features are based on statistical functionals computed over (1) the raw pressure signal $(p[n])$, (2) changes in pressure signal $(\Delta p = p[n+1] - p[n])$, (3) the rate of pressure changes over time $\left(p'[n] = \frac{\Delta p}{\Delta t}\right)$, (4) the rate of pressure variability $\left(p''[n] = \frac{\Delta^2 p}{\Delta t^2}\right)$, and (5) the pressure jerk $\left(p'''[n] = \frac{\Delta^3 p}{\Delta t^3}\right)$. Additionally, we can measure the number of changes in pressure (NCP) and the relative number of changes in pressure $\left(RNCP = \frac{NCP}{time}\right)$, using $(\Delta p, p'[n], \text{and } p''[n])$. The resulting feature set includes a total of 26 pressure features.

Kinematic features: According to the status of the *z-axis* signal, handwriting signals can be grouped into on-surface and in-air movements. On-surface samples correspond to digits' strokes; conversely, in-air samples correspond to hand movements during the transition between digits. To compute kinematic features from on-surface and in-air movements, we employed the set of signals $\{x, y, azimuth, altitud\}$. Notice that features computed from the *z-axis* signal contain samples of in-air movements only. Furthermore, we employ the x and y axes to compute the pen trajectory $r[n]$ defined in Equation (1), and the pen displacement $Di[n]$ defined in Equation (2). Then, the set of kinematic features contains (1) movement descriptors as $\{\Delta x, \Delta y, \Delta azimuth, \Delta altitud, \Delta z, r[n], Di[n]\}$, (2) velocity descriptors computed as changes of the previous signals over time $\left(sig_{vel}[n] = \frac{\Delta sig}{\Delta t}\right)$, (3) acceleration descriptors as changes of velocity over time $\left(sig_{acc}[n] = \frac{\Delta sig_{vel}}{\Delta t}\right)$, (4) jerk as the changes of acceleration over time $\left(sig_{jerk}[n] = \frac{\Delta sig_{acc}}{\Delta t}\right)$, and (5) number of changes of velocity and acceleration, NCV and NCA, respectively. Finally, we extracted a total of 120 and 140 kinematic features from on-surface and in-air movements, respectively. Table 2 presents a comprehensive summary of the features extracted in this work.

$$r[n] = \sqrt{x[n]^2 + y[n]^2} \quad (1)$$

$$Di[n] = \sqrt{(x[n+1] - x[n])^2 + (y[n+1] - y[n])^2} \quad (2)$$

Table 2. Summary of the computed feature in each set. s = scalar value, and v = vector of elements.

Set	Feature	s/v	Description
Pressure	$p[n], \Delta p, p'[n], p''[n], \text{and } p'''[n]$	v	Raw pressure, pressure changes, first, second and third derivatives
	NCP, and RNCP	s	Number of local extrema of pressure
Kinematic	$r[n], Di[n], \Delta x, \Delta y, \Delta azimuth, \Delta altitud, \Delta z$	v	Trajectory, displacements, and signal changes.
	Velocity	v	Velocity computed as changes in signals w.r.t. time
	Acceleration	v	Acceleration computed as changes in signal velocity w.r.t. time
	Jerk	v	Jerk computed as changes in signal acceleration w.r.t. time
	NCV and RNCV	s	Number of local extrema for velocity
	NCA and RNCA	s	Number of local extrema for acceleration

3.2. Statistical Modeling

The feature computation process introduced above can result in either a scalar value or a vector (see the third column in Table 2). The resulting vectors generate a feature matrix per subject. To obtain a static vector representation per subject, we consider two statistical modeling strategies, one based on statistical functionals and the other one based on Gaussian Mixture Models (GMMs). Scalar values are concatenated with resulting statistical representations.

Dynamic feature vectors that change over time are commonly represented using statistical functionals to describe their statistical distribution. However, there exist other robust methods like the GMM that can be applied to represent dynamic phenomena. In this section, we compare classical statistical modeling based on functionals vs. GMM modeling.

3.2.1. Statistical Functionals

Statistical functionals are used to describe properties of data distributions. These functionals capture specific characteristics such as central tendency, variability, or higher-order moments. This strategy is commonly used to obtain fixed representations from time- dependent signals. We consider 4 statistical fuctionals, namely, mean, standard deviation, skewness, and kurtosis, forming a static representation per feature vector. The dimensionality of the kinematic feature vector is now $4 \times 52 = 208$, while the dimensionality of of the pressure feature vector is $4 \times 5 = 20$.

3.2.2. Gaussian Mixture Models (GMMs)

GMM representations enable modeling complex dynamics of time-dependent signals. GMM is a probabilistic model that combines multiple Gaussian distributions to obtain a tighter representation of the data distribution. Equation (3) defines a GMM with M Gaussians, where each Gaussian's contribution is weighted by the parameter c. The parameters μ_m and Σ_m represent the mean vector and covariance matrix of the m-th Gaussian, respectively.

$$f(x) = \sum_{m=1}^{M} c_m \mathcal{N}(x; \mu_m, \Sigma_m), \qquad (3)$$

The idea behind the GMM model is that each Gaussian in the mixture models a sub-population along the temporal dynamics. Once the GMM is calculated, a fixed representation is obtained by combining the mean vectors and covariance matrices of all the Gaussians in the mixture. This representation is known as the GMM supervector (λ) [36]. The dimension of the supervector depends on the number of features in the input matrix and the number of Gaussians, where $\lambda_{dimension} = M \times F \times 2$. M is the number of Gaussian components, and F is the number of vector measurements in the feature matrix. We optimized the number of Gaussians based on the obtained accuracy during training. The dimensionality of the supervector that results to represent a given phenomenon or feature vector is computed as follows: optimal number of Gaussians × number of feature vectors × 2. This last number appears because the supervector is formed with the entries of the mean vector and the diagonal of the covariance matrix. For instance, when the optimal number of Gaussians is GMM with $M = 4$, the cardinality of the resulting λ is 416-dimensional ($4 \times 52 \times 2$).

4. Experiments and Results

4.1. Experimental Setup

We conducted two experiments in this work: image-based analysis and dynamic analysis. The image-based analysis involved fine-tuning a pre-trained CNN model, described in Section 3.1.1. The dynamic analysis is based on two feature sets: pressure and kinematic. Each feature set was modeled considering two approaches for comparison purposes, statistical funtionals and GMMs. All models were trained, fine-tuned, and tested following the same partitions according to a 5-fold cross-validation strategy. The hyperparameters of the SVM classifier, namely C, γ, and the *kernel*, were optimized using a grid-search, where C and $\gamma \in \{1e^{-3}, 1e^{-2}, \cdots, 1e^3\}$, and *kernel* $\in$ {linear, rbf}). Notice that we evaluated two more classification methods, namely Random Forest and Gradient Boosting (GB); however, we decided to report only the ones obtained with the SVM because all accuracies with that classifier were higher.

4.2. Experiment 1: Image-Based Analysis

The pre-trained CNN architecture used to discriminate between non-modified and modified sequences was further used as a feature extractor for images in the Hw-DB corpus. We took the flattened output of the last convolutional layer as a feature vector to feed an SVM classifier to distinguish between PD patients and HC subjects. To improve the characterization capability of the pre-trained CNN, we considered four fine-tuning schemes over the base model using data from Hw-DB: fully frozen, partially frozen, semi-frozen, and unfrozen. In the fully frozen schema, the weights and biases of all layers in the CNN were fixed during the training process; therefore, the pre-trained CNN only used the weights and biases obtained with the synthetic data. In the partially frozen schema, the first convolutional layer is unfrozen; thus, only the weights and biases of this layer can be fine-tuned with the Hw-DB data. In the semi-frozen schema, the first and second convolutional layers were fine-tuned. Finally, in the unfrozen schema, the weights and bias of all convolutional layers were fine-tuned. Results of the image-based experiments are shown in Table 3.

Table 3. Results from the image-based analysis of the digit sequences using a pre-trained CNN. Values reported in terms of ($\mu \pm \sigma$).

Fine-Tuning	Accuracy (%)	Specificity (%)	Sensitivity (%)	F1-Score (%)
Fully frozen	55.7 ± 9.3	59.6 ± 19.9	50.7 ± 13.3	0.52 ± 0.10
Partially frozen	57.6 ± 8.4	61.5 ± 19.8	52.9 ± 13.3	0.54 ± 0.09
Semi-frozen	**62.3 ± 11.8**	**65.5 ± 18.2**	**58.7 ± 18.5**	**0.60 ± 0.13**
Unfrozen	61.4 ± 9.4	63.6 ± 17.8	58.7 ± 13.5	0.59 ± 0.09

Results indicate a progressive improvement in terms of accuracy when more convolutional layers are unfrozen. This suggests that the pre-trained model needs more knowledge from Parkinson's data (i.e., the Hw-DB corpus). However, a slight decrease in the model's accuracy is observed when the three convolutional layers are unfrozen. This could be attributed to the limited amount of data in the Hw-DB, which may not be sufficient to properly fine-tune all filters in the layers. The semi-frozen schema shows the best results, with an accuracy of up to 62.3%.

4.3. Experiment 2: Dynamic Analysis

Pressure and kinematics features, extracted from the time series provided by the digital tablet, are used in this experiment. An early fusion of these two feature sets was also considered. We consider two strategies to obtain a fixed representation from these time-dependent characterization strategies, namely statistical functionals and GMMs. Although the first strategy is simple, it constitutes a well-established approach to statically represent phenomena that originate from time-dependent feature sets. Concerning the GMM-based strategy, the number of Gaussians was optimized according to the accuracy obtained in training such that $M = 2, 4, 6, \ldots, 30$. Figure 3 shows the results obtained in the training process with each number of Gaussians per feature set. Notice that they are sorted from the lowest to the highest accuracy. Therefore, the optimal number of Gaussians is the one indicated at the right-hand side of each figure.

Table 4 summarizes the results obtained in this experiment with both strategies (statistical functionals and GMMs). Results indicate that pressure is the feature set with the best performance, achieving an accuracy of 75% when using the statistical functionals. Notice that results based on statistical functionals outperformed those obtained with GMMs when the pressure feature set was considered. In contrast, when only kinematic features were considered, both strategies showed similar results. Finally, results with the early fusion strategy did not show improvement.

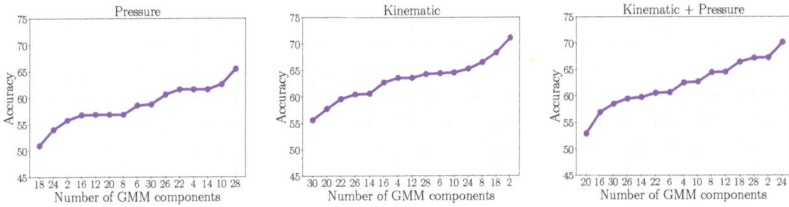

Figure 3. Accuracy mean obtained in training folds with different feature sets when changing the number of Gaussians in the GMM models.

Table 4. Values are reported as ($\mu \pm \sigma$).

Features	Accuracy (%)	Specificity (%)	Sensitivity (%)	F1-Score (%)
Statistical fuctionals				
Pressure	75.0 ± 5.2	79.3 ± 12.1	70.5 ± 7.2	73.4 ± 5.1
Kinematic	71.3 ± 12.4	73.8 ± 21.4	68.5 ± 15.0	69.9 ± 11.7
Kinematic + Pressure	71.3 ± 14.1	70.1 ± 19.2	72.5 ± 13.0	71.4 ± 12.7
GMMs				
Pressure (with 28 Gaussians)	65.5 ± 8.2	62.2 ± 15.7	68.5 ± 4.9	66.3 ± 3.3
Kinematic with 28 Gaussians	71.1 ± 7.1	73.5 ± 15.5	68.4 ± 13.5	69.5 ± 8.3
Kinematic + Pressure (with 28 Gaussians)	70.2 ± 15.6	69.5 ± 17.4	71.1 ± 21.8	69.5 ± 17.1

5. Discussion

Three different approaches were presented in this paper: one based on images resulting from the handwriting process and two based on time-dependent signals collected from a digital tablet. This discussion includes remarkable aspects of each approach and a comparison among them.

Our experiments show that classification results with the image-based features improve as the architecture adjusts more weights. The best result is obtained in the semi-frozen schema, where we allowed the fine-tuning of weights in two convolutional layers. The unfrozen schema shows slightly less accuracy. This behavior suggests that the CNN needs more real samples from the database to obtain better classification results.

The dynamic analysis yields the best results when considering features extracted from the pressure signal. These results outperform those obtained with the kinematic feature set, suggesting that vertical control of hand movement while writing is more challenging for PD patients than the horizontal ones.

When comparing models based on statistical functionals vs. GMMs, we found that the first approach is more accurate when considering the pressure feature set. Kinematic features yielded similar results with both statistical modeling strategies.

Figure 4 shows the ROC curves and their corresponding distribution of scores for the best results achieved with each modeling approach. The AUC values confirm the aforementioned claims. Image-based features are outperformed by the dynamic analyses with the pressure feature set using statistical functionals. This result is in line with the findings reported in Tables 3 and 4, where the best accuracy obtained with the dynamic approach outperformed by up to 13% the best accuracy obtained with the image-based approach. We believe that the low performance of the imaged-based approach is because, although micrographia is a key feature in handwriting deficiencies, the writing process itself (i.e., the dynamic of handwriting over time) is the one that reveals motor symptoms more clearly.

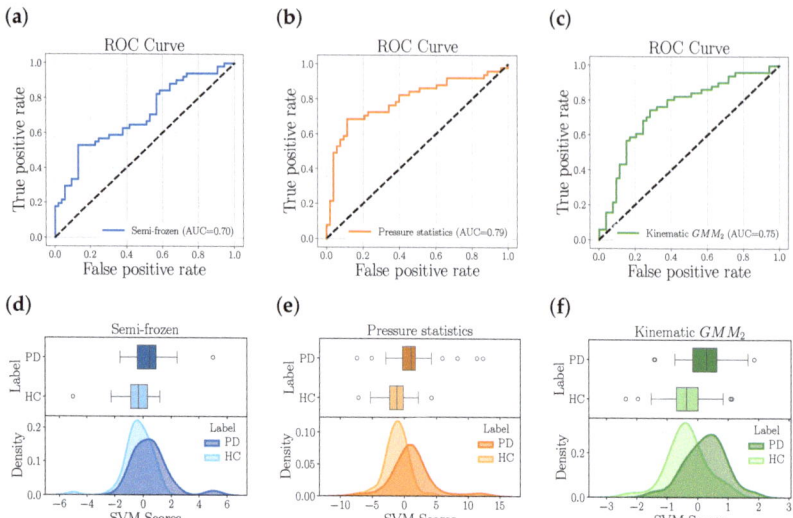

Figure 4. Results of the image-based analysis and the two dynamic analyses (modeled with statistical functionals and GMMs). The first row presents the ROC curves for (**a**) semi-frozen scheme, (**b**) pressure features modeled by statistical functionals, and (**c**) kinematic features modeled by two GMM components. The second row (**d**–**f**) depicts the distribution of the corresponding SVM decision scores resulting from the classification with the three feature sets.

We believe that this study constitutes a step forward in the development of automated systems that could be used to diagnose and monitor PD progression. For future work, we will focus on modeling transitions that occur while writing because our previous works show promising results [37] and because other studies have recently reported interesting insights towards this direction in neurodegenerative and immune diseases [38].

6. Conclusions

The present study showed that time-dependent feature sets extracted from digital tablets (namely, pressure and kinematic) are more accurate than those features extracted from images resulting from the writing process, when discriminating between PD patients and HC subjects. Additionally, our results show that the fusion of pressure and kinematic features does not improve the accuracy. Time-dependent features are represented following two strategies, one based on statistical functionals and another one based on GMMs. The comparison between using statistical functionals and using GMMs showed that the first is more suitable and yields higher accuracies. The main advantage of using statistical functionals is their direct interpretability, while the use of GMMs requires more sophisticated computations and their interpretation is not as easy, therefore limiting their use in clinical practice. This paper only considered the writing of numbers from 0 to 9; we believe that the results will stay the same when considering other tasks, like those based on words or sentences, because all these tasks are natural and belong to the set of daily living activities. Therefore, findings reported in this paper constitute a step forward in the process of creating clinically informative methods to model Parkinson's symptoms. Further research is required considering more writing tasks and also a larger number of patients to make it possible to create more sophisticated models like those based on recurrent neural networks or long short-term memory (LSTM) models.

Author Contributions: Conceptualization, D.E.-G., J.F.V.-B., A.M.G. and J.R.O.-A.; Methodology, D.E.-G., C.D.R.-U., A.M.G. and J.R.O.-A.; Software, J.D.G.-A., D.E.-G. and C.D.R.-U.; Validation, J.D.G.-A. and D.E.-G.; Formal analysis, J.D.G.-A., D.E.-G. and J.R.O.-A.; Investigation, J.D.G.-A. and D.E.-G.; Data curation, J.D.G.-A. and C.D.R.-U.; Writing—original draft, J.D.G.-A. and D.E.-G.; Writing—review & editing, D.E.-G. and J.R.O.-A.; Visualization, J.D.G.-A.; Supervision, D.E.-G., A.M.G. and J.R.O.-A.; Project administration, J.F.V.-B. and J.R.O.-A.; Funding acquisition, J.F.V.-B. and J.R.O.-A. All authors have read and agreed to the published version of the manuscript.

Funding: This work has been funded by the School of Engineering at UdeA and Pratech Group S.A.S. grants # IAPFI23-1-01 and # PI2023-58010. Adolfo M. García is an Atlantic Fellow at the Global Brain Health Institute (GBHI) and is partially supported by the National Institute On Aging of the National Institutes of Health (R01AG075775, 2P01AG019724); ANID (FONDECYT Regular 1210176, 1210195); DICYT-USACH (032351G-DAS); Agencia Nacional de Promoción Científica y Tecnológica (01-PICTE-2022-05-00103); Agencia Nacional de Investigación e Innovación (EI-X-2023-1-176993); and the Multi-partner Consortium to Expand Dementia Research in Latin America (ReDLat), which is supported by the Fogarty International Center and the National Institutes of Health, the National Institute on Aging (R01AG057234, R01AG075775, R01AG21051, and CARDS-NIH), Alzheimer's Association (SG-20- 725707), Rainwater Charitable Foundation's Tau Consortium, the Bluefield Project to Cure Frontotemporal Dementia, and the Global Brain Health Institute.

Institutional Review Board Statement: Not applicable.

Informed Consent Statement: Not applicable.

Data Availability Statement: The original contributions presented in this study are included in the article. Further inquiries can be directed to the corresponding author.

Conflicts of Interest: The authors declare no conflicts of interest.

References

1. Hornykiewicz, O. Biochemical aspects of Parkinson's disease. *Neurology* **1998**, *51*, S2–S9. [CrossRef] [PubMed]
2. Meder, D.; Herz, D.M.; Rowe, J.B.; Lehéricy, S.; Siebner, H.R. The role of dopamine in the brain-lessons learned from Parkinson's disease. *Neuroimage* **2019**, *190*, 79–93. [CrossRef] [PubMed]
3. Sveinbjornsdottir, S. The clinical symptoms of Parkinson's disease. *J. Neurochem.* **2016**, *139*, 318–324. [CrossRef] [PubMed]
4. Thomas, M.; Lenka, A.; Kumar Pal, P. Handwriting analysis in Parkinson's disease: Current status and future directions. *Mov. Disord. Clin. Pract.* **2017**, *4*, 806–818. [CrossRef]
5. Letanneux, A.; Danna, J.; Velay, J.; Viallet, F.; Pinto, S. From micrographia to Parkinson's disease dysgraphia. *Mov. Disord.* **2014**, *29*, 1467–1475. [CrossRef]
6. D'Alessandro, T.; Carmona-Duarte, C.; De Stefano, C.; Diaz, M.; Ferrer, M.; Fontanella, F. A Machine Learning Approach to Analyze the Effects of Alzheimer's Disease on Handwriting Through Lognormal Features. In Proceedings of the Graphonomics in Human Body Movement: Bridging Research and Practice from Motor Control to Handwriting Analysis and Recognition (IGS), Évora, Portugal, 16–19 October 2023; pp. 103–121.
7. D'Alessandro, T.; De Stefano, C.; Fontanella, F.; Nardone, E.; Pace, C. From Handwriting Analysis to Alzheimer's Disease Prediction: An Experimental Comparison of Classifier Combination Methods. In Proceedings of the Document Analysis and Recognition—ICDAR 2024, Athens, Greece, 30 August–4 September 2024; pp. 334–351.
8. Impedovo, D.; Pirlo, G. Dynamic Handwriting Analysis for the Assessment of Neurodegenerative Diseases: A Pattern Recognition Perspective. *IEEE Rev. Biomed. Eng.* **2019**, *12*, 209–220. [CrossRef]
9. Aouraghe, I.; Khaissidi, G.; Mrabti, M. A literature review of online handwriting analysis to detect Parkinson's disease at an early stage. *Multimed. Tools Appl.* **2023**, *82*, 11923–11948. [CrossRef]
10. Vessio, G. Dynamic Handwriting Analysis for Neurodegenerative Disease Assessment: A Literary Review . *Appl. Sci.* **2019**, *9*, 4666. [CrossRef]
11. Pereira, C.R.; Weber, S.A.; Hook, C.; Rosa, G.H.; Papa, J.P. Deep learning-aided Parkinson's disease diagnosis from handwritten dynamics. In Proceedings of the 2016 29th SIBGRAPI Conference on Graphics, Patterns and Images (SIBGRAPI), Sao Paulo, Brazil, 4–7 October 2016; pp. 340–346.

12. Kotsavasiloglou, C.; Kostikis, N.; Hristu-Varsakelis, D.; Arnaoutoglou, M. Machine learning-based classification of simple drawing movements in Parkinson's disease. *Biomed. Signal Process. Control* **2017**, *31*, 174–180. [CrossRef]
13. Mucha, J.; Zvoncak, V.; Galaz, Z.; Faundez-Zanuy, M.; Mekyska, J.; Kiska, T.; Smekal, Z.; Brabenec, L.; Rektorová, I.; Lopez-de Ipina, K. Fractional derivatives of online handwriting: A new approach of parkinsonic dysgraphia analysis. In Proceedings of the 2018 41st International Conference on Telecommunications and Signal Processing (TSP), Athens, Greece, 4–6 July 2018; pp. 1–4.
14. Zham, P.; Arjunan, S.P.; Raghav, S.; Kumar, D.K. Efficacy of guided spiral drawing in the classification of Parkinson's disease. *IEEE J. Biomed. Health Inform.* **2017**, *22*, 1648–1652. [CrossRef]
15. Valla, E.; Nomm, S.; Medijainen, K.; Taba, P.; Toomela, A. Tremor-related feature engineering for machine learning based Parkinson's disease diagnostics. *Biomed. Signal Process. Control* **2022**, *75*, 103551. [CrossRef]
16. Pereira, C.R.; Pereira, D.R.; Rosa, G.H.; Albuquerque, V.H.; Weber, S.A.; Hook, C.; Papa, J.P. Handwritten dynamics assessment through convolutional neural networks: An application to Parkinson's disease identification. *Artif. Intell. Med.* **2018**, *87*, 67–77. [CrossRef] [PubMed]
17. Gil-Martín, M.; Montero, J.M.; San-Segundo, R. Parkinson's disease detection from drawing movements using convolutional neural networks. *Electronics* **2019**, *8*, 907. [CrossRef]
18. Kamran, I.; Naz, S.; Razzak, I.; Imran, M. Handwriting dynamics assessment using deep neural network for early identification of Parkinson's disease. *Future Gener. Comput. Syst.* **2021**, *117*, 234–244. [CrossRef]
19. Drotár, P.; Mekyska, J.; Rektorová, I.; Masarová, L.; Smékal, Z.; Faundez-Zanuy, M. Evaluation of handwriting kinematics and pressure for differential diagnosis of Parkinson's disease. *Artif. Intell. Med.* **2016**, *67*, 39–46. [CrossRef]
20. Pereira, C.R.; Pereira, D.R.; Silva, F.A.; Masieiro, J.P.; Weber, S.A.; Hook, C.; Papa, J.P. A new computer vision-based approach to aid the diagnosis of Parkinson's disease. *Comput. Methods Programs Biomed.* **2016**, *136*, 79–88. [CrossRef]
21. Li, Z.; Yang, J.; Wang, Y.; Cai, M.; Liu, X.; Lu, K. Early diagnosis of Parkinson's disease using Continuous Convolution Network: Handwriting recognition based on off-line hand drawing without template. *J. Biomed. Inform.* **2022**, *130*, 104085. [CrossRef]
22. Galaz, Z.; Drotar, P.; Mekyska, J.; Gazda, M.; Mucha, J.; Zvoncak, V.; Smekal, Z.; Faundez-Zanuy, M.; Castrillon, R.; Orozco-Arroyave, J.R.; et al. Comparison of CNN-Learned vs. Handcrafted Features for Detection of Parkinson's Disease Dysgraphia in a Multilingual Dataset. *Front. Neuroinform.* **2022**, *16*, 877139. [CrossRef]
23. Gazda, M.; Hireš, M.; Drotár, P. Multiple-fine-tuned convolutional neural networks for Parkinson's disease diagnosis from offline handwriting. *IEEE Trans. Syst. Man Cybern. Syst.* **2021**, *52*, 78–89. [CrossRef]
24. Miler Jerkovic, V.; Kojic, V.; Dragasevic Miskovic, N.; Djukic, T.; Kostic, V.S.; Popovic, M.B. Analysis of on-surface and in-air movement in handwriting of subjects with Parkinson's disease and atypical parkinsonism. *Biomed. Eng. Tech.* **2019**, *64*, 187–194. [CrossRef]
25. Angelillo, M.T.; Impedovo, D.; Pirlo, G.; Vessio, G. Performance-driven handwriting task selection for Parkinson's disease classification. In Proceedings of the AI*IA 2019–Advances in Artificial Intelligence: XVIIIth International Conference of the Italian Association for Artificial Intelligence, Rende, Italy, 19–22 November 2019; Proceedings 18. Springer: Cham, Switzerland, 2019; pp. 281–293.
26. Aouraghe, I.; Alae, A.; Ghizlane, K.; Mrabti, M.; Aboulem, G.; Faouzi, B. A novel approach combining temporal and spectral features of Arabic online handwriting for Parkinson's disease prediction. *J. Neurosci. Methods* **2020**, *339*, 108727. [CrossRef] [PubMed]
27. Rios-Urrego, C.D.; Vásquez-Correa, J.C.; Vargas-Bonilla, J.F.; Nöth, E.; Lopera, F.; Orozco-Arroyave, J.R. Analysis and evaluation of handwriting in patients with Parkinson's disease using kinematic, geometrical, and non-linear features. *Comput. Methods Programs Biomed.* **2019**, *173*, 43–52. [CrossRef] [PubMed]
28. Diaz, M.; Ferrer, M.A.; Impedovo, D.; Pirlo, G.; Vessio, G. Dynamically enhanced static handwriting representation for Parkinson's disease detection. *Pattern Recognit. Lett.* **2019**, *128*, 204–210. [CrossRef]
29. Moetesum, M.; Siddiqi, I.; Vincent, N.; Cloppet, F. Assessing visual attributes of handwriting for prediction of neurological disorders—A case study on Parkinson's disease. *Pattern Recognit. Lett.* **2019**, *121*, 19–27. [CrossRef]
30. Li, Z.; Liu, F.; Yang, W.; Peng, S.; Zhou, J. A survey of convolutional neural networks: Analysis, applications, and prospects. *IEEE Trans. Neural Netw. Learn. Syst.* **2021**, *33*, 6999–7019. [CrossRef]
31. Tan, C.; Sun, F.; Kong, T.; Zhang, W.; Yang, C.; Liu, C. A survey on deep transfer learning. In Proceedings of the Artificial Neural Networks and Machine Learning–ICANN 2018: 27th International Conference on Artificial Neural Networks, Rhodes, Greece, 4–7 October 2018; Proceedings, Part III 27; Springer: Cham, Switzerland, 2018; pp. 270–279.
32. Shorten, C.; Khoshgoftaar, T.M. A survey on image data augmentation for deep learning. *J. Big Data* **2019**, *6*, 60. [CrossRef]
33. Cilia, N.; D'Alessandro, T.; De Stefano, C.; Fontanella, F. Deep transfer learning algorithms applied to synthetic drawing images as a tool for supporting Alzheimer's disease prediction. *Mach. Vis. Appl.* **2022**, *33*, 49. [CrossRef]
34. Cohen, G.; Afshar, S.; Tapson, J.; Van Schaik, A. EMNIST: Extending MNIST to handwritten letters. In Proceedings of the Proceedings of IJCNN, Anchorage, AK, USA, 14–19 May 2017; pp. 2921–2926.

35. Gallo-Arisitizábal, J.; Escobar-Grisales, D.; Ríos-Urrego, C.; Pérez-Toro, P.; Nöth, E.; Maier, A.; Orozco-Arroyave, J. Assessment of handwriting in patients with Parkinson's disease using non-intrusive tasks. In Proceedings of the International Symposium on Biomedical Imaging (ISBI), Cartagena, Colombia, 18–21 April 2023; pp. 1–4.
36. Rios-Urrego, C.; Rusz, J.; Nöth, E.; Orozco-Arroyave, J. Automatic Classification of Hypokinetic and Hyperkinetic Dysarthria based on GMM-Supervectors. In Proceedings of the Annual Conference of the International Speech Communication Association, Dublin, Ireland, 20–24 August 2023; INTERSPEECH 2023.
37. Vásquez-Correa, J.; Arias-Vergara, T.; Orozco-Arroyave, J.; Eskofier, B.; Klucken, J.; Nöth, E. Multimodal assessment of Parkinson's disease: A deep learning approach. *IEEE J. Biomed. Health Inform.* **2019**, *23*, 1618–1630. [CrossRef]
38. Romijnders, R.; Atrsaei, A.; Rehman, R.Z.U.; Strehlow, L.; Massoud, J.; Hinchliffe, C.; Macrae, V.; Emmert, K.; Reilmann, R.; van der Woude, C.J.; et al. Association of real life postural transitions kinematics with fatigue in neurodegenerative and immune diseases. *npj Digit. Med.* **2025**, *8*, 12. [CrossRef]

Disclaimer/Publisher's Note: The statements, opinions and data contained in all publications are solely those of the individual author(s) and contributor(s) and not of MDPI and/or the editor(s). MDPI and/or the editor(s) disclaim responsibility for any injury to people or property resulting from any ideas, methods, instructions or products referred to in the content.

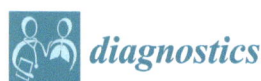

Article

Reliable Autism Spectrum Disorder Diagnosis for Pediatrics Using Machine Learning and Explainable AI

Insu Jeon [1], Minjoong Kim [2], Dayeong So [2], Eun Young Kim [2], Yunyoung Nam [2], Seungsoo Kim [3], Sehoon Shim [4], Joungmin Kim [2,5,*] and Jihoon Moon [1,2,6,*]

1. Department of Medical Science, Soonchunhyang University, Asan 31538, Republic of Korea; jis601@sch.ac.kr
2. Department of ICT Convergence, Soonchunhyang University, Asan 31538, Republic of Korea; wooni3804@sch.ac.kr (M.K.); sodayeong@sch.ac.kr (D.S.); eykim@sch.ac.kr (E.Y.K.); ynam@sch.ac.kr (Y.N.)
3. Department of Pediatrics, Soonchunhyang University Cheonan Hospital, Cheonan 31151, Republic of Korea; equalkss@schmc.ac.kr
4. Department of Psychiatry, Soonchunhyang University Cheonan Hospital, Cheonan 31151, Republic of Korea; shshim@schmc.ac.kr
5. College of Hayngsul Nanum, Soonchunhyang University, Asan 31538, Republic of Korea
6. Department of AI and Big Data, Soonchunhyang University, Asan 31538, Republic of Korea
* Correspondence: nicki123@sch.ac.kr (J.K.); jmoon22@sch.ac.kr (J.M.)

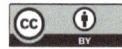

Citation: Jeon, I.; Kim, M.; So, D.; Kim, E.Y.; Nam, Y.; Kim, S.; Shim, S.; Kim, J.; Moon, J. Reliable Autism Spectrum Disorder Diagnosis for Pediatrics Using Machine Learning and Explainable AI. *Diagnostics* 2024, 14, 2504. https://doi.org/10.3390/diagnostics14222504

Academic Editor: Dechang Chen

Received: 27 September 2024
Revised: 31 October 2024
Accepted: 6 November 2024
Published: 8 November 2024

Copyright: © 2024 by the authors. Licensee MDPI, Basel, Switzerland. This article is an open access article distributed under the terms and conditions of the Creative Commons Attribution (CC BY) license (https://creativecommons.org/licenses/by/4.0/).

Abstract: Background: As the demand for early and accurate diagnosis of autism spectrum disorder (ASD) increases, the integration of machine learning (ML) and explainable artificial intelligence (XAI) is emerging as a critical advancement that promises to revolutionize intervention strategies by improving both accuracy and transparency. **Methods:** This paper presents a method that combines XAI techniques with a rigorous data-preprocessing pipeline to improve the accuracy and interpretability of ML-based diagnostic tools. Our preprocessing pipeline included outlier removal, missing data handling, and selecting pertinent features based on clinical expert advice. Using *R* and the *caret* package (version 6.0.94), we developed and compared several ML algorithms, validated using 10-fold cross-validation and optimized by grid search hyperparameter tuning. XAI techniques were employed to improve model transparency, offering insights into how features contribute to predictions, thereby enhancing clinician trust. **Results:** Rigorous data-preprocessing improved the models' generalizability and real-world applicability across diverse clinical datasets, ensuring a robust performance. Neural networks and extreme gradient boosting models achieved the best performance in terms of accuracy, precision, and recall. XAI techniques demonstrated that behavioral features significantly influenced model predictions, leading to greater interpretability. **Conclusions:** This study successfully developed highly precise and interpretable ML models for ASD diagnosis, connecting advanced ML methods with practical clinical application and supporting the adoption of AI-driven diagnostic tools by healthcare professionals. This study's findings contribute to personalized intervention strategies and early diagnostic practices, ultimately improving outcomes and quality of life for individuals with ASD.

Keywords: autism spectrum disorder; clinical diagnosis; data preprocessing; healthcare analytics; machine learning; patient outcomes; personalized intervention; explainable artificial intelligence

1. Introduction

Autism spectrum disorder (ASD) is a complex neurodevelopmental disorder affecting approximately 1 in 54 children worldwide [1]. It is marked by ongoing challenges in social communication and interaction, along with restricted and repetitive behaviors and interests [2]. The wide range of symptoms varies greatly among individuals, making diagnosis difficult and necessitating personalized intervention strategies to effectively support each child. ASD's profound impact extends beyond individuals to families, educational systems, and healthcare infrastructures, resulting in significant social and economic burdens [3].

Early and accurate diagnosis is crucial, as early intervention can greatly and significantly improve developmental outcomes and quality of life for children with ASD [4].

Identifying ASD is essential, as initial signs typically appear between 2 and 3 years of age, a critical period for brain development [5]. In this period, the brain's increased plasticity makes it ideal for interventions that can positively influence developmental paths [6]. However, early symptoms are often subtle and diverse, encompassing a range of behavioral and communication issues that can be easily overlooked or misinterpreted [7]. Traditional diagnostic methods rely primarily on subjective behavioral assessments by clinicians, such as the Autism Diagnostic Observation Schedule and the Autism Diagnostic Interview—Revised (ADI-R) [8]. In addition, standardized assessment tools such as the Childhood Autism Rating Scale (CARS), the Social Responsiveness Scale (SRS), and the Autism Spectrum Quotient 10 (AQ10) are commonly used to evaluate ASD symptoms [9–11].

While these assessments are invaluable, their reliance on clinical expertise introduces variability and potential bias, causing inconsistencies in diagnosis [12]. Furthermore, due to the nature of ASD assessments and surveys, there may be an overwhelming representation of individuals with ASD compared to non-ASD individuals in the datasets. This imbalance can lead to decreased diagnostic accuracy when relying solely on traditional methods, as models may be biased toward overrepresented classes. In addition, shortages of trained professionals and high demand for diagnostic services exacerbate identification delays, highlighting the need for more efficient and scalable diagnostic approaches.

In recent years, artificial intelligence (AI) and machine learning (ML) has become pivotal in advancing early ASD diagnosis and intervention. ML algorithms, including support vector machines (SVMs), random forest (RF), and extreme gradient boosting (XGBoost), are highly effective in analyzing large and complex datasets [13], uncovering patterns that are undetectable by traditional methods. For example, RF and XGBoost have successfully classified ASD using behavioral and clinical data, achieving high accuracy [14,15]. These algorithms enable predictive models that improve diagnostic accuracy and support personalized intervention plans tailored to each child's developmental [16]. In this study, we focus on survey-based behavioral and clinical data and use R for our analyses, prioritizing accessibility and ease of use for clinicians. By not including imaging data, we aim to develop a more streamlined and interpretable diagnostic approach, suitable for initial assessments prior to specialized testing by clinicians.

Even when AI models achieve high accuracy, it is critical to understand their decision-making processes, especially what variables they consider important beyond known factors, such as CARS, SRS, and AQ10 scores. Adopting ML in ASD diagnosis faces challenges, notably the 'black-box' nature of models, which lack transparency in their predictions [17]. This opacity can undermine clinician confidence and hinder AI integration in healthcare [18]. Understanding the importance of different variables, including those not typically emphasized in clinical assessments, may provide new insights and previously overlooked factors in ASD diagnosis. In addition, the absence of rigorous validation of data reliability affects the accuracy and generalizability of ML models [19]. Issues such as missing data, outliers, and biased feature selection can distort predictions [20].

To overcome these hurdles, this study incorporates explainable artificial intelligence (XAI) techniques [21], such as permutation feature importance (PFI), local interpretable model-agnostic explanations (LIMEs), and Shapley additive explanations (SHAP), to clarify ML model's decision-making processes. These methods aim to enhance transparency and trust, ensuring that models are both accurate and interpretable [22]. This dual emphasis on performance and explainability is critical for fostering collaboration between AI systems and healthcare professionals, facilitating the integration of ML-driven diagnostic tools into clinical practices [23]. In addition, by identifying and understanding the importance of variables beyond traditional assessment tools, we can improve diagnostic criteria and support the development of more comprehensive intervention strategies.

This study underscores the paramount importance of data reliability, implementing a meticulous data-preprocessing pipeline involving outlier removal, missing data handling, and feature selection based on clinical expert input [24]. This refinement ensures that our ML models are based on high-quality data, enhancing accuracy and credibility. Our rigorous approach addresses common oversights in previous research, improving the generalizability and real-world applicability of our findings [25]. Furthermore, we provide clear guidelines to help clinicians adopt AI tools effectively in diagnostics. In addition, by using *R*, which is widely used in medicine for statistical analysis and data modeling, we aim to provide accessible and practical AI tools for clinicians without requiring extensive programming expertise. Our current study does not include imaging data, but instead focuses on survey-based assessments to streamline the diagnostic process prior to specialized testing by clinicians.

This study is guided by the following research questions:

1. What is the impact of a rigorous data-preprocessing pipeline—including outlier removal, missing data handling, and expert-driven feature selection—on the performance, robustness, and generalizability of ML models for ASD diagnosis, especially in the context of data heterogeneity and imbalance?
2. How do different ML algorithms (e.g., SVMs, RFs, XGBoost, and neural networks) compare in terms of accuracy, interpretability, and computational efficiency in diagnosing ASD using the *R* programming language and the *caret* package, and what are the trade-offs between model complexity and practical usability in clinical settings?
3. How can the integration of advanced XAI techniques (e.g., PFI, LIME, and SHAP) improve the interpretability of ML models for ASD diagnosis, and what new insights do they provide into the relative importance of different features, including those not traditionally emphasized in clinical assessments, such as CARS, SRS, and AQ10?
4. How does the development of accessible ML tools using *R* and *caret* facilitate the adoption of AI-driven diagnostic methods by clinicians, and how does this accessibility impact the effectiveness and reliability of ASD diagnosis without requiring extensive programming expertise?

This study significantly advances ASD diagnosis and prediction through several key contributions:

- We implement a careful data-preprocessing pipeline that includes outlier removal, missing data handling, and feature selection based on input from clinical experts. This rigorous approach addresses common data challenges, such as heterogeneity and imbalance, and improves the validity, robustness, and generalizability of our ML models. Our results demonstrate the critical role of data quality in the development of reliable diagnostic tools.
- We develop and rigorously evaluate several ML models—including SVMs, RFs, XGBoost, and neural networks (NNETs)—for ASD diagnosis, using *R* and the *caret* package. Using 10-fold cross-validation and grid search hyperparameter tuning, we optimize model performance and thoroughly compare their accuracy, interpretability, and computational requirements. This comprehensive analysis provides valuable insight into the trade-offs between model complexity and diagnostic efficacy.
- We integrate advanced XAI techniques, such as PFI, LIME, and SHAP, into our ML models to improve interpretability. This integration allows us to dissect the decision-making processes of complex models and uncover the relative importance of different features, including those not traditionally emphasized in clinical evaluations. These insights can inform the development of more comprehensive diagnostic criteria and personalized intervention strategies for ASD.
- Using *R* programming and the *caret* package, we create practical and accessible ML tools tailored for clinicians. Our emphasis on user-friendly implementations and model interpretability through XAI techniques ensures that these tools can be effectively integrated into clinical practice. This enables healthcare professionals to use AI-driven diagnostics without extensive programming skills, thereby increasing the accessibility and effectiveness of ASD diagnosis.

The remainder of this paper is organized as follows: Section 2 reviews existing ASD diagnosis studies and challenges. Section 3 outlines our data-collection sources, preprocessing steps, and reliability checks and describes the ML algorithms and rationale for using R and the *caret* package for model training and evaluation. Section 4 presents the experimental setup, performance metrics, and results of our models, including XAI application. Section 5 discusses the cross-validation results and evaluates model generalizability, noting areas for further validation and improvement. Section 6 summarizes our key findings, clinical implications, and future research directions.

2. Related Work
2.1. Machine-Learning Approaches in ASD Diagnosis

Research on ASD diagnosis highlights the vital role of early detection in enhancing children's developmental outcomes. Table 1 summarizes previous studies' contributions and the distinct features of our study. While earlier research demonstrated effective diagnostic tools and ML models, they lacked explainable AI techniques and rigorous data preprocessing. Our study bridges this gap by integrating advanced ML algorithms prioritizing model interpretability and data reliability, enhancing both predictive performance and clinical applicability.

Table 1. Comparison between previous studies on autism spectrum disorder (ASD) diagnosis and intervention and the present study.

Authors	Year	Contributions	Differences from Present Study
Lord and Luyster [5]	2006	Demonstrated stability of ASD diagnosis from age 2 to 9; emphasized reliability of early diagnosis.	Does not incorporate ML or XAI; focuses on longitudinal stability rather than predictive modeling.
McCarty and Frye [6]	2020	Identified challenges in early diagnosis; proposed multi-stage screening to improve diagnostic accuracy.	Does not utilize ML algorithms or XAI techniques; focuses on screening methodologies.
Bryson et al. [7]	2003	Reviewed impact of early intervention on developmental outcomes; emphasized importance of early detection tools.	Lacks application of ML models and XAI; focuses on intervention strategies rather than predictive analytics.
Guthrie et al. [8]	2013	Examined stability of early diagnoses; highlighted need for multifaceted diagnostic approaches.	Does not apply ML or XAI; emphasizes clinical expertise and multi-source information integration.
Omar et al. [12]	2019	Developed ML models using RF-CART and RF-ID3; created a mobile diagnostic application for ASD.	Focuses on model development and application without integrating XAI techniques; limited interpretability of model predictions.
Usta et al. [13]	2019	Evaluated ML algorithms for predicting short-term ASD outcomes; found decision tree to be most effective.	Does not incorporate XAI for model interpretability; primarily focuses on prognosis prediction rather than diagnostic accuracy.
Alsuliman and Al-Baity [26]	2022	Developed optimized ML models for ASD classification using PBC and GE data with bio-inspired algorithms.	Does not integrate advanced XAI techniques to improve both the accuracy and interpretability of their models.
Ben-Sasson et al. [27]	2023	Developed a gradient boosting model for early ASD prediction using electronic health records.	Lacks integration of XAI techniques; focuses on predictive modeling using electronic health records.
Abbas et al. [28]	2023	Compared TPOT and KNIME for ASD detection, focusing on feature selection.	Does not include XAI techniques; focuses on comparing AutoML tools for ASD detection.
Reghunathan et al. [29]	2023	Used machine-learning classifiers for ASD detection, with logistic regression showing the highest accuracy.	Does not use XAI techniques; focuses on feature reduction and classifier accuracy.
Bala et al. [30]	2023	Built an ASD detection model across age groups, with SVM performing best.	Focuses on model performance across age groups without applying XAI for interpretability.
Batsakis et al. [31]	2023	Built a data-driven AI model for clinical ASD diagnosis, highlighting data limitations.	Emphasizes model development using AutoML without integrating XAI for improved interpretability.
Our Study	2024	Developed interpretable ML models using XAI techniques; implemented rigorous data preprocessing; provided guidelines for non-experts.	Integrates XAI for model transparency; emphasizes data reliability and preprocessing; offers practical guidelines for clinical use.

Lord and Luyster's [5] longitudinal studies demonstrated that ASD diagnoses made at age 2 remain stable through age 9, providing strong evidence for the reliability of early diagnosis. They noted that differentiating between narrowly defined autism and broader ASD categories is unnecessary owing to high variability in children's developmental trajectories. This study highlighted the importance of early diagnosis for predicting developmental trajectories and planning appropriate interventions. McCarty and Frye [6] noted challenges in identifying behavioral abnormalities that delay diagnosis, suggesting a multi-step screening to reduce false positives. Despite the high sensitivity and specificity of M-CHAT-R/F screening tool, it has a low positive predictive value owing to ASD's low prevalence. Bryson et al. [7] emphasized the importance of early identification and intervention in ASD, showing that early intervention can positively impact long-term developmental outcomes, enabling some children to achieve normal developmental paths. This underscores the necessity for effective early diagnostic tools and interventions.

Guthrie et al. [8] examined the stability of early ASD diagnoses and emphasized the importance of integrating clinical expertise with information from multiple sources to improve diagnostic accuracy. Their study supports a multifaceted diagnostic approach to ensure reliable and consistent ASD diagnoses. In ML for ASD, Omar et al. [12] developed a predictive model using classification and regression trees (RF-CARTs) and iterative dichotomizer 3 (RF-ID3) algorithms with the AQ-10 dataset and real-world data, achieving high accuracy across various age groups (4–11 years, 12–17 years, and 18 years and older). They also created a mobile application to make their model accessible for public use. Usta et al. [13] evaluated the performance of four ML algorithms, namely naive Bayes (NB), generalized linear model (GLM), logistic regression (LR), and decision tree (DT), in predicting ASD prognosis in 433 children, highlighting early diagnosis and intervention as key for positive outcomes. Among the models tested, the DT algorithm demonstrated the highest area under the curve (AUC) value.

Alsuliman and Al-Baity [26] developed 16 optimized ML models to improve the classification of ASD using personal and behavioral characteristics (PBCs) and gene expression (GE) data. The study applied bio-inspired algorithms, such as gray wolf optimization (GWO), flower pollination algorithm (FPA), bat algorithm (BA), and artificial bee colony (ABC), to improve feature selection and model accuracy. The GWO-SVM model achieved the highest accuracies of 99.66% (PBC) and 99.34% (GE). Ben-Sasson et al. [27] developed an ML model to predict ASD in infants using electronic health records from a national screening program. The model, validated with 3-fold cross-validation, used gradient-boosting machine (GBM) to achieve a mean AUC of 0.86 and identified developmental delay and parental concern as key predictors. Abbas et al. [28] compared the automated ML (AutoML) tools TPOT and KNIME for the detection of ASD in toddlers. TPOT achieved 85.23% accuracy, while KNIME achieved 83.89%, illustrating the benefit of feature-selection techniques for early diagnosis of ASD.

Reghunathan et al. [29] investigated different classifiers for the detection of ASD in different age groups. They used the cuckoo search algorithm for feature reduction and found key factors for ASD classification, with LR showing the highest accuracy. Bala et al. [30] developed an ML model to detect ASD across different age groups, including infants, children, adolescents, and adults. The study applied various feature selection techniques and evaluated several classifiers, with SVM performing best across all age datasets. Accuracy rates ranged from 95.87 to 99.61%. The authors used SHAP to analyze and rank the most important features to further improve classification accuracy. Batsakis et al. [31] describe an ongoing study using AI technologies to support diagnostic decision-making in clinical settings. They developed a data-driven prediction model by analyzing clinical data from past cases using an AutoML platform. Initial results are promising, but the study highlights the limitations of the available data and the need for further research to improve the model's capabilities.

2.2. Advanced Techniques in ASD Diagnosis: fMRI and NLP Applications

Research on ASD has used functional magnetic resonance imaging (fMRI) and natural language processing (NLP) to study its neurological and behavioral aspects. fMRI is a technique that maps brain activity with the objective of identifying neurological differences. In contrast, NLP is a method that assesses communication patterns with the goal of enhancing our comprehension and diagnosis of ASD. Mainas et al. [32] evaluated traditional ML classifiers, such as SVM and XGBoost, and compared them with deep learning (DL) models, such as TabNet and multilayer perceptrons (MLPs), for fMRI data analysis in ASD diagnosis. They found that SVMs with radial basis function (RBF) kernels outperformed DL models, achieving an AUC of 75%, and highlighted key brain regions involved in sensory perception and attention as critical for ASD classification.

Rodrigues et al. [33] used ML and resting-state fMRI (rs-fMRI) to classify ASD severity based on brain activity. Using Autism Diagnostic Observation Schedule (ADOS) scores as a measure of severity, their study identified potential brain region biomarkers and achieved an accuracy of 73.8% in the cingulum regions, suggesting the utility of rs-fMRI data in classifying ASD severity, although they noted the need for further validation. Helmy et al. [34] reviewed the role of AI and ML in the diagnosis of ASD using various brain imaging techniques, particularly magnetic resonance imaging (MRI). The focus was on diffusion tensor imaging (DTI) and fMRI, discussing how DL has improved the early, objective, and efficient diagnosis of ASD. The paper summarized advances in AI for ASD detection and discussed future trends in the integration of AI into clinical practice.

Themistocleous et al. [35] developed an ML model using NLP to discriminate children with ASD from typically developing peers based on narrative and vocabulary skills. The model achieved 96% accuracy, with histogram-based GBM and XGBoost outperforming DTs and GBM in terms of accuracy and F1 score. This study highlights the potential of AI tools for early diagnosis of ASD, especially in underserved communities. Toki et al. [36] used ML techniques to classify ASD in children using data from a serious game specifically designed for ASD assessment. Different NNETs, including MLPs and constructed NNETs, were used, with the constructed NNET performing best, achieving 75% accuracy and 66% recall. This suggests that these techniques can increase the efficiency of ASD screening and help clinicians provide better care.

2.3. R's Growing Importance in Medical Data Analysis: Paths and Perspectives

Recent studies have confirmed the growing importance of the *R* programming language in medical data analysis. Kaur and Kumari [37] used ML techniques on the Pima Indian diabetes dataset to detect patterns and risk factors. They developed predictive models using various supervised ML algorithms—linear kernel SVM, RBF kernel SVM, *k*-nearest neighbors (*k*-NN), artificial neural networks (ANNs), and multifactor dimensionality reduction (MDR)—to classify patients as diabetic or non-diabetic, demonstrating the utility of ML in early detection of diabetes. Li and Chen [38] applied classification models—DT, RF, SVM, NNET, and LR—to the Breast Cancer Coimbra Dataset (BCCD) and the Wisconsin Breast Cancer Database (WBCD). These models were evaluated using predictive accuracy, F-measure, and AUC values, with RF showing the strongest performance for breast cancer classification, highlighting its clinical relevance.

Leha et al. [39] investigated ML algorithms to predict pulmonary hypertension (PH) using echocardiographic data from 90 patients with measured pulmonary artery pressure (PAP). They applied models such as RF, lasso penalized LR, boosted classification trees, and SVMs and achieved high predictive accuracy, especially with the RF model (AUC 0.87), indicating the potential of ML to improve diagnostic support for PH. Miettinen et al. [40] investigated metabolic markers associated with chronic pain, sleep disturbance, and obesity in 193 patients undergoing pain management. Using ML and hypothesis-driven approaches, they identified key metabolites as significant for classifying patients with severe-pain phenotypes. The study found that metabolomic changes related to amino acid and methionine metabolism were associated with obesity and sleep problems, suggesting that co-occurring problems may influence chronic pain at the metabolic level.

Beunza et al. [41] compared several supervised ML algorithms, including DT, RF, SVM, NNET, and LR, to predict clinical events using data from the Framingham Heart Study. The study used two platforms, *R*-Studio and RapidMiner, and evaluated the models based on their AUC scores. NNET performed best in R-Studio (AUC = 0.71), while SVM had the highest AUC in RapidMiner (AUC = 0.75). The research highlights how ML algorithms can improve traditional regression techniques in clinical prediction. Despite these advances, previous studies often lack interpretability, posing a challenge for clinical adoption. Recognizing this gap, this study integrates XAI techniques, such as PFI, LIME, and SHAP, to improve model transparency. Improving model transparency using XAI techniques allows us to examine whether and how variables known to be important in clinical practice differ from those identified by the model.

We emphasize data reliability through a rigorous preprocessing pipeline that includes outlier removal, missing data handling, and feature selection based on input from clinical experts [31]. These enhancements increase analytical accuracy and reliability, ensuring that ML models are built on high-quality data. This approach improves the generalizability and practical applicability of research findings by addressing issues often overlooked in previous research [32]. This study provides clear guidance and best practices to help clinicians use ML tools for diagnosis in an accessible and effective manner through the R programming language, emphasizing improved data reliability, model interpretability, and practical use. This approach differentiates research and contributes to the development of more reliable and clinically applicable diagnostic tools for ASD.

3. Methods

This section outlines the framework and methods for developing ML models for the early diagnosis of ASD. It covers the rationale for selecting specific tools and techniques, model selection and configuration, hyperparameter optimization strategies, and XAI integration to ensure model interpretability and transparency. Figure 1 illustrates the overall flow of this process, highlighting the key stages, from data preprocessing to model evaluation, with a clear emphasis on how each step contributes to the goal of accurate and interpretable ASD predictions.

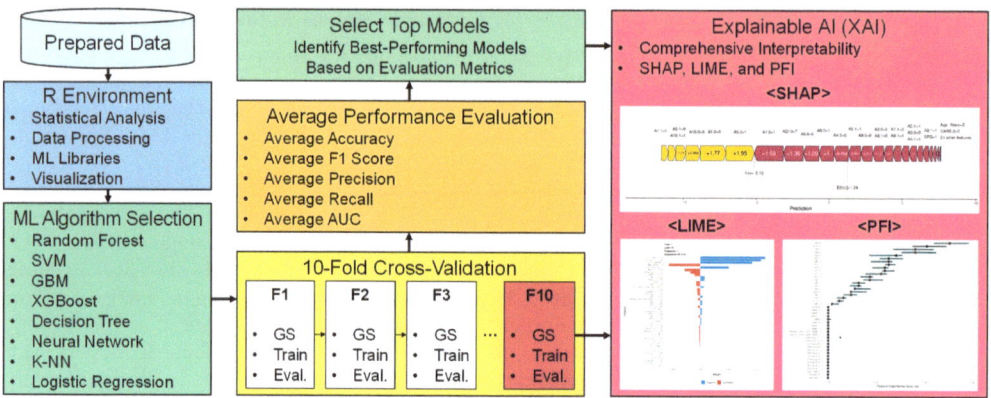

Figure 1. ML framework and methodology flowchart.

3.1. Data Acquisition and Preparation

This study uses the ASD children trait dataset, which comprehensively captures characteristics of children with ASD, including age, gender, diagnostic criteria, and socioeconomic status. Table 2 details these variables. The dataset features identifiers for 1985 cases under *CASE_NO_PATIENT'S*. The *Social_Responsiveness_Scale* scores range from 0 to 10, with some entries missing. *Age_Years* covers ages 1 to 18, consistently captured across all entries. The *Qchat_10_Score*, assessing certain ASD traits, also ranges from 0 to 10 but includes some missing values. Binary attributes such as *Speech Delay/Language Disorder*, *Learning Disorder*, and *Genetic_Disorders* are clearly marked as 'yes' or 'no', without missing data, while *Depression* and *Social/Behavioral Issues* have some missing entries. Ethnicity is categorized into 11 distinct types, fully represented. This table ensures a comprehensive view of the dataset's structure and content, aiding in the analysis of significant variables.

Table 2. Detailed overview of ASD children trait dataset with variable characteristics.

Variable	Description	Range/Values	Missing Data
CASE_NO_PATIENT'S	Unique identifier for each patient case	1 to 1985	No
A1–A10	Behavioral indicators, measured as binary values, reflecting certain autistic traits	0 or 1	No
Social_Responsiveness_Scale	Score measuring social responsiveness; higher values indicate more difficulties	0 to 10	Yes
Age_Years	The age of the child in years	1 to 18	No
Qchat_10_Score	Questionnaire score assessing autistic traits in young children	0 to 10	Yes
Speech Delay/Language Disorder	Whether the child has speech or language delays	Yes, no	No
Learning Disorder	Presence of learning disabilities	Yes, no	No
Genetic Disorders	Whether the child has any known genetic disorders	Yes, no	No
Depression	Indicates if the child has depression	Yes, no	Yes
Global Developmental Delay/Intellectual Disability	Indicates the presence of developmental delays or intellectual disabilities	Yes, no	No
Social/Behavioral Issues	Whether the child exhibits social or behavioral problems	Yes, no	Yes
Childhood Autism Rating Scale (CARS)	A clinical tool to rate autism severity (1 = nothing, 2 = little, 3 = medium, and 4 = severe)	1 to 4	No
Anxiety Disorder	Indicates if the child has been diagnosed with anxiety disorders	Yes, no	No
Sex	Gender of the child	M, F	No
Ethnicity	Ethnic background of the child	Asian, Black, Hispanic, Latino, Middle Eastern, Mixed, Native Indian, PaciFica, South Asian, White European, others	No
Jaundice	Whether the child had jaundice at birth	Yes, no	No
Family_mem_with_ASD	Indicates if a family member has been diagnosed with ASD	Yes, no	No
Who_completed_the_test	The person who completed the assessment	Family member, Healthcare professional, others	No
ASD_traits (dependent variable)	Final diagnostic classification for ASD	Yes, no	No

The data used in this study were carefully selected and restricted by clinical experts according to the following strict criteria:

1. Ensuring data completeness was a priority, and only datasets with no missing values were considered for analysis. Rather than simply excluding records with missing values, a transparent method for handling missing values was used. Missing values were handled through multiple imputations, and records were excluded from the analysis only when imputation was not feasible. For example, for the *SRS* records, data from 781 individuals—about 40% of the original 1985—were excluded because of incomplete items.
2. The analysis included only datasets that were appropriate for the age range specified by each test tool, with strict adherence to the age range specified by the test tool. For example, *QCHAT-10*, which targets infants and toddlers aged 18–24 months, required the exclusion of datasets outside this age range for reliability reasons. Similarly, *SRS* datasets that did not meet their specific age criteria were excluded. *Age* criteria for each instrument were determined based on the relevant literature in order to maintain validity and reliability.
3. To improve the reliability of the test responses, cases categorized as 'other', 'school and NGO', or 'self' were excluded from the analysis, as they were considered less reliable. This exclusion criterion was based on previous studies indicating that results can vary significantly depending on the respondent, making them statistically unreliable.
4. Any datasets that were likely to introduce prediction error or statistical bias were omitted during the analysis phase. For example, cases in which the responses to items A1–A10 were all zeros were excluded because they showed insufficient variability to effectively predict autism. This exclusion was considered justified because previous analyses confirmed a low correlation with autism prediction.

To identify the most effective ML model for ASD diagnosis, we first imported the dataset using *readxl* [42] and performed a thorough preprocessing to ensure compatibility with the different models. This preprocessing allowed us to test a variety of algorithms, each chosen for their ability to handle complex, high-dimensional data and provide insight into feature importance. Through these strict data-selection criteria, we ensured the consistency and reliability of the data, thereby guaranteeing the accuracy and validity of the analysis results. Figure 2 briefly illustrates the data-processing steps used to ensure accurate analysis.

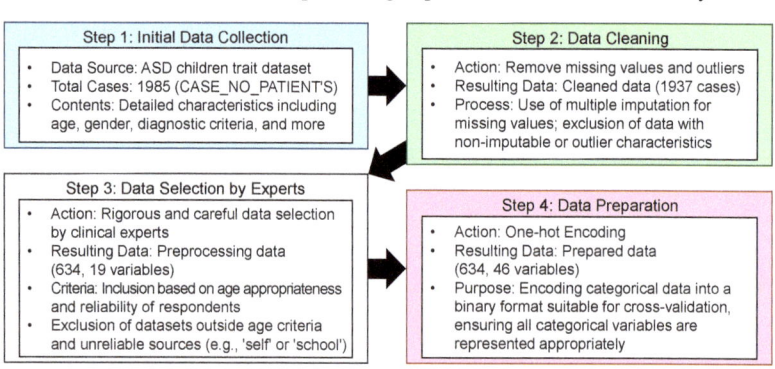

Figure 2. Flowchart of data selection and analysis process.

In our study, the dataset underwent a comprehensive transformation process to ensure its suitability for analyzing ASD traits. Key transformations included the following:

- Gender transformation: The original *Sex* variable ('F' for female; 'M' for male) was converted to numerical values (males as 1; females as 2) for easier analysis.
- Age preservation: The *Age_Years* variable remained unchanged to ensure reliable age-related analysis.

- Ethnicity recoding: The *Ethnicity* variable, initially comprising various ethnic descriptors, was recoded into numeric identifiers (e.g., Asian as 1, Black as 2, and Hispanic as 3) for standardized modeling inputs.
- Family history of ASD: The *Family_mem_with_ASD* variable, which originally documented responses as 'yes' or 'no', was transformed into a binary format (1 for 'yes'; 2 for 'no') to simplify familial ASD analysis.
- Rater categorization: The *Who_completed_the_test* variable was reclassified into *Rater*, encoding family members as 1 and healthcare professionals as 2.
- ASD traits: The *ASD_traits* variable retained its binary format, with 'yes' as 1 and 'no' as 2 for analysis.
- Social Responsiveness Scale (SRS): Scores from 1 to 10 were kept to measure social-responsiveness severity.
- Autism diagnostic scores: The *Childhood Autism Rating Scale* variable consolidated various diagnostic metrics into a single score, reflecting autism severity, categorizing symptoms from 'nothing' to 'severe', thereby standardizing ASD severity assessments.
- Autism Quotient Score: The *Qchat_10_Score* variable was renamed to AQ10 in the cleaned dataset. This score quantifies autism severity on a scale from 1 to 10, standardizing diagnostic outcomes across different assessments.
- Other ASD-relevant variables (A1–A10): ASD-relevant variables, labeled from A1 to A10, reflect diagnostic criteria or behavioral observations. These variables were standardized to ensure uniformity across datasets, enhancing their analytical use.

Meticulous data transformations enhanced analytical clarity and aligned the dataset with established standards, ensuring robust ASD-related analyses. Data reliability, crucial in social science research, was verified through statistical validation and expert review. Clinical experts identified inconsistencies, increasing dataset reliability by removing erroneous data. After preprocessing and reliability checks, the dataset was refined to 634 samples and 19 variables from 1985 samples and 28 variables, focusing on variables essential for ASD diagnosis. This refined dataset optimized predictive performance for ML models. Table 3 classifies each variable, detailing ranges and categories for clarity, while the preprocessed dataset used for our experiments, along with brief descriptions of the values and characteristics of each variable, is available in Table S1 (ASD_Preprocessed_Dataset.xlsx).

Table 3. Preprocessed dataset characteristics.

Variable	Description
Gender	Categorical variable: 1 = boy; 2 = girl.
Age_Years	Numeric variable. Represents the age of the child (range: 1–18 years).
Ethnicity	Categorical variable: 1 = Asian, 2 = Black, 3 = Hispanic, 4 = Latino, 5 = Middle Eastern, 6 = Mixed, 7 = Native Indian, 8 = Others, 9 = Pacifica, 10 = South Asian, and 11 = White European.
Family_mem_with_ASD	Binary variable: 1 = yes; 2 = no. Indicates if any family member has ASD.
Rater	Categorical variable indicating who completed the test. 1 = Family member, 2 = Healthcare professional, 3 = Others.
ASD_traits (Dependent Variable)	Binary variable: 1 = yes; 2 = no. Represents if ASD traits are present.
Social Responsiveness Scale (SRS)	Numeric variable ranging from 1 to 10. Measures the severity of social impairment. Missing values are present.
CARS	Numeric variable ranging from 1 to 10. Higher values indicate more severe symptoms. Missing values are present.
A1 to A10 (Autism Spectrum Quotient)	Binary variables (0 = no; 1 = yes). Represents responses to a series of questions related to autism traits.
AQ10 (Autism Quotient Score)	Numeric variable ranging from 1 to 10. Measures autism-trait severity.

3.2. R: A Robust Environment for Statistical Analysis and ML

The *R* programming language was chosen for ASD diagnostic models because of its strengths in statistical analysis, data manipulation, and ML [43]. Its user-friendly libraries facilitate complex analyses for non-experts, thus assisting healthcare professionals.

R excels in data processing, with packages such as *dplyr* and *data.table*, which are essential for preparing datasets for model training [44,45]. Visualization tools such as *ggplot2* and *lattice* libraries [46,47] have improved data interpretation for data scientists and clinicians. The *caret* package provided a unified interface for implementing a wide variety of ML algorithms [48], streamlining training and evaluation. In addition, specialized packages optimized for specific ML techniques, such as *xgboost*, *randomForest*, and *nnet*, integrate seamlessly with *R*, further enhancing model versatility and performance. *R* supports automated cross-validation and hyperparameter tuning, ensuring efficient model optimization and reproducibility. In summary, *R*'s comprehensive suite of statistical and ML tools, combined with its power and flexibility, made it an ideal platform for both data preprocessing and model development in this study.

3.3. Selection and Configuration of ML Algorithms

To identify the most effective ML model for ASD diagnosis, a diverse set of algorithms was tested for their ability to handle complex, high-dimensional data and provide insights into feature importance. The evaluated algorithms include the following:

- Random forest (RF) [49,50]: Utilized the *randomForest* package. This ensemble-learning method improves prediction performance and reduces overfitting by using multiple DTs. Equation (1) shows that the RF model predicts the output based on the majority vote from multiple DTs, thus improving accuracy and robustness.

$$y_{hat} = \text{majority\_vote}(T_1(x), T_2(x), \ldots, T_n(x)). \tag{1}$$

- Support vector machine (SVM) [51,52]: Implemented using the *e1071* package. SVM is effective in high-dimensional spaces and captures complex patterns by finding the optimal separating hyperplane. Equation (2) determines the classification of SVM by computing a hyperplane in high-dimensional space that best separates the classes. $alpha_i$, y_i, and K represent support vectors, labels, and the kernel function, respectively, enhancing SVM's ability to model complex relationships.

$$f(x) = \text{sign}(\text{sum}(alpha_i \times y_i \times K(x_i, x) + b)). \tag{2}$$

- Gradient-boosting machine (GBM) [53,54]: Operated using the *gbm* package. GBM increases model accuracy by sequentially correcting errors from previous models, effectively handling complex data relationships. Equation (3) updates the prediction model by incrementally improving errors, where $h_m(x)$ is the improvement term, and v is a scaling factor that helps fine-tune the correction.

$$F_m(x) = F_{(m-1)}(x) + v \times h_m(x). \tag{3}$$

- XGBoost [55,56]: Configured using the *xgboost* package. It is an optimized version of GBM that includes additional regularization and parallel processing to improve speed and performance. Equation (4) represents XGBoost's loss computation, which not only focuses on reducing the prediction error ($l(y_i, y_{hat\_i})$), but also includes a regularization term (*Omega*) to prevent overfitting.

$$L(theta) = \text{sum}(l(y_i, y_{hat\_i})) + \text{sum}(Omega(f_k))). \tag{4}$$

- C5.0 Decision Tree [57,58]: Facilitated by the *C50* package. C5.0 simplifies complex tree structures to improve interpretability and predictive accuracy. Equation (5) calculates the information gain from using attribute, *A*, to split set, *S*, which helps decide the best splits to improve tree accuracy and simplicity.

$$Gain(S, A) = Entropy(S) - \text{sum}((|S_v|/|S|) \times Entropy(S_v)). \tag{5}$$

- Neural network (NNET) [59,60]: Built with the *nnet* package. NNET models complex nonlinear relationships and is powerful for pattern recognition, although it is resource intensive. Equation (6) represents the activation of a neuron, where sigma is the activation function, w_{ij} is the weight, x_i is the input, and b_j is the bias, illustrating the computational process of the neuron.

$$a_j = \text{sigma}(\text{sum}(w_{ij} \times x_i + b_j)). \tag{6}$$

- *k*-nearest neighbors (*k*-NN) [61,62]: Implemented through the *class* package. *k*-NN classifies instances based on the proximity of the *k* nearest training data points. Equation (7) averages the labels yi of the *k*-nearest neighbors to predict the class, demonstrating *k*-NN's reliance on local data similarity.

$$y_{hat} = (1/k) \times \text{sum}(yi). \tag{7}$$

- Logistic regression [63,64]: Used the *glmnet* package. This model assumes a linear relationship between variables and outcomes, effectively modeling binary data. This logistic function (Equation (8)) calculates the probability that the outcome is 1 based on the linear combination of the input features, x, weighted by w, plus a bias term, b, illustrating a simple yet effective classification approach.

$$P(y = 1 | x) = 1/(1 + \exp(-(w \times x + b))). \tag{8}$$

Each model is selected to provide a comprehensive comparison that addresses both linear and nonlinear relationships and focuses on accuracy, reliability, and interpretability in ASD diagnosis.

3.4. Hyperparameter Optimization and Grid Search Using Caret

Hyperparameter optimization is critical for enhancing ML model performance [65], significantly affecting accuracy and generalizability. This study utilized a grid search approach to systematically explore the hyperparameter space for each algorithm, ensuring optimal performance [66]. The optimization process was integrated with ten-fold cross-validation to validate model performance and prevent overfitting.

3.4.1. The Caret Package: An Overview

The *caret* package in *R* is a comprehensive toolkit that simplifies training, tuning, and evaluating ML models [48]. It provides a consistent interface to a wide array of ML algorithms, facilitating the implementation of standardized workflows for model development. The key reasons for utilizing *caret* in this study are as follows:

- Unified interface for diverse models: *Caret* offers a consistent set of functions for training and evaluating different algorithms, streamlining workflows and simplifying model comparison.
- Automated cross-validation and resampling [67]: *Caret* automates cross-validation and resampling to assess model performance and ensure generalization to unseen data, reducing human error and enhancing reproducibility.
- Efficient hyperparameter tuning: A standout feature of *caret* is its ability to perform hyperparameter tuning through grid search and other optimization techniques. By automating hyperparameter space exploration, it boosts model performance with minimal manual effort.

- Feature engineering and preprocessing integration: *Caret* seamlessly integrates feature-engineering and data-preprocessing steps into the modeling pipeline, ensuring consistent data transformations and fair model comparisons.
- Performance metrics and model comparison: *Caret* provides built-in functions for calculating various performance metrics and supports side-by-side model comparisons to identify best-performing algorithms.
- Reproducibility and documentation: By encapsulating the entire modeling process within a single framework, *caret* enhances the reproducibility and allows comprehensive documentation for easy replication and validation.

3.4.2. Implementation of Hyperparameter Optimization with Caret

1. Setting up cross-validation and train control: A ten-fold cross-validation strategy was established using *trainControl* within *caret*. This setup involved the following:
    - Method: Cross-validation to partition the data into training and testing sets.
    - Number: Ten for ten-fold cross-validation, ensuring that each model was evaluated on ten different data subsets.
    - Search: Grid to perform grid search hyperparameter tuning.
    - Class Probabilities: Enabled (*TRUE*) to allow for probability-based metrics.
    - Summary Function: *multiClassSummary* to calculate various performance metrics suitable for multi-class classification problems.
2. Defining hyperparameter grids for each model: Specific hyperparameter grids were developed for each algorithm to explore different configurations. The following are examples:
    - RF: Tuned the *mtry* parameter, representing the number of variables considered at each split.
    - SVM: Adjusted the *C* (cost) and *sigma* parameters for the radial basis function kernel.
    - GBM: Modified parameters such as *n.trees*, *interaction.depth*, *shrinkage*, and *n.minobsinnode*.
    - XGBoost: Focused on *nrounds*, *max_depth*, *eta*, *gamma*, *colsample_bytree*, *min_child_weight*, and *subsample*.
    - C5.0 Decision Tree: Tuned *trials*, *model*, and *winnow*.
    - NNET: Tuned *size* (number of neurons in hidden layers) and *decay* (weight decay rate).
    - *k-nearest* neighbors (*k*-NN): Tuned the number of neighbors (*k*).
    - Logistic *regression* (GLMNET): Tuned the *lambda* parameter for regularization.
3. Training models with *caret*: Each ML model was trained using the train function from *caret*, which seamlessly integrated the defined hyperparameter grids and cross-validation strategy. This consistent approach was applied across all models, ensuring a standardized training process.
4. Evaluating model performance: After training, each model was evaluated using resampling techniques provided by *caret*. Metrics such as accuracy, F1 score, precision, recall, and AUC were calculated to assess their effectiveness [48].
5. Selecting top-performing models: Based on the evaluation metrics, the top-performing models were identified for further analysis and interpretation. This selection was crucial for focusing subsequent efforts on models demonstrating the highest potential for accurate and reliable ASD diagnosis.

3.4.3. Advantages of Using Caret for Hyperparameter Optimization

The use of the *caret* package in this study provided numerous advantages that significantly enhanced the efficiency and effectiveness of hyperparameter optimization:

- Streamlined workflow: *Caret's* unified interface enabled a seamless workflow for data preprocessing, model training, hyperparameter tuning, and evaluation within a single framework. This reduced the need for switching between different packages and functions, reducing complexity and potential errors.

- Comprehensive model tuning: Through grid search, *caret* enabled exhaustive exploration of hyperparameter spaces, optimizing configurations for each model. This is crucial for enhancing performance and adapting models to ASD dataset characteristics.
- Consistency across models: By providing a standardized approach, *caret* ensured consistency in evaluating and comparing algorithms, vital for unbiased and accurate model assessments.
- Efficiency and speed: *Caret's* ability to parallelize computations accelerated tuning, especially beneficial for large datasets and complex models requiring extensive tuning.
- Robust evaluation metrics: *Caret* offers a wide range of performance metrics and supports multi-class classification evaluations, essential for accurately assessing models in the context of ASD diagnosis.
- Reproducibility and documentation: *Caret* facilitates documenting and reproducing the modeling process, ensuring other researchers can replicate procedures and validate findings and thus enhancing credibility.
- Flexibility and extensibility: *Caret* is highly flexible, allowing customization to specific needs. Its extensibility helps integrate new models and techniques, aligning with the latest ML advancements.

In summary, *caret* was instrumental in efficiently managing hyperparameter optimization, ensuring meticulous model tuning for optimal performance. Its features and ability to standardize workflows rendered it an invaluable tool in developing reliable diagnostic models for ASD.

3.5. Enhancing Model Transparency with XAI

In healthcare, especially when diagnosing complex conditions like ASD, the transparency and interpretability of ML are crucial. Clinicians must not only trust the accuracy of these models but also understand the rationale behind their predictions to confidently integrate AI tools into clinical practice. This transparency is particularly important in high-stakes domains like healthcare, where decisions significantly impact patient outcomes. Without clear insights into model predictions, clinicians may hesitate to rely on AI-generated diagnoses. To address the 'black box' nature of sophisticated algorithms, such as NNETs and ensemble methods like XGBoost, this study incorporated various XAI techniques [68]. XAI provides tools to clarify the internal workings of these models, offering explanations understandable to clinicians and stakeholders [69]. By leveraging these techniques, we transformed ML models from opaque decision-makers into transparent and interpretable tools, enhancing their trustworthiness in clinical settings.

In this study, we employed three main XAI techniques: PFI [70], LIME [71], and SHAP [72]. Each method contributed to our understanding of the models' prediction processes. Below, we explain each technique and how it was used to enhance model interpretability. For clarity and transparency in our ML model analysis for ASD diagnosis, we used the following R packages to implement specific XAI techniques alongside our best models:

- *iml* package: Used for SHAP scores and PFI, which evaluates the impact of each feature on model predictions and helps identify the most important predictors.
- *lime* package: Applied for LIME, which provides local explanations that help clarify why certain predictions were made by the model.

These tools were integrated after selecting the best performing models based on accuracy, ensuring that our explanations are relevant and directly applicable to the most effective models.

3.5.1. PFI

PFI is a model-agnostic technique used to measure feature importance by observing performance degradation when feature values are randomly shuffled. If shuffling a feature causes a notable accuracy drop, the feature is crucial for predictions; if not, it likely has little impact. We applied PFI to identify key variables in predicting ASD. By shuffling values like

'Frequency of Eye Contact' or 'Family History of ASD', we gauged accuracy changes, ranking features by importance (Equation (9)).

$$\text{Delta Accuracy} = \text{Accuracy}_{original} - \text{Accuracy}_{permuted}. \qquad (9)$$

Our study found behavior-related variables, such as communication patterns and repetitive actions, to be more influential than demographic factors, like age or gender. This methodology ensures a comprehensive understanding of the impact of each feature on the accuracy of the model, thereby enhancing the interpretability of our results.

3.5.2. LIME

While PFI focuses solely on global feature importance, LIME focuses on generating localized explanations for individual predictions. LIME creates an interpretable surrogate model, typically a simpler, linear model that approximates the complex model's behavior near a particular prediction. This is especially useful for understanding why a model classified a specific patient as having ASD (Equation (10)).

$$y = wx + b. \qquad (10)$$

In clinical practice, LIME provides transparent explanations for each diagnosis, helping clinicians trust the model outputs. For example, if a model identifies a patient with ASD, LIME can show which features, like limited eye contact or repetitive behaviors, were most influential. Such case-by-case analyses allow clinicians to cross-check the model reasoning with their own clinical judgment, building confidence in AI-driven diagnoses.

3.5.3. SHAP

SHAP, rooted in cooperative game theory, provides a unified approach to measure each feature's contribution to a model's prediction. By calculating 'SHAP values', it assigns an importance score to each feature, reflecting its impact on the prediction for a specific data point. This is especially useful for understanding how variables like behavioral traits, family history, and demographic information affect the likelihood of an ASD diagnosis. A key advantage of SHAP is its consistent application across diverse ML models. Whether applied to tree-based models like RF and XGBoost or complex models like NNETs, SHAP offers a consistent framework for understanding feature importance. The contribution of each feature i to a prediction can be expressed quantitatively by Equation (11):

$$\text{Phi}(i) = \text{sum}((v(S \cup \{i\}) - v(S))). \qquad (11)$$

In this study, we used SHAP to analyze key variables, such as behavioral indicators (e.g., repetitive actions or communication challenges), and their effect on the model's ASD classification decisions. SHAP provided both global explanations, highlighting the most influential features across the dataset, and local explanations, offering insights into individual predictions.

3.5.4. Integrating XAI Techniques for Comprehensive Interpretability

The combination of PFI, LIME, and SHAP provided a comprehensive set of explanations for our ML models. PFI ranked features based on their impact on performance, providing an initial global understanding. LIME then added local insights, helping clinicians understand features that are important for specific diagnoses. Finally, SHAP provided both global and local explanations, deepening the understanding of model behavior at multiple levels. Together, these techniques transformed complex models into interpretable tools that clinicians could trust. This transparency is critical to the adoption of AI-based diagnostic tools in healthcare, ensuring that predictions are consistent with clinical reasoning and real-world observations. In addition, XAI methods emphasized the importance of behavioral factors in diagnosing ASD, highlighting the need to prioritize these features in clinical practice.

4. Results

This section analyzes the experimental results from evaluating multiple ML models for diagnosing ASD. We set the *tuneLength* parameter to 10 to optimize the hyperparameters of each ML model through a comprehensive grid search. The models were assessed using various performance metrics to compare their predictive capabilities in a robust way. XAI techniques were also employed to enhance model transparency and interpretability.

4.1. Model Performance Evaluation

Each model's performance was evaluated using several key metrics: accuracy, F1 score, area under the precision–recall curve (prAUC), precision, and recall. These metrics offer a comprehensive understanding of each model's effectiveness in diagnosing ASD. Accuracy, reflecting the proportion of correct predictions, is critical for understanding overall model success. The F1 score balances precision and recall, particularly valuable when class imbalance could skew accuracy calculations. The prAUC metric was vital in this study, as it evaluates the model ability to distinguish true positives from false positives, essential for early and accurate ASD detection.

Table 4 summarizes the overall performance metrics of the machine-learning models evaluated in our study for diagnosing ASD. The NNET and XGBoost models achieved the highest accuracy scores of 1 and 0.9984, respectively. These models also excelled in F1 score and prAUC, highlighting their effectiveness in discriminating between ASD and non-ASD cases. Such high performance suggests that these models are highly reliable for our diagnostic purposes. To statistically validate the performance differences among the models and to select the best one for our work, we performed the Wilcoxon signed-rank test and the Friedman test based on the fold-wise performance metrics obtained from the 10-fold cross-validation. The detailed performance metrics for each fold are presented in Appendix A (Tables A1–A10).

Table 4. Performance metrics for each model based on 10-fold cross-validation.

Model	Accuracy	F1 Score	prAUC	Precision	Recall
Random forest	0.9463	0.9642	0.9317	0.9409	0.9891
SVM	0.9874	0.9913	0.9545	0.9892	0.9934
GBM	0.9984	0.9989	0.9601	1	0.9978
XGBoost	0.9984	0.9989	0.9103	1	0.9978
C5.0	0.9701	0.9796	0.5358	0.9705	0.9892
NNET	1	1	0.9601	1	1
k-NN	0.8883	0.9231	0.5984	0.9156	0.9331
Logistic regression	0.9858	0.9903	0.9576	0.9873	0.9935

The Wilcoxon signed-rank test is a nonparametric statistical method used to compare two related samples to determine whether their population mean ranks differ [73,74]. In this context, it was used to compare the NNET model with each of the other models across all folds, testing the null hypothesis that there is no significant difference in performance between NNET and the compared model. Table 5 presents the *p*-values from the Wilcoxon signed-rank test comparing the NNET model to each of the other models on various performance metrics. A *p*-value less than 0.05 indicates a statistically significant difference in favor of the NNET model.

The results show that NNET significantly outperforms RF, C5.0, and *k*-NN for all performance metrics, as evidenced by *p*-values well below 0.05. When compared to SVM, GBM, XGBoost, and LR, the differences are not statistically significant for certain metrics, suggesting that these models perform comparably to NNET in some aspects. The Friedman test is another nonparametric test used to detect differences in treatments across multiple trials, especially when comparing more than two groups [74,75]. It assesses whether there are significant differences in the performance of all models across all folds. Table 6 shows the results of the Friedman test for each performance metric. The extremely low p-values (all less than 0.05) indicate that there are statistically significant differences between the models for each metric evaluated.

Table 5. Wilcoxon signed-rank test results (p-values) with NNET with other models based on fold-wise performance metrics.

Model	Accuracy	F1 Score	prAUC	Precision	Recall
Random forest	0.003	0.003	0.001	0.027	0.003
SVM	0.049	0.049	0.140	0.500	0.087
GBM	0.500	0.500	0.047	0.500	1.000
XGBoost	0.500	0.500	0.007	1.000	0.500
C5.0	0.007	0.007	0.001	0.024	0.007
k-NN	0.003	0.001	0.001	0.003	0.001
Logistic regression	0.091	0.087	0.248	0.500	0.186

Table 6. Friedman test results across all models based on fold-wise performance metrics.

Metric	Chi Squared	df	p-Value
Accuracy	56.161	7	8.775×10^{-10}
F1 Score	57.058	7	5.822×10^{-10}
prAUC	57.416	7	4.942×10^{-10}
Precision	42.265	7	4.623×10^{-7}
Recall	57.377	7	5.030×10^{-10}

These statistical analyses reinforce the results presented in Table 4, confirming that the NNET model consistently outperforms other models, especially RF, C5.0, and k-NN. The significant p-values from the Wilcoxon signed-rank test highlight the robustness of NNET's performance across multiple metrics. In addition, the Friedman test indicates overall significant differences among all models tested, further justifying the selection of NNET as the most effective model for our work. By demonstrating statistically significant improvements in key performance metrics, the NNET model proves to be highly effective in discriminating between ASD and non-ASD cases.

To achieve these optimal performance metrics, different neural network architectures were systematically tested, resulting in the architecture shown in Table 7 and Figure 3. Through a grid search on the NNET model, we found that a hidden layer size of 5 neurons and a decay of 0.1 provided the best performance and learning speed. The results for each combination of size and decay are detailed in Table 7. In addition, Figure 3 illustrates the architecture of the neural network used, which consists of an input layer with 45 nodes, a hidden layer with 5 nodes, and an output layer with 1 node.

Table 7. Optimization results for neural network (NNET) hyperparameters.

Size	Decay	Accuracy	F1 Score	prAUC	Precision	Recall
5	0.01	1	1	0.9600	1	1
5	0.1	1	1	0.9601	1	1
7	0.01	1	1	0.9524	1	1
7	0.1	1	1	0.9600	1	1
10	0.01	1	1	0.9600	1	1
10	0.1	1	1	0.9600	1	1
15	0.01	1	1	0.8900	1	1
15	0.1	1	1	0.9600	1	1
20	0.01	1	1	0.7354	1	1
20	0.1	1	1	0.9526	1	1

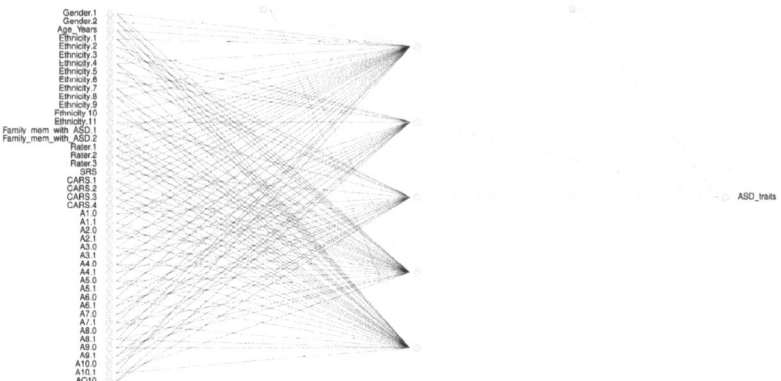

Figure 3. Neural network (NNET) architecture for ASD diagnosis.

GBM also demonstrated strong performance, achieving similarly high accuracy and precision, marking it another top-performing model. Conversely, k-NNs and C5.0 DTs demonstrated lower performance, particularly in prAUC and F1 scores, indicating that they may not be as suitable for ASD diagnosis within this dataset. Despite these differences, all models contributed valuable insights into handling ASD data complexities. To further understand the varying performance of k-NN, we analyzed how different k-values affect its accuracy, which helped to identify the optimal configuration for ASD diagnosis.

Table 8 provides a detailed analysis of the performance metrics of the k-NN model, including the accuracy, F1 score, and prAUC, for different k-values. The analysis shows that $k = 7$ achieves the best balance of sensitivity and specificity, establishing it as the optimal setting for the k-NN model in this study. Although $k = 7$ shows the best performance among the k-NN settings, it inherently lacks the robust predictive power of models such as XGBoost, NNET, and GBM, primarily due to its simpler, proximity-based algorithm, which may not capture complex patterns as effectively.

Table 8. Detailed evaluation of k-NN performance across different k-values.

k	Accuracy	F1 Score	prAUC	Precision	Recall
1	0.8380	0.8802	0.1145	0.8971	0.8672
2	0.8284	0.8749	0.1765	0.8829	0.8695
3	0.8680	0.9024	0.3057	0.9092	0.8977
4	0.8517	0.8890	0.3815	0.8994	0.8998
5	0.8695	0.9049	0.4465	0.8987	0.9127
6	0.8618	0.8983	0.4770	0.8976	0.9019
7	0.8883	0.9231	0.5984	0.9156	0.9331
8	0.8670	0.8969	0.5573	0.8905	0.9150
9	0.8601	0.8894	0.5818	0.8807	0.8993
10	0.8602	0.8893	0.6005	0.8834	0.9071

4.2. Results of XAI

In addition to evaluating performance metrics, we applied XAI techniques—specifically SHAP, LIME, and PFI—to our top-performing models, including GBM, XGBoost, and NNET, to improve our understanding of their decision-making processes. These techniques are used to interpret and explain the predictions made by these models. By using methods such as SHAP scores and variable importance scores provided by LIME and PFI, we can determine which variables significantly influence predictions. A higher value assigned to a variable indicates that it is more important to the model and therefore plays a critical role in the outcome of the predictions. This approach ensures a comprehensive analysis, providing a deeper insight into how these models process and analyze data and eliminating any ambiguity about their function.

Figure 4 shows the results of the PFI analysis, where the x-axis represents the 'Feature Importance (loss: ce)'. This figure illustrates the extent to which the cross-entropy loss of the model is amplified when the values of one feature are randomly shuffled while the values of other features remain unchanged. A higher value on the x-axis indicates that a given feature has a greater impact on the model's predictions. The y-axis displays the features in descending order of importance, with the most critical features listed first. The dots represent the estimated importance of each feature, while the horizontal lines show the variability, indicating the uncertainty in the importance of the feature across different permutations. Detailed explanations of the GBM, XGBoost, and NNET models are provided below:

- In the GBM model, as shown in Figure 4a, behavioral characteristics such as *A8.0*, *A10.0*, *A9.0*, and *A4.0* were the most influential, while demographic variables such as gender and ethnicity had little impact. *A8.0* emerged as the top variable, while other behavioral indicators played key roles.
- Similarly, as shown in Figure 4b, XGBoost highlighted significant behavioral variables such as *A7.0* and *A5.0*, while clinical and demographic variables such as *CARS*, *Family_mem_with_ASD*, and *gender* had little impact on model predictions, reinforcing the emphasis on behavioral characteristics.
- In the NNET model, as shown in Figure 4c, behavioral variables such as *A9.0*, *A10.1*, *A8.1*, and *A2.0* significantly influenced predictions, while traditional clinical variables such as *CARS*, *SRS*, and *Family_mem_with_ASD* were rarely used. Variables *A10.1* and *A6.0* contributed with a wide range of uncertainty, suggesting context-dependent importance.
- Behavioral characteristics are consistently shown to be highly influential in all models, while demographic variables have a comparatively small impact. The longer bars indicate greater uncertainty in the importance of some characteristics, but overall, the results highlight the critical role of behavioral characteristics in driving model predictions.

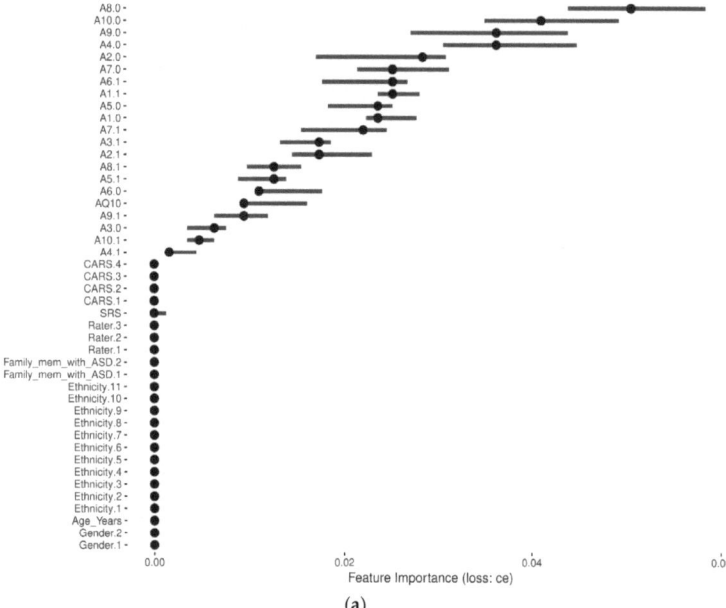

(a)

Figure 4. *Cont.*

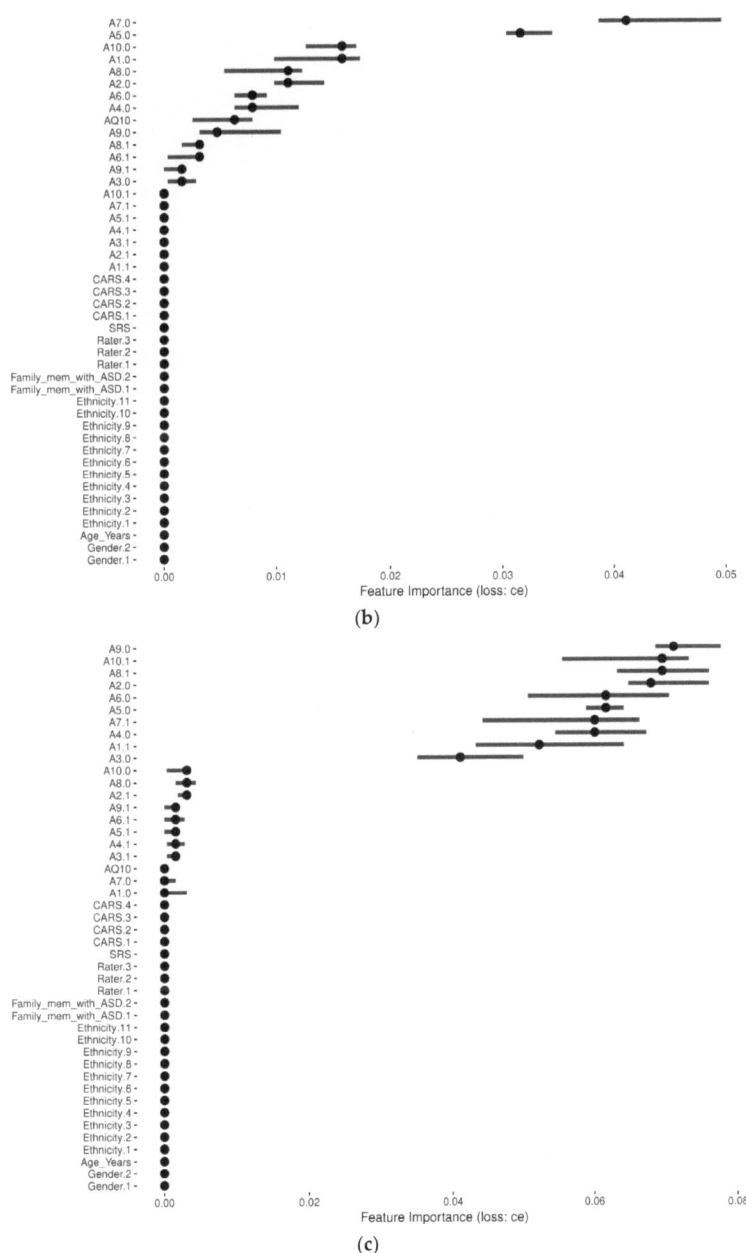

Figure 4. Permutation feature importance (PFI) results: (**a**) GBM, (**b**) XGBoost, and (**c**) neural network.

LIME provides localized explanations for individual diagnoses, showing probability and explanation fit. This helps to assess the reliability of the model predictions. When evaluating NNET and XGBoost with LIME, similar to the PFI and SHAP results, variables *A1* through *A10* have a high weight and contribute to the prediction of variables. In general, the likelihood and explanation fit were high, but occasionally they were low, and the feature contributions differed from SHAP and PFI, as shown in Figures 5 and 6.

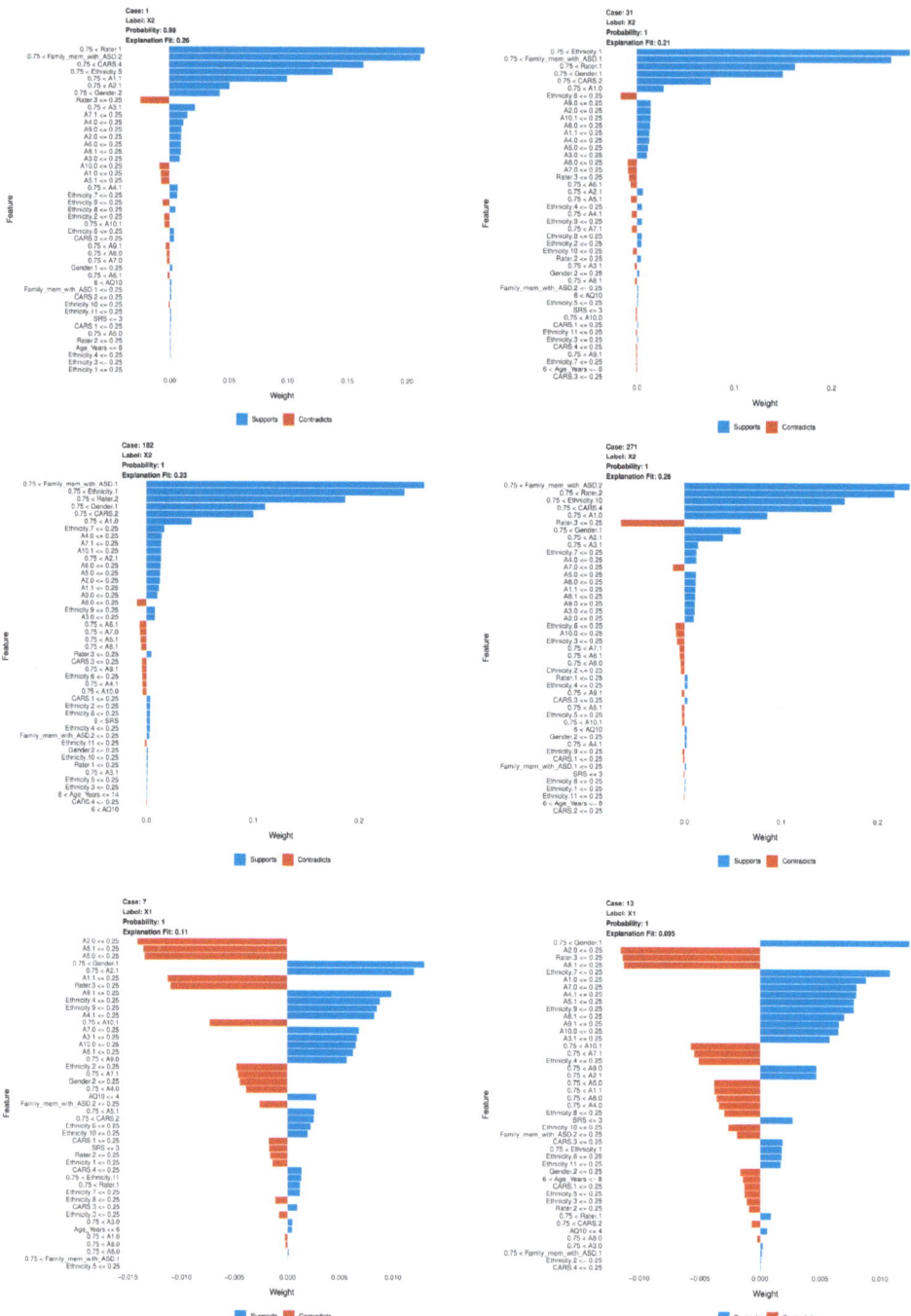

Figure 5. Local interpretable model-agnostic explanation (LIME) results in six different cases, using the NNET model.

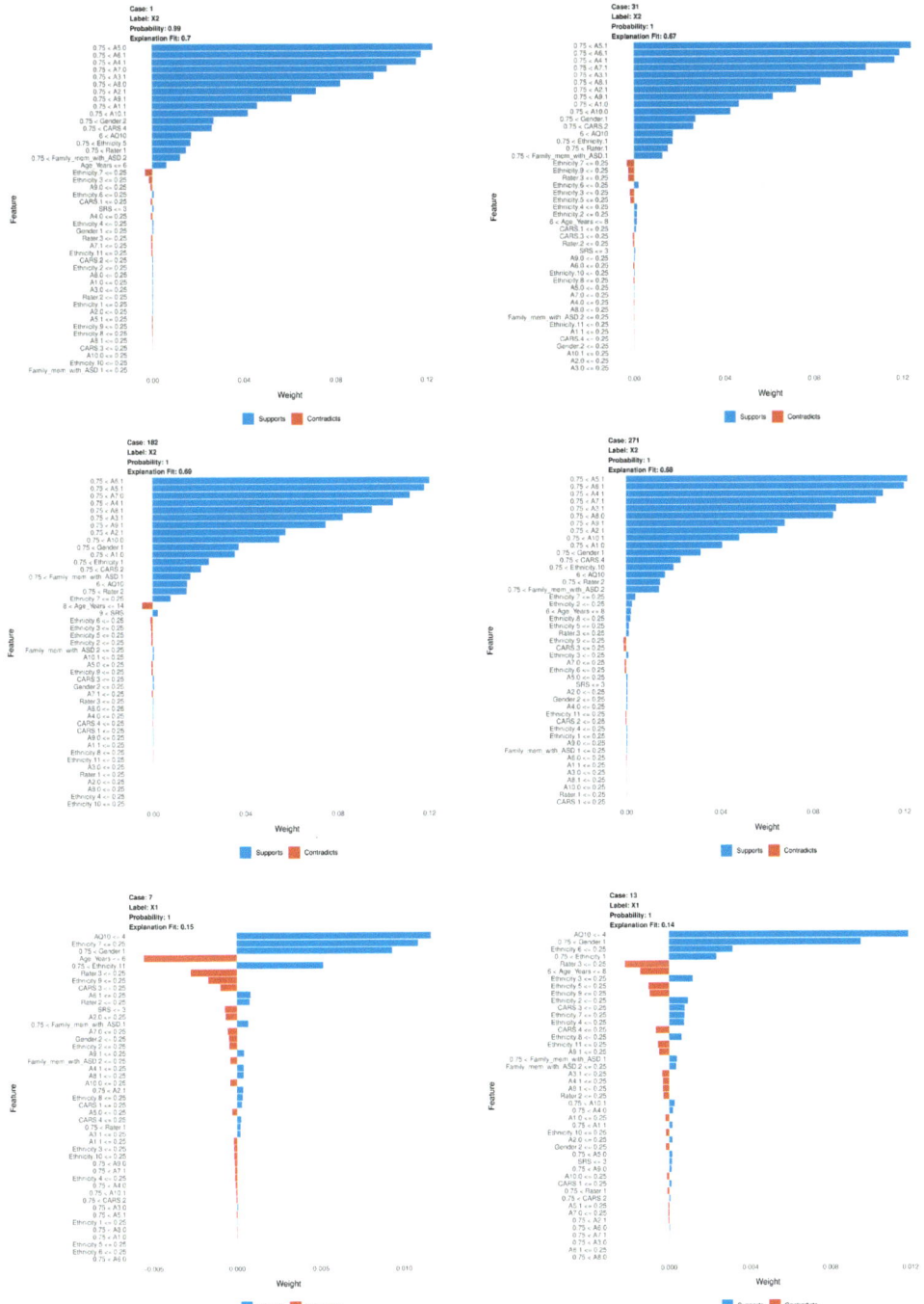

Figure 6. LIME results in six different cases using the XGBoost model.

In this context, the term 'case' is used to denote a specific observation derived from the dataset under consideration. The assignment of a case number represents a specific instance. For example, 'Case 1' denotes the first observation. The 'label' denotes the class predicted by the model, where 'label X2' indicates that the model assigned this instance to category X2. The 'probability' value represents the degree of confidence the model has in its prediction. Thus, a probability of 0.99 means that the model is 99% certain that the case belongs to the class X2. The 'explanation fit' metric quantifies the extent to which LIME's explanation matches the model's behavior for a given case. A higher value, approaching 1, indicates that LIME has a satisfactory fit to the model's decision.

Figure 5 shows the LIME for six cases using the NNET model. Below is a summary of each case, highlighting the main factors that support or contradict the model's predictions:

- In Case 1, the model predicted label *X2* with an accuracy of 0.99 and an explanation fit of 0.26, indicating a moderate level of interpretability. The LIME explanation shows that the most influential features in supporting the prediction are *Rater*, *Family_mem_with_ASD*, and *CARS*. These features played a significant role in the model's decision, with *Rater* being the most significant contributor. However, characteristics *A10* and *A1* slightly contradict the prediction, although their influence is less significant compared to the supporting factors.
- In Case 31, the model predicted label *X2* with an accuracy of 1 and an explanation fit of 0.21, showing lower interpretability. The LIME results indicate that *Ethnicity* was the most influential feature, followed by *Family_mem_with_ASD*, *Rater*, and *Gender*. The combination of these features primarily drove the model's prediction toward label *X2*, with *Ethnicity* being particularly influential. On the other hand, some ethnicity variables, as well as lower scores on traits *A8* and *A7*, contradict the prediction, although they have relatively small effects.
- In Case 182, the model also predicted Label X2 with an accuracy of 1 and an explanation fit of 0.23, which is relatively low. According to the LIME results, *Family_mem_with_ASD*, *Ethnicity*, and *Rater* were the main contributors to this prediction. The high importance of *Family_mem_with_ASD* and *Ethnicity* strongly biased the model toward the *X2* label. However, some ethnicity traits and lower scores on trait *A8* act as opposing factors, but their influence is comparatively weaker.
- In Case 271, the model predicted label *X2* with an accuracy of 1 and an explanation fit of 0.26, similar to Case 182. The LIME explanation shows that *Family_mem_with_ASD*, *Ethnicity*, and *Rater* were again the most influential features. This consistency across cases suggests that these features are critical to the model's decision to predict label *X2*. Conversely, certain ethnicity characteristics and a lower score on trait *A7* contradict the model's decision, although their influence is relatively small.
- In Case 7, the model predicted label *X1* with an accuracy of 1 and a relatively low explanation fit of 0.11. Here, *Gender* was a positive contributor to the prediction of X1, while *A2* and *Rater* were negative contributors, making the interpretation more complex due to the mixed influences of these features.
- In Case 13, the model, again, predicted label *X1* with an accuracy of 1 and an explanation fit of 0.095, indicating low interpretability. In this case, *Gender* contributed positively to the prediction, but *A2* and *Rater* had negative effects. This combination of opposing influences presents additional challenges in interpreting the model's decision for label *X1*.

Figure 6 shows the LIME for six cases using the XGBoost model. Below is a summary of each case, highlighting the main factors that support or contradict the model's predictions:

- For Case 1, the label is X2, the probability is 0.99, and the explanation fit is 0.7. The LIME explanation shows that several features, such as A5, A6, and A4, contribute significantly to the prediction of class X2. These features have the highest positive weights, supporting the model's decision. Although some smaller features, shown in red, contradict the prediction, their impact is negligible. The model has a very high confidence of 99%, and the explanation fit is relatively strong at 0.7, indicating that the LIME explanation for this case is in good agreement with the model's behavior.

- For Case 31, the label is also X2, with a probability of 1 and an explanation fit of 0.67. As in Case 1, the top features supporting classification into X2 include A5, A6, and A4. Although a few features related to ethnicity and CARS scores have a small negative impact on the prediction, their contribution is minimal compared to the top supporting features. The model's confidence is perfect, with a probability of 100%, although the explanation fit is slightly lower than in Case 1, at 0.67.
- In Case 182, the label remains X2 with a probability of 1 and an explanation fit of 0.69. The same key features as in the previous cases, such as A5, A6, and A7, play a large role in supporting the model's decision. There are small negative contributions from features such as ethnicity, but these are overshadowed by the stronger supporting features. The model's confidence is absolute, with a probability of 1, and the explanation fit is moderate, at 0.69, indicating reasonable agreement between LIME's explanation and the model's prediction.
- For Case 271, the label is X2, the probability is 1, and the explanation fit is 0.68. As with the other cases predicting X2, features A5, A6, and A4 contribute the most to the prediction. While some features related to ethnicity have a small negative influence, the overall prediction is overwhelmingly supported by the positively contributing features. The model again shows perfect confidence with a probability of 1, and the explanation fit is close to 0.7, indicating a high level of interpretability for this case.
- In contrast, Case 7 predicts label X1 with a probability of 1 and an explanation fit of 0.15. The low explanation fit of 0.15 suggests that LIME's explanation does not fit well with the model's decision process for this case. Several features, such as AQ10 and Ethnicity, contribute positively to the prediction of class X1, but there are also significant negative contributions from features such as Age_Years and Rater. This mix of support and contradiction makes the explanation more ambiguous and difficult to interpret compared to the earlier X2 cases.
- Finally, for Case 13, the model also predicts class X1 with a probability of 1 and an explanation fit of 0.14. Like Case 7, this case has a low explanation fit, which makes it more difficult to interpret the model's decision with confidence. The top features, such as AQ10 and Gender, provide strong positive support for the prediction of X1. However, many other features, particularly those related to Rater and Age_Years, provide negative contributions, complicating the overall explanation. This case, similar to Case 7, is less straightforward compared to the higher explanation fits seen in the X2 cases.

The LIME results for the NNET and XGBoost models show clear differences in feature influence and interpretability. In the NNET model, predictions for the *X2* label are strongly influenced by demographics such as *Family_mem_with_ASD*, *Ethnicity*, and *Rater*, but explanation fits are generally lower, indicating moderate interpretability and some ambiguity in understanding the model's decision process. For *X1* predictions, mixed positive and negative contributions from traits such as *Gender* and *A2* add complexity to interpretation. In contrast, the XGBoost model's LIME results for label *X2* consistently show high explanation fits (around 0.7), with top traits such as *A5*, *A6*, and *A4* providing strong support, making these explanations more interpretable and consistent with the model's decisions. However, for label *X1* predictions, XGBoost has lower explanation fits (around 0.15), indicating less agreement with the model's decision and a more difficult interpretation, similar to NNET's *X1* cases. In summary, while both models highlight key features for each label, XGBoost generally provides clearer explanations with higher fits for label *X2*, while NNET has more variation and lower overall interpretability.

Among the SHAP packages provided by *R*, *shapviz* [76] is notable for visualizing SHAP values, but it is limited to certain models, such as XGBoost and LightGBM. We applied the SHAP technique using the XGBoost model available in the built-in *caret* library. The visualization results of SHAP are shown in Figures 7–10. The SHAP summary plot, shown in Figure 7, highlights *A7.0*, *A10.0*, and *A9.0* as having the strongest positive effects on XGBoost predictions, while variables such as gender and ethnicity had minor effects. The SHAP swarm plot, shown in Figure 8, visually summarizes the feature contributions across data points. Positive SHAP values increase predictions, while negative values decrease predictions. The features at the top, such as *A7.0*, *A5.0*, and *A1.0*, significantly affect predictions, with *A7.0* typically decreasing and *A5.0* typically increasing the predicted value.

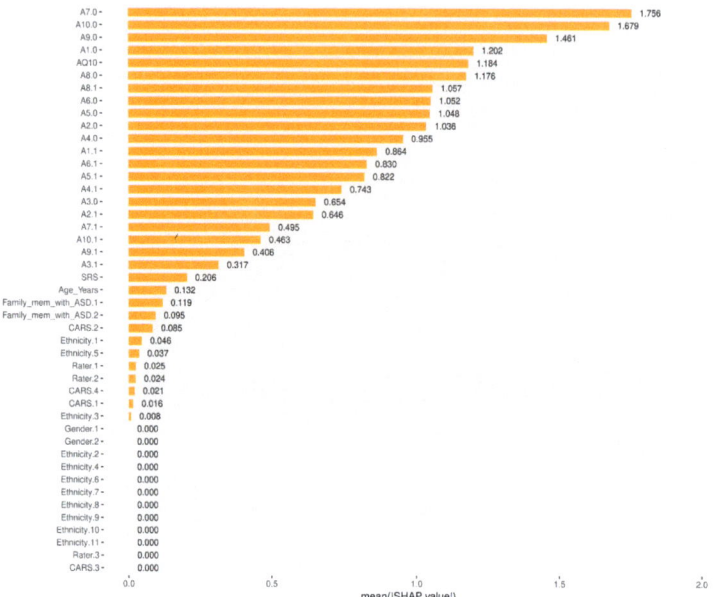

Figure 7. Shapley additive explanation (SHAP) absolute value bar plot. The x-axis represents the mean absolute SHAP value for each feature, showing how much each feature contributes to the model's predictions on average. The y-axis lists the features in descending order of importance, with the most important features at the top.

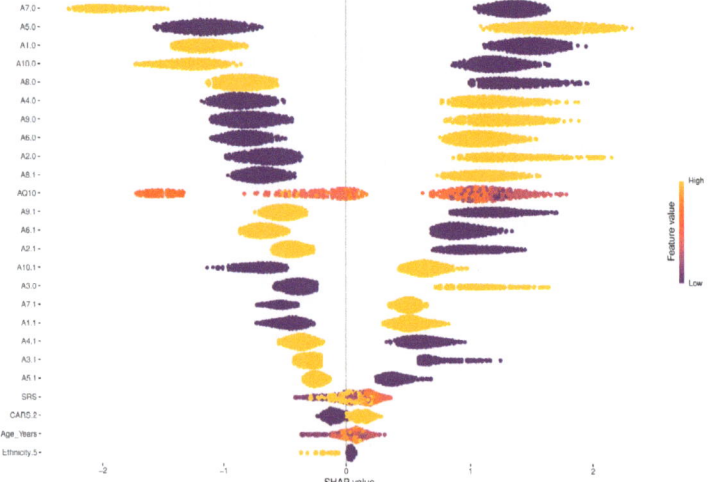

Figure 8. SHAP bee-swarm plot. The x-axis represents the SHAP value, which indicates the direction and magnitude of each feature's effect on the prediction. The y-axis lists the features in order of importance, with the most influential features at the top. The color of the dots represents the value of the feature, from low (purple) to high (yellow).

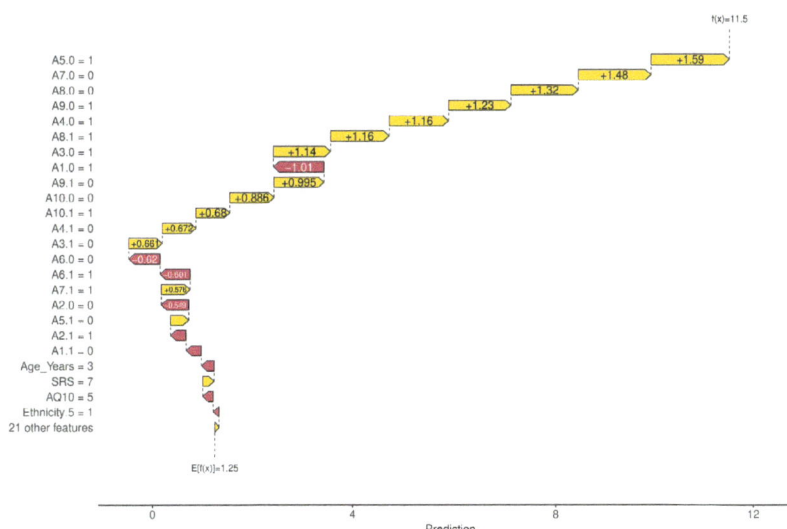

Figure 9. SHAP waterfall plot. The x-axis represents the cumulative contribution of each feature to the model's prediction, starting from the base value to the final prediction. The y-axis lists the features in descending order based on their contribution to the prediction for a given instance.

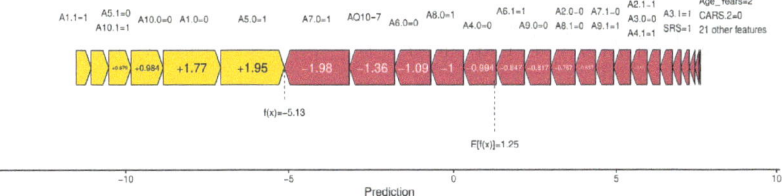

Figure 10. SHAP force plot. The x-axis represents the model's prediction, showing how different features contribute to the final predicted value. The y-axis is not explicitly labeled, but the plot visually shows the positive and negative contributions of each feature, represented by the color and direction of the forces.

The SHAP waterfall plot in Figure 9 shows the sequential feature contributions. For example, features $A5.0 = 1$, $A7.0 = 0$, and $A8.0 = 0$ positively influenced the predicted value to 11.5, while features $A1.0 = 1$ and $A6.0 = 0$ had a negative influence. The SHAP force plot shown in Figure 10 illustrates the predicted value of the model along the x-axis, with the feature contributions divided into positive or negative effects on the final predicted value ($f(x)$). $E[f(x)]$ is the standard predicted value, the average value when the model is predicted without features. The final predicted value of XGBoost is -5.13, influenced by features that either increase or decrease this value. Starting with a default of 1.25, features such as $A1.1 = 1$ and $A1.0 = 0$ increase the predicted value, while $A7.0 = 1$ and $AQ10 = 7$ decrease it to -5.13.

When comparing PFI, LIME, and SHAP, we see that PFI provides a broad, global understanding of the meaning of features throughout the model. However, it lacks the detailed, instance-specific explanations that SHAP provides. SHAP values provide a more granular interpretation that clearly shows the contribution of each feature to each prediction, allowing for both local and global interpretability. While LIME is useful for generating localized explanations for individual predictions, it lacks the consistency and additive properties of SHAP scores. SHAP's ability to explain both local and global behavior, while maintaining consistency with the model's overall predictions, makes it more reliable than LIME for understanding both feature importance and decision-making processes.

By integrating SHAP, LIME, and PFI, this study provides a comprehensive analysis of the inner workings of ML models. These techniques improve both model accuracy and interpretability, providing critical insights into the most influential features for predicting ASD outcomes. Among them, SHAP stands out for providing more comprehensive and reliable explanations compared to PFI and LIME. It excels at explaining both global and local model behavior, making it the preferred choice for understanding complex decision-making processes in the context of ASD prediction. For non-experts, this means that we can not only trust the predictions but also understand how these predictions are made, ensuring transparency in AI-driven healthcare.

5. Discussion

Because of the exceptionally high-performance metrics observed in our initial model evaluations, we were concerned about the potential for overfitting. To thoroughly investigate this possibility, we conducted additional cross-validation experiments using 2-fold, 4-fold, and 5-fold cross-validation, as detailed in Tables 9–11. These additional experiments were essential to ensure that the excellent performance of models such as NNET, XGBoost, and GBM was not simply a result of overfitting to the specific dataset used in this study.

Table 9. Model performance metrics using 2-fold cross-validation.

Model	Accuracy	F1 Score	prAUC	Precision	Recall
Random forest	0.9463	0.9642	0.9665	0.9408	0.9891
SVM	0.9605	0.9729	0.9832	0.9739	0.9718
GBM	0.9889	0.9924	0.9900	0.9913	0.9935
XGBoost	0.9968	0.9978	0.9871	1	0.9956
C5.0	0.9621	0.9741	0.7893	0.9679	0.9805
NNET	0.8691	0.9109	0.4091	0.9023	0.9199
k-NN	0.8691	0.9109	0.4091	0.9023	0.9199
Logistic regression	0.9684	0.9785	0.9882	0.9702	0.9870

Table 10. Model performance metrics using 4-fold cross-validation.

Model	Accuracy	F1 Score	prAUC	Precision	Recall
Random forest	0.9431	0.9623	0.9483	0.9374	0.9891
SVM	0.9842	0.9891	0.9821	0.9912	0.9870
GBM	0.9950	0.9967	0.9838	0.9957	0.9978
XGBoost	0.9952	0.9967	0.9506	0.9957	0.9978
C5.0	0.9526	0.8678	0.7735	0.9556	0.9804
NNET	1	1	0.9245	1	1
k-NN	0.8927	0.9273	0.6730	0.9157	0.9393
Logistic regression	0.9889	0.9924	0.9828	0.9914	0.9935

Table 11. Model performance metrics using 5-fold cross-validation.

Model	Accuracy	F1 Score	prAUC	Precision	Recall
Random forest	0.9385	0.9586	0.9353	0.9380	0.9804
SVM	0.9889	0.9923	0.9782	0.9934	0.9913
GBM	0.9984	0.9989	0.9800	1	0.9978
XGBoost	0.9968	0.9978	0.9700	0.9978	0.9870
C5.0	0.9763	0.9838	0.6667	0.9800	0.9870
NNET	1	1	0.9216	1	1
k-NN	0.8896	0.9259	0.6847	0.9100	0.9436
Logistic regression	0.9921	0.9946	0.9791	0.9914	0.9978

Table 9 shows the results of the 2-fold cross-validation. XGBoost achieved an impressive accuracy of 0.9968, an F1 score of 0.9978, and perfect precision and recall values of 1 and 0.9956, respectively. GBM also performed exceptionally well, with an accuracy of 0.9889 and an F1 score of 0.9924. In contrast, the NNET model showed an accuracy of 0.8691, indicating variability in performance depending on the cross-validation fold.

Table 10 details the results of the 4-fold cross-validation. Here, XGBoost maintained a high accuracy of 0.9952 and an F1 score of 0.9967, while GBM reached an accuracy of 0.9950 and an F1 score of 0.9967. Notably, the NNET model achieved perfect performance metrics (accuracy = 1; F1 score = 1) in this setting, raising concerns about potential overfitting to the specific data characteristics present in this fold.

Table 11 shows the performance metrics for a 5-fold cross-validation. XGBoost continued to show a strong performance, with an accuracy of 0.9968 and an F1 score of 0.9978. GBM continued to improve, with an accuracy of 0.9984 and an F1 score of 0.9989. The NNET model again showed perfect performance (accuracy = 1; F1 score = 1), consistent with the 4-fold results.

These consistent performance metrics across different cross-validation approaches suggest that XGBoost, NNETs, and GBM have some degree of generalizability, maintaining a stable performance despite variations in training and testing splits. However, the exceptionally high performance of the NNET model in certain folds, achieving perfect scores, indicates a potential risk of overfitting to specific data characteristics within those folds. This concern is further supported by the identical performance metrics observed in some cases for the NNET and k-NN models, as shown in Tables 7 and 8, which may indicate redundancy or overfitting in the model implementation or data processing.

The XGBoost and GBM models displayed a robust predictive performance, with high prAUC values, yet it is essential to acknowledge that their success may still be influenced by unique features of the dataset used in this study. To ensure that these models perform reliably in diverse real-world scenarios, future research should include validation on independent datasets with different demographic and clinical characteristics. This additional validation will help confirm the generalizability and reliability of the models outside of the specific dataset used in this study.

While this study demonstrates the effectiveness of ML models in diagnosing ASD, several limitations should be acknowledged. First, despite the extensive nature of our dataset, it may not be representative of all populations, as ASD symptoms vary widely across demographic groups. A larger, more diverse dataset would likely improve the generalizability and applicability of the models to broader clinical settings. Another important limitation concerns class imbalance: although we used prAUC to handle imbalanced data, models such as k-NN and C5.0 struggled to effectively discriminate between ASD and non-ASD cases. Future studies could employ techniques such as synthetic minority oversampling technique (SMOTE) or cost-sensitive learning to further improve performance with unbalanced data.

Moreover, while our study focused on using *R* due to its accessibility and widespread use in the medical field, we did not use the advanced deep-learning frameworks available in *Python*, such as *TensorFlow*, *Keras*, or *PyTorch*. This decision was primarily influenced by our emphasis on tabular datasets rather than image-based data, such as MRI scans, which were not available in our dataset. Complex models such as NNET and XGBoost achieved high accuracy but posed interpretability challenges even with XAI techniques. To mitigate this, we used SHAP and LIME, which provided valuable insights; however, simpler models such as logistic regression may be preferred where interpretability is critical, even at the expense of some accuracy.

Furthermore, we recognize the need for further discussion on the practical adoption and use of these tools, including the development of user-friendly interfaces and addressing potential clinician or caregiver resistance. This would facilitate a smoother integration of AI-based diagnostic tools into clinical practice. Integrating AI-driven diagnostic tools into clinical practice presents significant challenges beyond model performance, requiring a focus on user-friendly interface design and extensive clinician training. Developing intuitive interfaces ensures that healthcare professionals can easily navigate and interpret model output without requiring extensive technical expertise.

Overcoming clinician resistance requires demonstrating the practical utility and reliability of AI tools through evidence-based validation and aligning model predictions with established clinical guidelines. While XAI techniques such as SHAP and LIME increase model transparency by explaining feature contributions, these explanations must also be clinician-centric, translating complex model insights into actionable clinical knowledge. Balancing the computational complexity of advanced models with the need for real-time applicability in busy clinical environments is essential.

Finally, our current reliance on *R* limited our ability to implement more sophisticated deep-learning models that *Python*'s libraries facilitate, particularly those that could handle multimodal data integration. Therefore, future efforts should prioritize the creation of seamless integration workflows to ensure that AI tools complement, rather than disrupt, existing clinical processes. In addition, fostering collaboration between data scientists and clinicians can facilitate the development of models that are both technically robust and clinically relevant, ultimately promoting the widespread adoption and effective use of AI-driven diagnostic tools in healthcare settings.

Future research directions should emphasize the integration of multimodal data, including genetic, neuroimaging, and clinical data, to enrich datasets and provide a comprehensive view of ASD in children, thereby improving both diagnostic accuracy and personalized care. Incorporating imaging data, such as MRI scans, would likely improve the performance of both ML and DNN models by providing valuable structural and functional information about the brain. However, our current study did not include such data and instead focused on survey-based assessments. Another focus could be the real-time implementation of models in clinical settings, especially for childcare, which requires the development of user-friendly interfaces and mobile applications for healthcare professionals. Addressing class imbalance in rare conditions such as ASD through advanced methods such as SMOTE and ensemble learning could lead to more balanced and accurate results during model training. In addition, improving the interpretability of AI models for non-experts, such as parents and caregivers, is essential. Simplified AI output and visual aids can help these stakeholders understand and effectively use advanced models to support their child's care.

Future research should prioritize the development of AI-driven systems that facilitate early, personalized interventions for children with ASD. While *R* was used in this study due to its accessibility and widespread use in the medical field, we intend to explore *Python* in future studies to take advantage of its extensive libraries and community support, such as *TensorFlow*, *Keras*, and *PyTorch* for deep learning, and to incorporate a wider range of data, including MRI images [77,78], voice recordings, and video analysis. Additionally, we plan to integrate genetic expression data [79] and gut microbiome data [80]. This transition will enable the use of more advanced machine-learning and deep neural-network models, thereby expanding the scope and applicability of our research in clinical settings. While *R* was used in this study due to its accessibility and widespread use in the medical field, we are committed to exploring *Python* in future research to take advantage of its extensive libraries and community support. This transition will enable the use of more advanced machine-learning libraries and foster greater collaboration within the childcare research community.

6. Conclusions

This study was guided by four primary research questions, which we addressed through a comprehensive ML framework using *R* and the *caret* package.

- First, to evaluate the impact of a rigorous data-preprocessing pipeline—including outlier removal, missing data handling, and expert-driven feature selection—we meticulously implemented these steps to improve the performance, robustness, and generalizability of ML models for ASD diagnosis. This approach was particularly critical in the context of data heterogeneity and imbalance, ensuring that the models could effectively handle diverse and imbalanced datasets.

- Second, we compared different ML algorithms (e.g., SVMs, RFs, XGBoost, and NNETs) in terms of accuracy, interpretability, and computational efficiency, using *R*. The results highlighted trade-offs between model complexity and practical usability in clinical settings. For example, while complex models such as NNET and XGBoost showed superior accuracy, simpler models such as logistic regression offered greater interpretability, which is essential for clinical decision-making.
- Third, we integrated advanced XAI techniques (e.g., PFI, LIME, and SHAP) to improve the interpretability of ML models for ASD diagnosis. These methods revealed that some features traditionally emphasized in clinical assessments, such as *CARS*, *SRS*, and *AQ10*, were less significant in the ML models, likely due to data imbalance, with a higher number of ASD patient interviews. This finding helps to improve communication between clinicians and AI models, promoting trust and usability.
- Finally, we developed accessible ML tools using *R* and the *caret* package to facilitate the adoption of AI-driven diagnostic methods by clinicians. By leveraging *R*'s accessibility and widespread use in the medical field, we aimed to ensure that these tools could be used effectively without requiring extensive programming expertise, thereby improving the effectiveness and reliability of ASD diagnosis in clinical practice.

A major contribution of this study is the use of XAI techniques, which provided clearer insights into the decision-making processes of the models. These techniques revealed that specific behavioral characteristics, such as social communication patterns, were more important than demographic factors or family history in diagnosing ASD in children. This finding is consistent with the multifaceted nature of ASD, where individual behavioral indicators in children are critical. By increasing transparency, XAI enabled clinicians to better understand the models' predictions, thereby increasing confidence in AI-based diagnostic tools. This study demonstrates the potential of ML models to improve early diagnosis of ASD in children by emphasizing both interpretability and accuracy.

Moving forward, it is imperative to validate these models in diverse clinical settings, particularly pediatric-care settings, to ensure robustness and generalizability. In addition, the exploration of advanced regularization techniques and the use of cross-validation methods will be critical to further improve accuracy and reduce the risk of overfitting. By refining these models, we can significantly improve diagnostic tools for ASD in children, leading to more effective intervention planning and improved quality of life for children and their families. These efforts will not only advance healthcare analytics but also foster greater trust in AI applications in childcare, contributing to emotionally intelligent, child-focused clinical practices.

Supplementary Materials: The following supporting information can be downloaded at: https://www.mdpi.com/article/10.3390/diagnostics14222504/s1, Table S1: ASD_Preprocessed_Dataset.xlsx, which is the preprocessed dataset used for our experiments, including brief descriptions of each variable's values and characteristics.

Author Contributions: Conceptualization, I.J., J.K., and J.M.; methodology, I.J. and M.K.; software, I.J., M.K., and D.S.; validation, S.K., S.S., and E.Y.K.; formal analysis, S.K., S.S., and J.K.; investigation, I.J., M.K., and J.K.; resources, E.Y.K. and J.K.; data curation, I.J., M.K., D.S., E.Y.K., and J.K.; writing—original draft preparation, I.J.; writing—review and editing, J.K. and J.M.; visualization, D.S. and M.K.; supervision, Y.N. and J.M.; project administration, Y.N.; funding acquisition, Y.N. All authors have read and agreed to the published version of the manuscript.

Funding: This work was supported by the National Research Foundation of Korea (NRF) grant funded by the Korean government (MSIT) (No. RS-2023-00218176) and the Soonchunhyang University Research Fund.

Institutional Review Board Statement: Ethical review and approval were waived for this study due to the use of publicly available data without any identifiable information.

Informed Consent Statement: Patient consent was waived due to the use of a widely accepted, publicly available dataset. This dataset has been used in numerous research studies, establishing a general consensus regarding its use for research purposes. In addition, all patient information has been de-identified, ensuring that individual identities cannot be traced back to the dataset. Therefore, individual consent is not required to use this dataset.

Data Availability Statement: The dataset utilized in this study, titled 'ASD Children Traits', is publicly accessible and can be obtained from Kaggle at the following URL: https://www.kaggle.com/datasets/uppulurimadhuri/dataset (accessed on 1 June 2024). Additional data supporting the findings of this research are available from the corresponding author upon reasonable request.

Acknowledgments: We would like to express our sincere gratitude to all the researchers who contributed to this project. In particular, we thank Chomyong Kim, MinKyung Hong, Gyung Hun Hong, Jiyoung Woo, Ji Young Na, Jung-Yeon Kim, Sungjun Choi, Mi-Sun Yoon, Yongwon Cho, and Jung Ki Kim for their invaluable support and collaboration. Their dedication and expertise have been instrumental in advancing our research on early screening for developmental disabilities and the development of innovative childcare solutions. This work was made possible through the collaborative efforts of the Convergent Research Center for Emotionally Intelligent Child Care Systems, led by Yunyoung Nam. We are deeply grateful for their commitment to creating a new paradigm in childcare research and contributing to the well-being of children and families. We also sincerely thank the four anonymous reviewers for their valuable feedback and the editor for expertly guiding the review process, which greatly improved this manuscript.

Conflicts of Interest: The authors declare no conflicts of interest, and the funders had no role in the design of the study; in the collection, analyses, or interpretation of data; in the writing of the manuscript; or in the decision to publish the results.

Appendix A

The following tables present the detailed performance metrics for each cross-validation fold used in the evaluation of multiple ML models for diagnosing ASD. These metrics complement the main text and provide comprehensive insights necessary to understand and replicate the research. In addition, these detailed results facilitate the application of statistical tests to assess the significance of performance differences between models.

Table A1. Performance metrics for fold 1.

Model	Accuracy	F1 Score	prAUC	Precision	Recall
Random forest	0.9523	0.9677	0.9405	0.9782	0.9574
SVM	0.9687	0.9791	0.9493	1	0.9591
GBM	1	1	0.9597	1	1
XGBoost	1	1	0.9287	1	1
C5.0	1	1	0.6323	1	1
NNET	1	1	0.9599	1	1
k-NN	0.8281	0.8705	0.7232	0.8043	0.9487
Logistic regression	1	1	0.9597	1	1

Table A2. Performance metrics for fold 2.

Model	Accuracy	F1 Score	prAUC	Precision	Recall
Random forest	0.9523	0.9684	0.9271	1	0.9387
SVM	1	1	0.9599	1	1
GBM	0.9841	0.9890	0.9557	0.9782	1
XGBoost	0.9682	0.9787	0.9340	1	0.9583
C5.0	0.9687	0.9782	0.5509	0.9782	0.9782
NNET	1	1	0.9597	1	1
k-NN	0.8095	0.8750	0.5080	0.9130	0.8400
Logistic regression	0.9841	0.9892	0.9578	1	0.9787

Table A3. Performance metrics for fold 3.

Model	Accuracy	F1 Score	prAUC	Precision	Recall
Random forest	0.9687	0.9791	0.9117	1	0.9591
SVM	1	1	0.9613	1	1
GBM	1	1	0.9613	1	1
XGBoost	1	1	0.9599	1	1
C5.0	0.9843	0.9892	0.7222	1	0.9787
NNET	1	1	0.9613	1	1
k-NN	0.9375	0.9583	0.6450	0.9787	0.9387
Logistic regression	1	1	0.9597	1	1

Table A4. Performance metrics for fold 4.

Model	Accuracy	F1 Score	prAUC	Precision	Recall
Random forest	0.9523	0.9684	0.9587	1	0.9387
SVM	0.9841	0.9892	0.9597	1	0.9787
GBM	1	1	0.9597	1	1
XGBoost	1	1	0.9597	1	1
C5.0	0.9682	0.9782	0.6953	0.9782	0.9782
NNET	1	1	0.9597	1	1
k-NN	0.8730	0.9111	0.6264	0.8913	0.9318
Logistic regression	1	1	0.9597	1	1

Table A5. Performance metrics for fold 5.

Model	Accuracy	F1 Score	prAUC	Precision	Recall
Random forest	0.9375	0.9583	0.9291	0.9787	0.9387
SVM	1	1	0.9597	1	1
GBM	1	1	0.9194	1	1
XGBoost	1	1	0.9173	1	1
C5.0	0.9523	0.9648	0.6030	1	0.9387
NNET	1	1	0.9615	1	1
k-NN	0.9206	0.9462	0.6924	0.9565	0.9361
Logistic regression	0.9843	0.9892	0.9560	0.9787	1

Table A6. Performance metrics for fold 6.

Model	Accuracy	F1 Score	prAUC	Precision	Recall
Random forest	0.9047	0.9361	0.8983	0.9565	0.9166
SVM	1	1	0.9597	1	1
GBM	1	1	0.9597	1	1
XGBoost	1	1	0.9271	1	1
C5.0	0.9531	0.9684	0.6547	0.9787	0.9583
NNET	1	1	0.9597	1	1
k-NN	0.9206	0.9450	0.6106	0.9347	0.9555
Logistic regression	1	1	0.9599	1	1

Table A7. Performance metrics for fold 7.

Model	Accuracy	F1 Score	prAUC	Precision	Recall
Random forest	0.9682	0.9787	0.9162	1	0.9583
SVM	0.9841	0.9892	0.9560	1	0.9787
GBM	1	1	0.9198	1	1
XGBoost	1	1	0.9597	1	1
C5.0	1	1	0.4561	1	1
NNET	1	1	0.9597	1	1
k-NN	0.9062	0.9361	0.6021	0.9565	0.9166
Logistic regression	1	1	0.9613	1	1

Table A8. Performance metrics for fold 8.

Model	Accuracy	F1 Score	prAUC	Precision	Recall
Random forest	0.9365	0.9574	0.9201	0.9782	0.9375
SVM	1	1	0.9597	1	1
GBM	1	1	0.9613	1	1
XGBoost	1	1	0.9488	1	1
C5.0	0.9682	0.9782	0.6529	0.9782	0.9782
NNET	1	1	0.9597	1	1
k-NN	0.9206	0.9473	0.6730	0.9782	0.9183
Logistic regression	1	1	0.9597	1	1

Table A9. Performance metrics for fold 9.

Model	Accuracy	F1 Score	prAUC	Precision	Recall
Random forest	0.9687	0.9787	0.9437	1	0.9583
SVM	1	1	0.9597	1	1
GBM	1	1	0.9305	1	1
XGBoost	1	1	0.8836	1	1
C5.0	0.9682	0.9787	0.7966	1	0.9583
NNET	1	1	0.9597	1	1
k-NN	0.9365	0.9565	0.5708	0.9565	0.9565
Logistic regression	0.9687	0.9787	0.9613	1	0.9583

Table A10. Performance metrics for fold 10.

Model	Accuracy	F1 Score	prAUC	Precision	Recall
Random forest	0.9531	0.9677	0.9015	0.9782	0.9574
SVM	0.9843	0.9890	0.9613	0.9782	1
GBM	1	1	0.9597	1	1
XGBoost	1	1	0.9178	1	1
C5.0	0.9365	0.9574	0.6453	0.9782	0.9375
NNET	1	1	0.9597	1	1
k-NN	0.8750	0.9200	0.5928	0.9787	0.8679
Logistic regression	1	1	0.9597	1	1

References

1. Lauritsen, M.B. Autism Spectrum Disorders. *Eur. Child Adolesc. Psychiatry* **2013**, *22*, S37–S42. [CrossRef] [PubMed]
2. Webb, S.J.; Jones, E.J.H. Early Identification of Autism: Early Characteristics, Onset of Symptoms, and Diagnostic Stability. *Infants Young Child* **2009**, *22*, 100–118. [CrossRef] [PubMed]
3. Fernell, E.; Eriksson, M.A.; Gillberg, C. Early Diagnosis of Autism and Impact on Prognosis: A Narrative Review. *Clin. Epidemiol.* **2013**, *5*, 33–43. [CrossRef] [PubMed]
4. Hinnebusch, A.J.; Miller, L.E.; Fein, D.A. Autism Spectrum Disorders and Low Mental Age: Diagnostic Stability and Developmental Outcomes in Early Childhood. *J. Autism Dev. Disord.* **2017**, *47*, 3967–3982. [CrossRef]
5. Lord, C.; Luyster, R. Early Diagnosis of Children with Autism Spectrum Disorders. *Clin. Neurosci. Res.* **2006**, *6*, 189–194. [CrossRef]
6. McCarty, P.; Frye, R.E. Early Detection and Diagnosis of Autism Spectrum Disorder: Why Is It So Difficult? In *Seminars in Pediatric Neurology*; W. B. Saunders: Philadelphia, PA, USA, 2020; Volume 35, p. 100831.
7. Bryson, S.E.; Rogers, S.J.; Fombonne, E. Autism Spectrum Disorders: Early Detection, Intervention, Education, and Psychopharmacological Management. *Can. J. Psychiatry* **2003**, *48*, 506–516. [CrossRef]
8. Guthrie, W.; Swineford, L.B.; Nottke, C.; Wetherby, A.M. Early Diagnosis of Autism Spectrum Disorder: Stability and Change in Clinical Diagnosis and Symptom Presentation. *J. Child Psychol. Psychiatry* **2013**, *54*, 582–590. [CrossRef]
9. Thabtah, F.; Peebles, D. Early Autism Screening: A Comprehensive Review. *Int. J. Environ. Res. Public Health* **2019**, *16*, 3502. [CrossRef]
10. Fekar Gharamaleki, F.; Bahrami, B.; Masumi, J. Autism Screening Tests: A Narrative Review. *J. Public Health Res.* **2022**, *11*, 2308. [CrossRef]
11. Sappok, T.; Heinrich, M.; Underwood, L. Screening Tools for Autism Spectrum Disorders. *Adv. Autism* **2015**, *1*, 12–29. [CrossRef]
12. Omar, K.S.; Mondal, P.; Khan, N.S.; Rizvi, M.R.K.; Islam, M.N. A Machine Learning Approach to Predict Autism Spectrum Disorder. In Proceedings of the 2019 International Conference on Electrical, Computer and Communication Engineering (ECCE), Cox's Bazar, Bangladesh, 7–9 February 2019; IEEE: New York, NY, USA, 2019; pp. 1–6.

13. Usta, M.B.; Karabekiroglu, K.; Sahin, B.; Aydin, M.; Bozkurt, A.; Karaosman, T.; Aral, A.; Cobanoglu, C.; Kurt, A.D.; Kesim, N.; et al. Use of Machine Learning Methods in Prediction of Short-Term Outcome in Autism Spectrum Disorders. *Psychiatry Clin. Psychopharmacol.* **2019**, *29*, 320–325. [CrossRef]
14. Uddin, M.J.; Ahamad, M.M.; Sarker, P.K.; Aktar, S.; Alotaibi, N.; Alyami, S.A.; Kabir, M.A.; Moni, M.A. An Integrated Statistical and Clinically Applicable Machine Learning Framework for the Detection of Autism Spectrum Disorder. *Computers* **2023**, *12*, 92. [CrossRef]
15. Hasan, M.; Ahamad, M.M.; Aktar, S.; Moni, M.A. Early Stage Autism Spectrum Disorder Detection of Adults and Toddlers Using Machine Learning Models. In Proceedings of the 2021 5th International Conference on Electrical Information and Communication Technology (EICT), Khulna, Bangladesh, 17–19 December 2021; IEEE: New York, NY, USA, 2021; pp. 1–6.
16. Bhuyan, F.; Lu, S.; Ahmed, I.; Zhang, J. Predicting Efficacy of Therapeutic Services for Autism Spectrum Disorder Using Scientific Workflows. In Proceedings of the 2017 IEEE International Conference on Big Data (Big Data), Boston, MA, USA, 11–14 December 2017; IEEE: New York, NY, USA, 2017; pp. 3847–3856.
17. Farooq, M.S.; Tehseen, R.; Sabir, M.; Atal, Z. Detection of Autism Spectrum Disorder (ASD) in Children and Adults Using Machine Learning. *Sci. Rep.* **2023**, *13*, 9605. [CrossRef] [PubMed]
18. Alanazi, A. Clinicians' Views on Using Artificial Intelligence in Healthcare: Opportunities, Challenges, and Beyond. *Cureus* **2023**, *15*, e45255. [CrossRef]
19. Mohanty, A.S.; Patra, K.C.; Parida, P. Toddler ASD Classification Using Machine Learning Techniques. *Int. J. Online Biomed. Eng.* **2021**, *17*, 156–171. [CrossRef]
20. Ferrari, E.; Bosco, P.; Calderoni, S.; Oliva, P.; Palumbo, L.; Spera, G.; Fantacci, M.E.; Retico, A. Dealing with Confounders and Outliers in Classification Medical Studies: The Autism Spectrum Disorders Case Study. *Artif. Intell. Med.* **2020**, *108*, 101926. [CrossRef]
21. Alam, M.N.; Kaur, M.; Kabir, M.S. Explainable AI in Healthcare: Enhancing Transparency and Trust upon Legal and Ethical Consideration. *Int. Res. J. Eng. Technol.* **2023**, *10*, 828–835.
22. Abdullah, T.A.A.; Zahid, M.S.M.; Ali, W. A Review of Interpretable ML in Healthcare: Taxonomy, Applications, Challenges, and Future Directions. *Symmetry* **2021**, *13*, 2439. [CrossRef]
23. Hulsen, T. Explainable Artificial Intelligence (XAI): Concepts and Challenges in Healthcare. *AI* **2021**, *4*, 652–666. [CrossRef]
24. Akter, T.; Khan, M.I.; Ali, M.H.; Satu, M.S.; Uddin, M.J.; Moni, M.A. Improved Machine Learning Based Classification Model for Early Autism Detection. In Proceedings of the 2021 2nd International Conference on Robotics, Electrical and Signal Processing Techniques (ICREST), Dhaka, Bangladesh, 5–7 January 2021; IEEE: New York, NY, USA, 2021; pp. 742–747.
25. Maadi, M.; Akbarzadeh Khorshidi, H.A.; Aickelin, U. A Review on Human–AI Interaction in Machine Learning and Insights for Medical Applications. *Int. J. Environ. Res. Public Health* **2021**, *18*, 2121. [CrossRef]
26. Alsuliman, M.; Al-Baity, H.H. Efficient Diagnosis of Autism with Optimized Machine Learning Models: An Experimental Analysis on Genetic and Personal Characteristic Datasets. *Appl. Sci.* **2022**, *12*, 3812. [CrossRef]
27. Ben-Sasson, A.; Guedalia, J.; Nativ, L.; Ilan, K.; Shaham, M.; Gabis, L.V. A Prediction Model of Autism Spectrum Diagnosis from Well-Baby Electronic Data Using Machine Learning. *Children* **2024**, *11*, 429. [CrossRef] [PubMed]
28. Abbas, R.T.; Sultan, K.; Sheraz, M.; Chuah, T.C. A Comparative Analysis of Automated Machine Learning Tools: A Use Case for Autism Spectrum Disorder Detection. *Information* **2024**, *15*, 625. [CrossRef]
29. Reghunathan, R.K.; Palayam Venkidusamy, P.N.; Kurup, R.G.; George, B.; Thomas, N. Machine Learning-Based Classification of Autism Spectrum Disorder Across Age Groups. *Eng. Proc.* **2024**, *62*, 12. [CrossRef]
30. Bala, M.; Ali, M.H.; Satu, M.S.; Hasan, K.F.; Moni, M.A. Efficient Machine Learning Models for Early Stage Detection of Autism Spectrum Disorder. *Algorithms* **2022**, *15*, 166. [CrossRef]
31. Batsakis, S.; Adamou, M.; Tachmazidis, I.; Antoniou, G.; Kehagias, T. Data-driven decision support for autism diagnosis using machine learning. In Proceedings of the 13th International Conference on Management of Digital EcoSystems (MEDES '21), Virtual Event Tunisia, 1–3 November 2021; Association for Computing Machinery: New York, NY, USA, 2021; pp. 30–34.
32. Mainas, F.; Golosio, B.; Retico, A.; Oliva, P. Exploring Autism Spectrum Disorder: A Comparative Study of Traditional Classifiers and Deep Learning Classifiers to Analyze Functional Connectivity Measures from a Multicenter Dataset. *Appl. Sci.* **2024**, *14*, 7632. [CrossRef]
33. Rodrigues, I.D.; de Carvalho, E.A.; Santana, C.P.; Bastos, G.S. Machine Learning and rs-fMRI to Identify Potential Brain Regions Associated with Autism Severity. *Algorithms* **2022**, *15*, 195. [CrossRef]
34. Helmy, E.; Elnakib, A.; ElNakieb, Y.; Khudri, M.; Abdelrahim, M.; Yousaf, J.; Ghazal, M.; Contractor, S.; Barnes, G.N.; El-Baz, A. Role of Artificial Intelligence for Autism Diagnosis Using DTI and fMRI: A Survey. *Biomedicines* **2023**, *11*, 1858. [CrossRef]
35. Themistocleous, C.K.; Andreou, M.; Peristeri, E. Autism Detection in Children: Integrating Machine Learning and Natural Language Processing in Narrative Analysis. *Behav. Sci.* **2024**, *14*, 459. [CrossRef]
36. Toki, E.I.; Pange, J.; Tatsis, G.; Plachouras, K.; Tsoulos, I.G. Utilizing Constructed Neural Networks for Autism Screening. *Appl. Sci.* **2024**, *14*, 3053. [CrossRef]
37. Kaur, H.; Kumari, V. Predictive Modelling and Analytics for Diabetes Using a Machine Learning Approach. *Appl. Comput. Inform.* **2022**, *18*, 90–100. [CrossRef]
38. Li, Y.; Chen, Z. Performance Evaluation of Machine Learning Methods for Breast Cancer Prediction. *Appl. Comput. Math.* **2018**, *7*, 212–216. [CrossRef]
39. Leha, A.; Hellenkamp, K.; Unsöld, B.; Mushemi-Blake, S.; Shah, A.M.; Hasenfuß, G.; Seidler, T. A machine learning approach for the prediction of pulmonary hypertension. *PLoS ONE* **2019**, *14*, e0224453. [CrossRef] [PubMed]

40. Miettinen, T.; Nieminen, A.I.; Mäntyselkä, P.; Kalso, E.; Lötsch, J. Machine Learning and Pathway Analysis-Based Discovery of Metabolomic Markers Relating to Chronic Pain Phenotypes. *Int. J. Mol. Sci.* **2022**, *23*, 5085. [CrossRef]
41. Beunza, J.J.; Puertas, E.; García-Ovejero, E.; Villalba, G.; Condes, E.; Koleva, G.; Hurtado, C.; Landecho, M.F. Comparison of Machine Learning Algorithms for Clinical Event Prediction (Risk of Coronary Heart Disease). *J. Biomed. Inform.* **2019**, *97*, 103257. [CrossRef]
42. Wickham, H.; Bryan, J.; Posit, P.B.C.; Kalicinski, M.; Valery, K.; Leitienne, C.; Colbert, B.; Hoerl, D.; Miller, E. Readxl: Read Excel Files, Version 13. R [Software]. Available online: https://cran.r-project.org/package=readxl (accessed on 24 September 2024).
43. Chambers, J.M. *Software for Data Analysis: Programming with R*; Springer: New York, NY, USA, 2008; Volume 2, No. 1.
44. Wickham, H.; François, R.; Henry, L.; Müller, K. Dplyr: A Grammar of Data Manipulation. R [Software]. Available online: https://CRAN.R-project.org/package=dplyr (accessed on 24 September 2024).
45. Dowle, M.; Barrett, T.; Srinivasan, A.; Gorecki, J.; Chirico, M.; Hocking, T.; Schwendinger, B.; Stetsenko, P.; Short, T.; Lianoglou, S.; et al. Data.Table: Extension of Data.Frame. R [Software]. Available online: https://CRAN.R-project.org/package=data.table (accessed on 24 September 2024).
46. Wickham, H.; Chang, W. Ggplot2: Create Elegant Data Visualisations Using the Grammar of Graphics, Version 2.1. R [Software]. Available online: https://CRAN.R-project.org/package=ggplot2 (accessed on 24 September 2024).
47. Sarkar, D. Lattice (Version 0.20-33, 2015). R [Software]. Available online: https://CRAN.R-project.org/package=lattice (accessed on 24 September 2024).
48. Kuhn, M. Caret: Classification and Regression Training. *Astrophys. Source Code Libr.* **2020**, *12*, 48.
49. Rigatti, S.J. Random Forest. *J. Insur. Med.* **2017**, *47*, 31–39. [CrossRef]
50. Liaw, A. randomForest. R [Software]. University of California Berkeley, CA, USA, 2018. Available online: https://cran.r-project.org/package=randomForest (accessed on 24 September 2024).
51. Suthaharan, S. Support Vector Machine. In *Machine Learning Models and Algorithms for Big Data Classification: Thinking with Examples for Effective Learning*; Springer: Berlin/Heidelberg, Germany, 2016; pp. 207–235.
52. Dimitriadou, E.; Meyer, D.; Hornik, K.; Weingessel, A.; Leisch, F.; Chang, C.-C.; Lin, C.-C. e1071 R Software Package. R [Software]. Available online: http://cran.r-project.org/web/packages/e1071/index.html (accessed on 24 September 2024).
53. Ayyadevara, V.K. Gradient Boosting Machine. In *Pro Machine Learning Algorithms: A Hands-On Approach to Implementing Algorithms in Python and R*; Apress: Berkeley, CA, USA, 2018; pp. 117–134.
54. Greenwell, B.; Ridgeway, G.; Edwards, D.; Kriegler, B.; Schroedl, S.; Southworth, H.; Boehmke, B.; Cunningham, J.; GBM Developers. GBM: Generalized Boosted Regression Models, Version 2.5. R [Software]. Available online: https://cran.r-project.org/package=gbm (accessed on 24 September 2024).
55. Chen, T.; Guestrin, C. XGBoost: A Scalable Tree Boosting System. In Proceedings of the 22nd ACM SIGKDD International Conference on Knowledge Discovery and Data Mining, San Francisco, CA, USA, 13–17 August 2016; ACM: New York, NY, USA, 2016; pp. 785–794.
56. Chen, T.; Guestrin, C. XGBoost: Extreme Gradient Boosting, Version 90.1-66. R [Software]. Available online: https://cran.r-project.org/package=xgboost (accessed on 24 September 2024).
57. Pandya, R.; Pandya, J. C5.0 Algorithm to Improved Decision Tree with Feature Selection and Reduced Error Pruning. *Int. J. Comput. Appl.* **2015**, *117*, 18–21.
58. Kuhn, M.; Weston, S.; Culp, M.; Coulter, N.; Quinlan, R.; RuleQuest Research; Rulequest Research Pty Ltd. C50: Classification and Regression Trees. R [Software]. Available online: https://cran.r-project.org/package=C50 (accessed on 24 September 2024).
59. Dongare, A.D.; Kharde, R.R.; Kachare, A.D. Introduction to Artificial Neural Network. *Int. J. Eng. Innov. Technol.* **2012**, *2*, 189–194.
60. Ripley, B.; Venables, W. Nnet: Feed-Forward Neural Networks and Multinomial Log-Linear Models, Version 7.3-12. R [Software]. Available online: https://cran.r-project.org/package=nnet (accessed on 24 September 2024).
61. Peterson, L.E. K-Nearest Neighbor. *Scholarpedia* **2009**, *4*, 1883. [CrossRef]
62. Ripley, B.; Venables, W. Class: Classification, Version 11. R [Software]. Available online: https://cran.r-project.org/package=class (accessed on 24 September 2024).
63. LaValley, M.P. Logistic Regression. *Circulation* **2008**, *117*, 2395–2399. [CrossRef] [PubMed]
64. Friedman, J.; Hastie, T.; Tibshirani, R.; Narasimhan, B.; Tay, K.; Simon, N.; Qian, J.; Yang, J. Glmnet: Lasso and Elastic-Net Regularized Generalized Linear Models, Version 595. R [Software]. Available online: https://cran.r-project.org/package=glmnet (accessed on 24 September 2024).
65. Yang, L.; Shami, A. On Hyperparameter Optimization of Machine Learning Algorithms: Theory and Practice. *Neurocomputing* **2020**, *415*, 295–316. [CrossRef]
66. Ndiaye, E.; Le, T.; Fercoq, O.; Salmon, J.; Takeuchi, I. Safe Grid Search with Optimal Complexity. In Proceedings of the International Conference on Machine Learning, Long Beach, CA, USA, 10–15 June 2019; pp. 4771–4780.
67. Browne, M.W. Cross-Validation Methods. *J. Math. Psychol.* **2000**, *44*, 108–132. [CrossRef] [PubMed]
68. Dwivedi, R.; Dave, D.; Naik, H.; Singhal, S.; Omer, R.; Patel, P.; Qian, B.; Wen, Z.; Shah, Y.; Morgan, G.; et al. Explainable AI (XAI): Core Ideas, Techniques, and Solutions. *ACM Comput. Surv.* **2023**, *55*, 1–33. [CrossRef]
69. Thunki, P.; Reddy, S.R.B.; Raparthi, M.; Maruthi, S.; Dodda, S.B.; Ravichandran, P. Explainable AI in Data Science—Enhancing Model Interpretability and Transparency. *Afr. J. Artif. Intell. Sust. Dev.* **2021**, *1*, 1–8.
70. Altmann, A.; Toloşi, L.; Sander, O.; Lengauer, T. Permutation Importance: A Corrected Feature Importance Measure. *Bioinformatics* **2010**, *26*, 1340–1347. [CrossRef]

71. Dieber, J.; Kirrane, S. Why Model Why? Assessing the Strengths and Limitations of LIME. *arXiv* **2020**, arXiv:2012.00093. Available online: https://arxiv.org/abs/2012.00093 (accessed on 24 September 2024).
72. Lundberg, S.M.; Erion, G.; Chen, H.; DeGrave, A.; Prutkin, J.M.; Nair, B.; Katz, R.; Himmelfarb, J.; Bansal, N.; Lee, S.I. From Local Explanations to Global Understanding with Explainable AI for Trees. *Nat. Mach. Intell.* **2020**, *2*, 56–67. [CrossRef]
73. Min, H.; Hong, S.; Song, J.; Son, B.; Noh, B.; Moon, J. SolarFlux Predictor: A Novel Deep Learning Approach for Photovoltaic Power Forecasting in South Korea. *Electronics* **2024**, *13*, 2071. [CrossRef]
74. So, D.; Oh, J.; Jeon, I.; Moon, J.; Lee, M.; Rho, S. BiGTA-Net: A Hybrid Deep Learning-Based Electrical Energy Forecasting Model for Building Energy Management Systems. *Systems* **2023**, *11*, 456. [CrossRef]
75. Moon, J. A Multi-Step-Ahead Photovoltaic Power Forecasting Approach Using One-Dimensional Convolutional Neural Networks and Transformer. *Electronics* **2024**, *13*, 2007. [CrossRef]
76. Mayer, M. Shapviz: SHAP Visualizations, Version 0.9.0. [Software]. Available online: https://cran.r-project.org/package=shapviz (accessed on 24 September 2024).
77. ASD-fMRI Dataset (Kaggle). Available online: https://www.kaggle.com/datasets/mhkoosheshi/asdfmri (accessed on 31 October 2024).
78. Autism Brain Imaging Data Exchange (ABIDE). Available online: http://fcon_1000.projects.nitrc.org/indi/abide/ (accessed on 31 October 2024).
79. ASD Children Blood Gene Expression Data (Kaggle). Available online: https://www.kaggle.com/datasets/gokulbabyalex/asdchildrenbloodgeneexpressiondata (accessed on 31 October 2024).
80. Human Gut Microbiome with ASD Dataset (Kaggle). Available online: https://www.kaggle.com/datasets/antaresnyc/human-gut-microbiome-with-asd (accessed on 31 October 2024).

Disclaimer/Publisher's Note: The statements, opinions and data contained in all publications are solely those of the individual author(s) and contributor(s) and not of MDPI and/or the editor(s). MDPI and/or the editor(s) disclaim responsibility for any injury to people or property resulting from any ideas, methods, instructions or products referred to in the content.

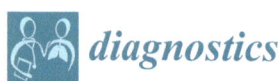

Article

Enhancing Medical Image Retrieval with UMLS-Integrated CNN-Based Text Indexing

Karim Gasmi [1,*], Hajer Ayadi [2] and Mouna Torjmen [3]

[1] Department of Computer Science, College of Computer and Information Sciences, Jouf University, Sakaka 72388, Saudi Arabia
[2] Information Retrieval and Knowledge Management Research Laboratory, York University, Toronto, ON M3J 1P3, Canada; hajaya1@yorku.ca
[3] Research Laboratory on Development and Control of Distributed Applications (REDCAD), National Engineering School of Sfax, Sfax University, Sfax 3029, Tunisia; mouna.torjmen@redcad.org
* Correspondence: kgasmi@ju.edu.sa

Abstract: In recent years, Convolutional Neural Network (CNN) models have demonstrated notable advancements in various domains such as image classification and Natural Language Processing (NLP). Despite their success in image classification tasks, their potential impact on medical image retrieval, particularly in text-based medical image retrieval (TBMIR) tasks, has not yet been fully realized. This could be attributed to the complexity of the ranking process, as there is ambiguity in treating TBMIR as an image retrieval task rather than a traditional information retrieval or NLP task. To address this gap, our paper proposes a novel approach to re-ranking medical images using a Deep Matching Model (DMM) and Medical-Dependent Features (MDF). These features incorporate categorical attributes such as medical terminologies and imaging modalities. Specifically, our DMM aims to generate effective representations for query and image metadata using a personalized CNN, facilitating matching between these representations. By using MDF, a semantic similarity matrix based on Unified Medical Language System (UMLS) meta-thesaurus, and a set of personalized filters taking into account some ranking features, our deep matching model can effectively consider the TBMIR task as an image retrieval task, as previously mentioned. To evaluate our approach, we performed experiments on the medical ImageCLEF datasets from 2009 to 2012. The experimental results show that the proposed model significantly enhances image retrieval performance compared to the baseline and state-of-the-art approaches.

Keywords: text-based medical image retrieval; Convolutional Neural Network; Medical-Dependent Features; UMLS metathesaurus

Citation: Gasmi, K.; Ayadi, H.; Torjmen, M. Enhancing Medical Image Retrieval with UMLS-Integrated CNN-Based Text Indexing. *Diagnostics* **2024**, *14*, 1204. https://doi.org/10.3390/diagnostics14111204

Academic Editors: Wan Azani Mustafa and Hiam Alquran

Received: 3 May 2024
Revised: 30 May 2024
Accepted: 4 June 2024
Published: 6 June 2024

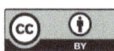

Copyright: © 2024 by the authors. Licensee MDPI, Basel, Switzerland. This article is an open access article distributed under the terms and conditions of the Creative Commons Attribution (CC BY) license (https://creativecommons.org/licenses/by/4.0/).

1. Introduction

Medical information retrieval has a range of applications and solutions connected with better health care. At a basic level, it encompasses image retrieval, retrieval of reports, and natural language queries to databases containing both images and text. However, image retrieval is a challenging task as it can be very subjective, requiring high-level cognitive processing. There are two main types of image retrieval used clinically. One is where the medical professional has a clear idea of what they are looking for and uses the image to seek specific information. The second is a case in which the medical professional has an image and desires to find all similar images to aid diagnosis or as a teaching aid. Step one carries manual work, as tags need to be manually attached to the image usually as metadata. When the images are stored in large databases such as Picture Archiving and Communication Systems (PACS), this can be a highly disorganized and time-consuming task. Step two involves searching using the image as the query and algorithmic methods using visual features of the image attempt to retrieve similar images. As technology advances, there has been increasing support to move to automatic image annotation and content-based retrieval. It is within content-based image retrieval (CBIR) that the model CNNMIR seeks to improve the current state of the art.

Usually in medical domain, images constitute a reference set of previously evaluated cases, that physicians may use to make the right decisions. With the massive growth of medical images, it becomes hard for domain experts to find relevant images in large medical datasets. Thus, the need for an efficient and effective medical image retrieval system becomes urgent [1]. Two main approaches for medical image retrieval are widely used: text- and content-based retrievals. These approaches search for relevant images by using different principles: the text-based approach relies on the high-level semantic features of the images, however, the content-based approach relies on the low-level visual features (e.g., color, shape, and texture) of the image. Comparing both approaches, the Content-Based Medical Image Retrieval (CBMIR) performance is less favorable due to the gap between low-level visual features and high-level semantic features [2,3]. Therefore, several medical image retrieval systems apply the Text-Based Medical Image Retrieval (TBMIR) approach to search for images [4]. Most of these approaches are: either, traditional simple keyword-based approaches; where the meanings of medical entities are ignored, or concept-based approaches; that are time and disk-space consuming. According to our previous works [5,6], the presence of specific medical information, namely Medical-Dependant Features (MDF) in the textual descriptions of medical images has a positive impact on the performance of TBMIR approaches.

In these last years, Convolutional Neural Network (CNN) [7,8] models have shown significant performance improvement in several fields as Natural Language Processing (NLP) [9] and computer vision [10]. Given their success in such fields, it seems to be efficient for image retrieval. Unfortunately, until now, the CNN models have not a significant positive impact on medical image retrieval, especially on text-based medical image retrieval (TBMIR) [11]. It may be due to the complexity of the ranking process: it is not obvious how to consider TBMIR tasks as an image retrieval task [12] and not as a traditional information retrieval task, nor an NLP task. Indeed, the traditional information retrieval systems identify the relevance of a document to a given query; however, the NLP systems deduce the semantic relations between the query and the document. These two systems do not take into account the specificity of images in their processes.

In our previous work [13], we proposed a personalized CNN model that considers the specificity of images in its retrieval process. In that model, we consider the Word2Vec model for word embedding. However, it is well known that the Word2Vec model considers general terminologies, which are not specific for any domain. As our work fits in the medical image retrieval field, we believe that using medical semantic resources, such as UMLS, for converting textual words is more appropriate.

In this paper, we propose a deep matching process for TBMIR that is different from traditional information retrieval and NLP described as follows: first, it takes into account the specificity of images, by mapping the textual queries and the image metadata (document) into MDF. Second, it extracts the semantic relations between MDF, using UMLS, to build a good representation of query and document, and third, it computes the document relevance to the query by using the extracted relations.

In the literature, a variety of deep matching models have been proposed; however, most of them are designed for NLP, rather than information retrieval. Indeed, they consider the semantic matching instead of relevance matching. These models can be categorized, according to their architecture, into two types [14]: the first one is the interaction-focused models [15,16]. These models extract the relationships between queries and documents and then integrate them into a deep neural network to create new matching models. The second one is the representation-focused models [15,17]. These models apply the deep neural network to extract the best representations for both query and document, and then integrate them into a matching process.

In this paper, we propose a new medical image re-ranking process based on a deep matching model (DMM) for TBMIR. Overall, our model is a new representation-focused model that builds a good representation of queries and documents using MDF, UMLS and a personalized CNN for relevance matching. Specifically, we first create the semantic similarity matrix by extracting the UMLS relationships between each pair of MDF. Each query/document MDF is mapped into a similarity vector representing the relationships between the corresponding MDF and all MDF. As each query/document is composed of MDF, the resulting representation of the query/document will be a similarity matrix. Using these matrixes, our model tries to find the best representations for both query and document. Indeed, It applies a personalized CNN which is composed of retrieval filters taking into account some ranking features. Finally, an overall matching score is computed.

We evaluate the effectiveness of the proposed DMM using the ImageCLEF datasets from 2009 to 2012. For comparison, we take into account three well-known traditional retrieval models. The empirical results show that our model significantly outperforms the baseline models in terms of all the evaluation metrics.

This paper is structured as follows: Section 2 summarizes related work. Section 3 describes the proposed DMM model. Section 4 describes, first, how to represent MDF as a semantic similarity matrix using UMLS similarity, and second, our personalized CNN model with specific filters and finally the matching function. Experiments and results are presented and discussed in Section 7. Finally, Section 8 concludes the paper and gives some future work.

2. Related Work

Text-based indexing opens the possibility of indexing medical images by utilizing the associated reports, thereby providing a crucial way to access the exponentially growing clinical image databases. Current methods to retrieve images from medical databases are either based on attribute image content or non-image content. The content-based image retrieval (CBIR) method relies on image features such as shape, texture, or (in most successful cases) a previously assigned semantic feature to retrieve similar images. Non-image content retrieval methods often deal with text-based searches of databases, where a search query is submitted to an image database and text associated with images is compared to the query. However, both methods do not consider the actual medical knowledge relevant to an image and more traditional methods of organizing medical records which are indexed by keywords. Text-based image retrieval by and large builds upon retrieval technique that aims at finding all images relevant to a given query out of large database of images. In most textbook studies in proposed system, a specific image is given as an entry and the user wants to retrieve all images relevant to the given query. Though it is actually a subtype of text-based image retrieval where actual text-based images are not available and it is limited by the availability of some keyword-based annotation of the image. But this method has been shown to be very effective in retrieving images relevant to a given query and hence can be generalized to retrieval systems where text is the main modality. The creation of 'indexes of associated features' from images is effectively the creation of a searchable database that links images to text.

In the literature, several works studied the use of CNN and semantics in medical image retrieval. This section briefly summarizes some of these works.

2.1. CNN for Medical Image Retrieval

The use of CNN models in the medical image retrieval domain has received great attention [18–20]. Authors in [21] used the CNN model based on the bag-of-word (BoW) technique to index biomedical articles. In this particular model, the input is a matrix of numbers that stand for the various medical terms that are contained in the input text. After that, a system of hidden layers is utilized to assign categories to the document. The authors of [22] developed yet another method for the classification of medical texts that may be put to use for retrieval operations. It does this by employing CNN training to extract the semantics of an input sentence; more specifically, it uses the Word2vec technique to represent the input sentences. This method is based on the use of CNNs. During the training of the CNN model, which is comprised of numerous hidden layers, it additionally maintains the list of stop-words. The CNN model was employed by the authors in the cited article [23] to remove the background noise from clinical notes that were going to be used for medical literature retrieval. They represented the input questions by using GloVe vectors, which are cited in the following reference: [24]. The CNN model's primary purpose in this study is to make predictions about the relative relevance of search query phrases.

Despite the success of CNN for computer vision and NLP, employing CNN to search for relevant documents in TBMIR is not effective; and this may be due to the complexity of the ranking process. Moreover, most existing CNN models represent queries and documents without taking into account the specificity of the medical domain. This latter requires semantic extraction using external medical resources.

2.2. Semantics in Medical Image Retrieval

The integration of semantic knowledge in the medical image retrieval domain has received great attention, such as [25–27]. Authors in [28] used UMLS meta-thesaurus in the medical domain to improve queries and converting words to medical terms. They integrated the semantics in the retrieval process to map the text into concepts using UMLS meta-thesaurus [29]. The authors of the cited paper [30] developed a retrieval method to discover discriminative qualities between various medical photos using a Pruned Dictionary that was based on a description of a Latent Semantic Topic. They did this by calculating the topic-word relevance, which allowed them to make a prediction about the word's relationship to the underlying topic. The latent themes are learned based on the association between the images and the words, and they are used to bridge the gap between low-level visual features and high-level semantic characteristics. This is accomplished by bridging the gap between low-level visual features and high-level semantic features. Moreover, in [31], an image retrieval framework that is based on semantic features has been proposed by the authors. This framework relies on (1) the automatic prediction of ontological terms that define the image content and (2) the retrieval of similar images by analyzing the similarity between annotations. The study of this system demonstrated that it is beneficial to make use of ontology while retrieving medical images.

Despite the large number of works using CNN and semantic resources in medical image retrieval, there is a lack of studies that investigate the integration of semantic knowledge on the CNN model to enhance the medical image retrieval performance. Therefore, we propose a new deep matching model based on personalized CNN and semantic resources (MDF, UMLS) to improve retrieval accuracy.

3. Overview of Our Approach

It is well known that medical images and their associated reports are not usually in agreement. For example, a patient who has a slipped disc, but displays no symptoms, will not have many abnormalities in his MR scan but will have many associated words or phrases about his condition. This inconsistency is a major problem for medical image retrieval systems, which rely on the images and associated text being "about the same thing". With this in mind, and the fact that we have indexed the images and text separately, we need to devise a way where a text query can be used to aid the image query and vice-versa, without the user having to switch between the two.

Our proposed solution leverages relevance feedback to integrate information from both image and text queries using the other modality. For instance, if a user seeks to locate an image corresponding to a report about 'left lung cancer', the current system requires them to separately index the text using a natural language processing (NLP) tool and formulate a query, then repeat the process for the image. This method is inefficient and requires users to switch between modalities. In contrast, our system enables users to use an NLP tool to index the text or query, subsequently identifying relevant images that correspond to the text. Modality-specific technology subsequently ranks the images based on their similarity to the text. This approach automates the task of 'finding images matching this report,' enhancing efficiency and accuracy.

Due to the positive impact of MDF on both retrieval performance [6,13] and query classification [32,33], we choose to integrate them into a deep matching model. In this study, we utilized the Unified Medical Language System (UMLS) as our semantic resource to construct a semantic similarity matrix, which represents the relationships between pairs of Medical Dependent Features (MDF). The literature [34–36] widely recognizes UMLS as a comprehensive thesaurus and ontology of biomedical concepts, designed to link various biomedical terminologies. By leveraging UMLS, we ensure a robust semantic framework for our analysis. Additionally, our system allows users to index text or queries using natural language processing (NLP) tools, facilitating more accurate and efficient retrieval of relevant medical information.

A new personalized CNN model using MDFs is proposed to build the best representation for both queries and documents, that are used to compute their matching score. In this paper, Figure 1 presents an overview of our approach:

- The preliminary step:

We represent each query/document as a set of features, then, for each MDF (F_i), we assign the corresponding vector extracted from the similarity matrix. Hence, each query/document is represented as a Matrix.

- The Deep Matching Model Process:

First, we build a good representation of the query/document with a personalized CNN model that takes into account the interaction between query and document. Indeed, several personalized filters have been proposed and integrated into this model. Then, a matching function is applied to measure the matching degree between the query and the document representations. More precisely, we use the cosine similarity function as a matching function.

Second, we combine the obtained score with the corresponding baseline score to form a new re-ranking score. The re-ranking process is achieved by sorting the images according to their new scores.

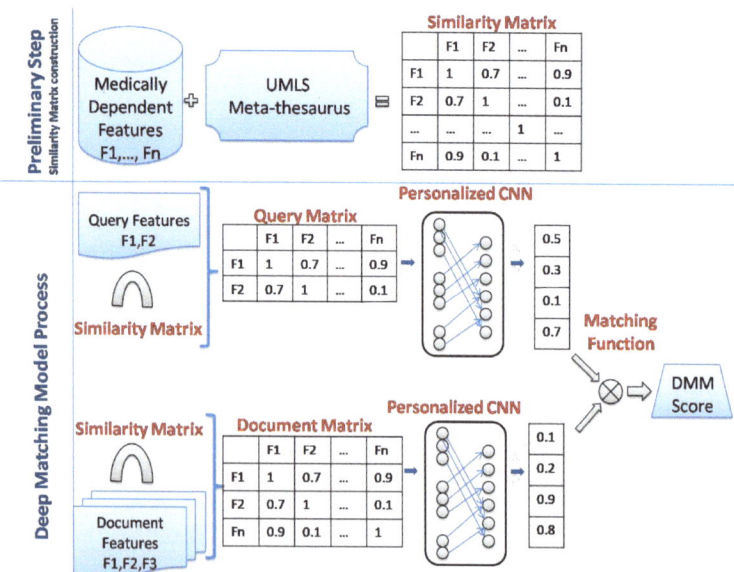

Figure 1. Overview of the Deep Matching Model.

4. Deep Matching Model: Preliminary Step
4.1. Medical Dependent Features

As our work falls into the medical image retrieval field, we propose to integrate the MDFs [6,32], that are a set of categorical medical features, into a new deep matching model to enhance the retrieval performance. A medical dependent features presented in the Figure 2.

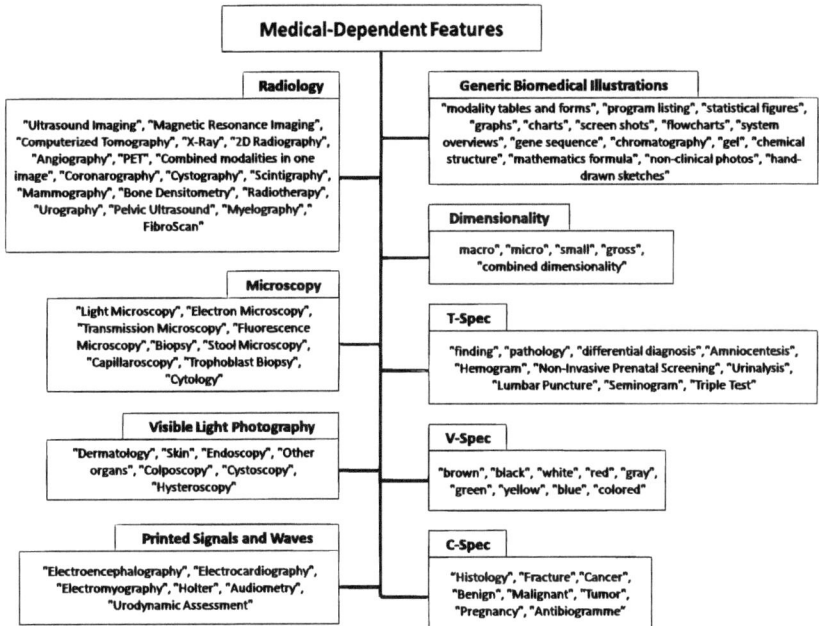

Figure 2. Medical -Dependent Features.

Each MDF f_i has m associated values v defined by $f_i = \{v1, v2, \ldots vm\}$. The set of MDF used in our work is detailed as follows:

- **Radiology** = "Ultrasound Imaging", "Magnetic Resonance Imaging", "Computerized Tomography", "X-Ray", "2D Radiography", "Angiography", "PET", "Combined modalities in one image", "Coronarography", "Cystography", "Scintigraphy", "Mammography", "Bone Densitometry", "Radiotherapy", "Urography", "Pelvic Ultrasound", "Myelography", "FibroScan"
- **Microscopy** = "Light Microscopy", "Electron Microscopy", "Transmission Microscopy", "Fluorescence Microscopy", "Biopsy", "Stool Microscopy", "Capillaroscopy", "Trophoblast Biopsy", "Cytology"
- **Visible light photography** = "Dermatology", "Skin", "Endoscopy", "Other organs", "Colposcopy", "Cystoscopy", "Hysteroscopy"
- **Printed signals and waves** = "Electroencephalography", "Electrocardiography", "Electromyography", "Holter", "Audiometry", "Urodynamic Assessment"
- **Generic Biomedical Illustrations** = "modality tables and forms", "program listing", "statistical figures", "graphs", "charts", "screen shots", "flowcharts", "system overviews", "gene sequence", "chromatography", "gel", "chemical structure", "mathematics formula", "non-clinical photos", "hand-drawn sketches"
- **Dimensionality** = "macro", "micro", "small", "gross", "combined dimensionality"
- **V-Spec** = "brown", "black", "white", "red", "gray", "green", "yellow", "blue", "colored"

- **T-spec** = "finding", "pathology", "differential diagnosis", "Amniocentesis", "Hemogram", "Non-Invasive Prenatal Screening", "Urinalysis", "Lumbar Puncture", "Seminogram", "Triple Test"
- **C-spec** = "Histology", "Fracture", "Cancer", "Benign", "Malignant", "Tumor", "Pregnancy", "Antibiogramme"

4.2. Semantic Matrix Construction

In this section, we present a new semantic mapping method using two semantic resources: MDF and UMLS. Frequently in NLP, the text data is converted into a vector of numbers, which deep models can process as input. Several approaches, such as Word2Vec, Glove, and one-hot-encoding, have been proposed for word embedding. Usually, these models consider general terminologies, which are not specific for any domain, to derive similarities and relations between words. As our work fits in the medical image retrieval field, we believe that retrieval performance could be improved if we use medical semantic resources such as UMLS for converting textual words. We represent the queries and documents as a set of MDF to keep only semantic information related to the medical domain. Then, each MDF is transformed into a concept using the MetaMap tool, then the UMLS Similarity tool [37] is used to calculate the similarities between each pair of concepts and then construct the similarity matrix as shown in Figure 1.

As shown in the preliminary step of Figure 1, all features are transformed into a similarity matrix and thus by following the next steps:

- Step 1: the MetaMap tool [38] is used to transform each MDF into a concept.
- Step 2: the similarities between each pair of medical concepts are calculated using the UMLS Similarity tool [37,39]. These semantic similarity scores are arranged in a semantic matrix. More precisely, we use the Resnik measure to determine the semantic relations between extracted concepts, as according to [40], it performs better than Path-based measures.

5. Deep Matching Model Construction

The new DMM model is a representation focused model that should build a good representation for a query and document with a deep neural network and conduct matching between the corresponding representations. Moreover, this model should take into account the specificity of information retrieval, NLP and medical image retrieval.

The inputs to our DMM model are a set of queries and documents presented with MDFs; each MDF is transformed into concepts then to a vector of numbers to be processed by the subsequent layers of the network. In the following, we detail the main components of our DMM model: the query/document matrix extraction, the personalized CNN and the matching function.

5.1. Query and Document Matrix Extraction

As our work fits in the medical image retrieval field, we represent the queries and the documents as a set of MDF in order to keep only semantic information related to the medical domain. In this paper, we propose to convert each query and document into an MDF vector. Then, each vector is converted to a semantic similarity matrix as presented in Figure 3:

- Step 1: For each query/document vector, we assign a binary value for each MDF depending on whether the query/document contains the feature value or not. The length of the resulting vector V equals n where n is the number of MDFs. This vector is transformed into a $n*n$ matrix M /$\forall i \in n, \forall j \in n, M[i][j] = V[i]$ where i represents the row index and j represents the column index.
- Step 2: we multiply the resulting matrix M with the semantic similarity matrix SSM to obtain a new query matrix NQM as follows:
$NQM[i][j] = M[i][j] * SSM[i][j]$
The illustration of the calculation is done in Figure 3.

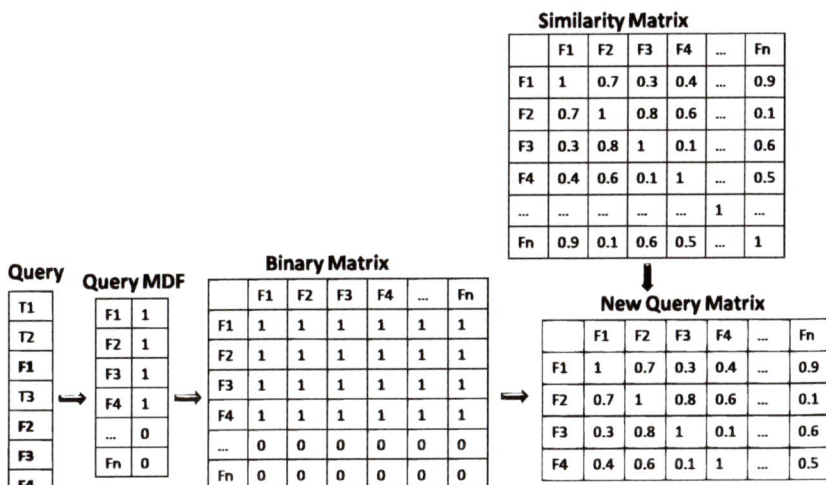

Figure 3. Query matrix extraction process.

5.2. Personalized CNN

We present, in this section, the personalized CNN that explicitly addresses the three specificities mentioned above. Indeed, the filters are designed to extract the best representation of queries and documents. In each representation, the network considers several retrieval features such as the MDF co-occurrence, the document ranking, and the IPM score. Moreover, it considers the NLP features for each query/document representation as it extracts the interaction between document and query. Indeed, according to [14], most of NLP models extract the interaction between two texts.

In the following, we present the layers of our network: convolutional, activations, pooling and fully connected layers.

Figure 4 Presents the architecture of the personalized CNN model.

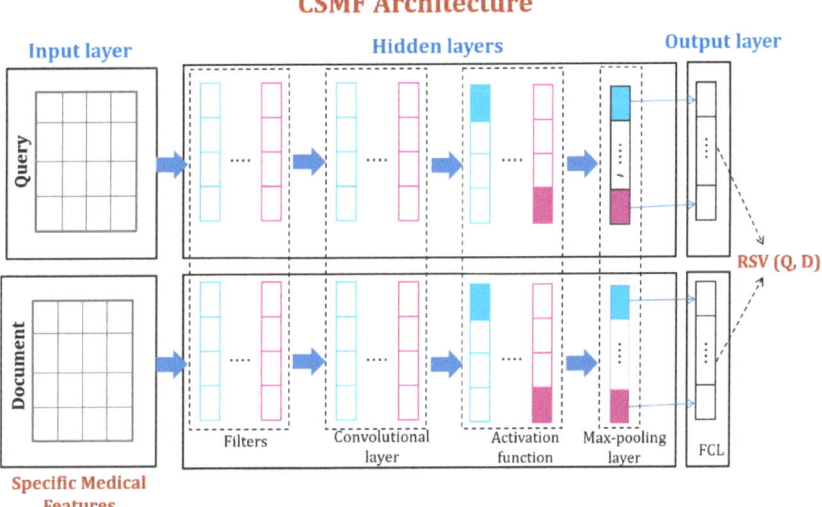

Figure 4. The architecture of the personalized CNN model.

5.2.1. Convolutional Layer

In this layer, a set of filters $F \in \mathbb{R}^d$ are applied to the query and document vectors to produce different feature maps. In our model, the query filters are distinct from the document filters. Below, we provide detailed information on the filters used for each component (document and query).

Query Filters:

The query filters aim to extract the best representation of the queries by considering the relationship between the document and the query. The more relevant the document is to the query, the higher the resulting vector values will be.

- Confidence Query Filter (CoQF): The idea consists of calculating the co-occurrences of query MDFs with all MDFs.

$$CoQF = \frac{\sum_{j \in Q} \sum_{i \in D} fr(f_i, f_j)}{\sum_{i \in D} fr(f_i)} \quad (1)$$

where Q is the query MDF, D is the document MDFs, $fr(f_j)$ is the cooccurrence of query MDFs in the collection, $fr(f_i)$ is the cooccurrence of document MDFs in the collection and $fr(f_i, f_j)$ is the cooccurrence of query MDF and document MDF in the collection.
In order to take into consideration, the length of the document, we use this filter. A document having only the query MDF should be more relevant than a document having other MDF in addition to the query ones. In fact, both documents are specific but the first document is more exhaustive. For that, we propose to divide the number of MDF in both document and query, with the number of document MDF. If the document did not include any query MDF, then the value will 0.

- Length Query Filter (LQF): For each query, if the document contains all query MDF, then we divide the number of MDF in both document and query, with the number of document MDF. Else, the value will be equal 0.

$$LQF = \frac{|MDF \in (Q, D)|}{|MDF \in D|} \quad (2)$$

where $|MDF \in (Q, D)|$ is the number of MDFs in both query MDF Q and document MDF D and $|MDF \in D|$ is the number of MDF in the document containing all query MDF.

- Rank Query Filter (RQF): We calculate the inverse document rank. If the document did not appear in the first search, the RQF will be equal.

$$RQF = \frac{1}{docrank} \quad (3)$$

- Proximity Query Filter (PQF): IIn the event that a document has query MDFs, we will compute the inverse of the distances that separate these MDFs in the document. In this instance, the distance between two features is represented by the total number of features that are located between them.

$$PQF = \frac{1}{1 + \sum distMDF \in D} \quad (4)$$

where $distMDF \in D$ is the distances between document MDFs.

- PMI Query Filter (PMIQF): The PMI (Pointwise Mutual Information) [41] is a proposed metric to find features with a close meaning. Indeed, the PMI of the MDFs f_i and f_j is defined using the occurrences of f_i ($fr(f_i)$) and f_j ($fr(f_j)$), the co-occurrences $fr(f_i, f_j)$ within a vector of features, and N is the collection size.

$$PMIF(QF) = \log \frac{N \times fr(f_i, f_j)}{fr(f_i) \times fr(f_j)} \qquad (5)$$

This equation calculates the semantically closest MDFs of the collection to f_i and f_j.

- Feature Difference Query Filter (FDQF): The more the query MDFs not found is small, the more the document is relevant. For each query, we compute the inverse of number of query MDFs not in document MDFs.

$$FDQF = \frac{1}{\sqrt{1 + |MDF \in \{Q \cap D\}|}} \qquad (6)$$

Document Filters:

Similar to the query filters, document filters try to extract the best representation of documents. They are based on the relationship between document and query. The more the document is relevant to the query, the highest is the resulting vector values.

- Confidence Document Filter (CoDF): This document filter determines the total amount of MDF documents that are included in the query. The relevance of the document will increase in proportion to the number of query MDFs it contains.

$$CoDF = \sum \left(f_i \underline{q} \cap f_j \underline{d} \right) \qquad (7)$$

where $\left(f_i \underline{q} \cap f_j \underline{d} \right)$ is the number of common MDF in query.

- Length Document Filter (LDF): When it comes to documents, first we determine the number of document MDFs that are included in the related query, and after we have that amount, we divide it by the document length (LD). In point of fact, the relevance of the document will increase if it is of a modest size and if it shares several characteristics with the query being conducted.

$$LDF = \frac{|MDFdocinquery|}{LD} \qquad (8)$$

where $|MDFdocinquery|$ is the number of MDF in both document and query and LD is the document length using the MDF features.

- Rank Document Filter (RDF):

$$RDF = \sum_{i \in q} fr(f_i indoc) \times \gamma \qquad (9)$$

The variable $fr(f_i)$ represents the frequency of query MDFs in the document, while γ represents the organization factor of the query in the document. The value of γ is 1 if the query preserves its organization in the document, and 0.5 if it does not.

- Proximity Document Filter (PDF): The more the document's features existing in the query are closer, the more it is relevant.

$$PDF = \frac{1}{|f_i \in Q|} \qquad (10)$$

where $FD \in Q$ is the documents MDFs in the query.

- PMI Document Filter (PMIDF): Similar to PMI in query filter, PMI in document filter try to find MDFs with a close meaning. It has the same equation except the N in this filter is the document size.

$$PMIF(DF) = \log \frac{N \times fr(f_i, f_j)}{fr(f_i) \times fr(f_j)} \quad (11)$$

This equation calculates the semantically closest MDFs in the document.
- Feature Difference Document Filter (FDDF): The more the number of document MDFs not in the query is small, the more the document is relevant.

$$FDDF = \frac{1}{\sqrt{1 + |MDF \in D - Q|}} \quad (12)$$

where D is the document MDFs and Q is the query MDFs.

The input of the DMM model is a matrix $S \in \mathbb{R}^{n \times n}$, and the convolutional filters are also matrices $F \in \mathbb{R}^n$. It is important to note that these filters have the same dimensionality, denoted as n, as the input matrix. In addition, these filters scan the vector representations and produce an output vector $C \in \mathbb{R}^m$. Each component c_i of the vector C is obtained by multiplying a vector V with a filter F, and then summing the resulting values to obtain a single value.

$$c_i = \sum_{k=1}^{n} V_k F_k \quad (13)$$

5.2.2. Activation Function

Immediately after the convolutional layer comes a non-linear activation function called *alpha* that is applied to the output of the layer that came before it. Through the use of this function, it is possible for a neuron's input signal to be transformed into an output signal. In the research that has been done, a number of different activation functions have been proposed [42]. One of these functions is called the Rectified Linear Unit (ReLU) function, and it assures that positive values are passed on to the subsequent layer. The authors in [43] demonstrated that this function is effective, uncomplicated, and has the capacity to lower the amount of complexity as well as the amount of time required for calculations. As a result, we have decided to include this function in our model in the capacity of an activation function.

5.2.3. Pooling Layer

The pooling layer's goal is to do three things: aggregate information, minimize the amount of representation used, and derive global features from the convolutional layer's local ones. There are two functions that can be found in the body of literary work: (1) the average consists of computing the average of each feature map of the convolutional layer to consider all the elements of the input are even if many of them have low weights [44], and (2) the Max consists of selecting the maximum value of each feature map of the convolutional layer. Both of these operations are performed in order to take into consideration all of the elements of the input are. We have decided to adopt max-pooling for our research because it takes into account only neurons with high activation values, which ultimately results in a high level of semantic abstraction of the input data.

5.2.4. Fully Connected Layer

In order to produce a final vector representation of the query or document, a Fully Connected Layer (FCL) is applied to the vector that was generated as a result of the previous step.

5.3. Matching Function

According to [14], the most significant challenge associated with the retrieval of information is the matching problem, which refers to the process of determining a document's relevancy in light of a query. If we have a document denoted by *d* and a query denoted by *q*, then the matching function is a mechanism for assigning a score to the representation of *d* and *q*:

$$RSV(d,q) = F(\Phi(d), \Phi(q)) \tag{14}$$

where *F* stands for the scoring function and *Phi* is the mapping function that converts each *d* | *q* pair into a vector representation. In the research that has been done on the subject, a number of different deep matching models have been suggested for the overall matching process. These silhouettes fall primarily into one of two categories when grouped together. The representation-focused model is the first one, and in this model, *Phi* is a complicated mapping function while *F* is a straightforward scoring function. A deep neural network is utilized by this model in order to construct an accurate representation for the document as well as the query. After that, it does some sort of matching between these different representations. The second one is the interaction-focused model where Φ is simple mapping function and *F* is complex scoring function.

We use a representation-focused model in which *Phi* is a sophisticated mapping function between representations and *F* is a straightforward matching function. Since the sophisticated *Phi*-based mapping function of the individualized CNN is what drives our selection, we resort to the more elementary *F*-based cosine similarity. The formal definition of a document's relevance to a query is as follows:

$$RSV(Q,D) = cosine(\vec{Q}, \vec{D}) = \frac{\vec{Q} \cdot \vec{D}}{\|\vec{Q}\| \cdot \|\vec{D}\|} \tag{15}$$

where $\vec{Q}$ and $\vec{D}$ are the query and the document vectors respectively. In the IR, for a given query, the documents are ranked by their relevance scores.

6. SemRank: Semantic Re-Ranking Model Based on DMM

In the last part of this article, we discussed our MDF-based deep matching model, which calculates the DMM score of the document *d* with respect to the query *q*. However, doing a search of relevant documents by utilizing MDF alone is insufficient; certain phrases could not be mapped to MDF, and as a result, such keywords should be eliminated from the search. As a result, we recommend combining the findings of the DMM with those of the baseline, taking into consideration all of the query terms. To be more specific, we suggest modeling the SemRank score using the most common type of late fusion approach, which is known as a straightforward linear combination. Before adding the two scores together, we first standardize the initial score and the DMM score in the following manner:

$$SemRank_{score} = \alpha * \frac{InitialScore}{\max InitialScores} + (1-\alpha) * \frac{DMMScore}{\max DMMScore} \tag{16}$$

where α is a balancing parameter $\alpha \in [0\ldots 1]$, InitialScore represents the initial ranking score of the document and DMM score of the same document. The normalized score is obtained by dividing the relevance score for a given document *d* by the highest relevance score in the whole collection. As a baseline, we propose to use the BM25 model which is well known for its efficiency and its performance in many retrieval tasks

7. Experiments and Results

In this section, we describe the experimental datasets, then we present our several experiments released to evaluate the accuracy of our model and we compare it to some existing approaches.

7.1. Experimental Datasets

In order to assess the effectiveness of our suggested method, it is imperative to utilize medical image datasets that include both images and textual descriptions, together with queries and ground truth. The majority of medical data sets currently available do not fulfill these criteria. Some sources lack assessment protocols, such as OHSUMED [45], while others focus on textual analysis and evaluation, like TREC. On the other hand, the ImageCLEFmed evaluation campaign offers specific medical picture collections for the purpose of assessing medical image retrieval. From 2011 onwards, the quantity and extent of the collections were comparable to those seen in real-world applications [46]. Due to copyright restrictions, the redistribution of the ImageCLEFmed collections to research groups is only allowed through a special agreement with the original copyright holders [47]. Therefore, we are restricted to conducting experiments using only the five collections for which we have obtained copyrights. The collections are shown in Table 1 and consist of two relatively small data sets: 74,902 and 77,495 images for the 2009 [48] and 2010 [49] data sets, respectively. After the evolution of ImageCLEF, three additional data sets were added: 230,088 images for the 2011 [50] data set, and 306,539 images for both the 2012 [51] and 2013 [52] data sets.

Each image in these data sets is accompanied by a textual description. An image can have the text from its caption or a hyperlink to the HTML page that has the complete text of the article [53], together with the title of the article [48]. Furthermore, the queries were chosen from a collection of themes suggested by physicians and clinicians in order to precisely mimic the information requirements of a clinician involved in diagnostic tasks. The images in the 2009 and 2010 data sets were sourced from the RSNA journals Radiology and Radiographics [48] and consist of a portion of the Goldminer data set. Nevertheless, the photos in the data sets from 2011, 2012, and 2013 are derived from studies that were published in open-access journals and may be accessed through PubMed Central. The later data sets have a wider range of images, including charts, graphs, and other nonclinical images, resulting in more visual variety.

To evaluate the proposed SemRank model, we conducted experiments using the ImageCLEF collections in Medical Retrieval Task from 2009 to 2012. These collections are composed of images and queries. Each image has a textual description. Each query is composed of text representation and a few sample images. In our work, we use only text representation of the queries and textual description of the images. The 2009 and the 2010 datasets are relatively small (74,902 and 77,495 images respectively). The 2011 and the 2012 datasets are significantly bigger (230,088 and 306,539 images respectively). Indeed, these datasets contain a greater image diversity and also include charts, graphs and other non-clinical images [32]. Also, we are limited to these datasets as we do not have the 2013 dataset, the last dataset in the medical image retrieval task of imageCLEF. Figure 5 illustrates 3 images of the used datasets, respectively with their associated MDF, extracted using the Medical-Dependent Features. We observe here that MDF features represent specific characteristics of medical images but not a body part (brain) or a pathology (cancer) and this due to the nature of medical textual queries aiming to find medical images.

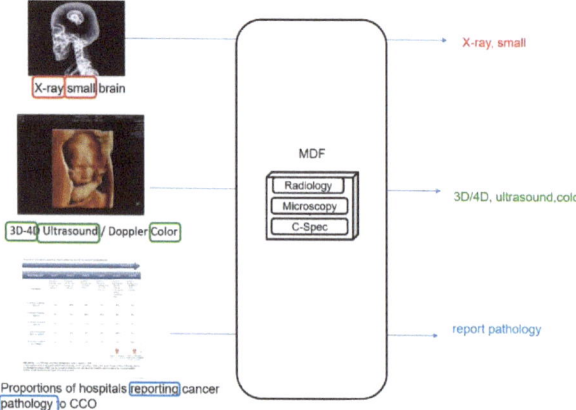

Figure 5. Some examples of ImageCLEF medical images and their extracted MDF.

7.2. Effectiveness of the SemRank Model in Image Reranking

In this section, we present a set of experiments carried out to the SemRank model. To achieve the best linear combination, we use several values of α. $\alpha = 0$ means that only the DMM score is used and $\alpha = 1$ means that only the BM25 score is used. Figure 6 presents the MAP, the P@5 and the P@10 values when: $\alpha \in [0:1]$ in datasets from 2009 to 2012.

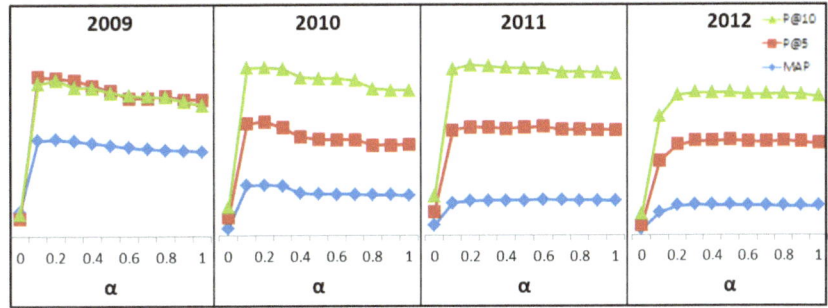

Figure 6. Results according to α using 4 ImageCLEF datasets 2009, 2010, 2011 and 2012.

According to Figure 6, we notice that using only DMM model to retrieve relevant documents gives the worst ranking results. However, the combination of the baseline and the DMM models gives better results. This proves our assumption that using only MDF to search for relevant documents is not sufficient; the combining models is a solution. According to MAP, P@5 and P@10 values, the best results are obtained when $\alpha \in [0.1:0.5]$. In the remaining experiments, we chose to set $\alpha = 0.3$.

7.3. Comparison of the SemRank Model with Literature Models

In this section, we propose to compare our model with BM25, DLM (Dirichlet Language Model) [54] and Bo1PRF (Bo1 Pseudo Relevance Feedback) [55] models. Table 1 summarizes this comparison according to the P@5, P@10 and MAP measures. The best result of all models and for each metric is presented in bold.

Table 1. Comparative results with the previous state-of-the-art approaches using ImageCLEF datasets.

		BM25	DLM	Bo1PRF	SemRank ($\alpha = 0.3$)
ImageClef-2009	P@5	0.608	0.592	0.608	**0.696**
	P@10	0.584	0.524	0.568	**0.664**
	MAP	0.379	0.327	0.371	**0.425**
ImageClef-2010	P@5	0.400	0.436	0.361	**0.453**
	P@10	0.420	0.375	0.330	**0.453**
	MAP	0.312	0.313	0.305	**0.389**
ImageClef-2011	P@5	0.393	0.240	0.386	**0.406**
	P@10	0.313	0.223	0.326	**0.340**
	MAP	0.193	0.138	**0.211**	0.195
ImageClef-2012	P@5	0.418	0.281	**0.554**	0.427
	P@10	0.313	0.241	**0.409**	0.322
	MAP	0.193	0.146	**0.361**	0.201

For the 2009 and the 2010 ImageClef datasets, the results show that our SemRank model performs better than the existing models in terms of MAP, P@5 and P@10. For the 2011 dataset, the SemRank model gives better results than the BM25 and the DLM models in terms of P@5 and P@10, but do not outperform the Bo1PRF model in term of MAP. Moreover, For the 2012 dataset, the Bo1PRF model outperforms our model in terms of MAP, P@5 and P@10. This can be explained by the high number of non-clinical images in these datasets which contain a diversity of images (tables, shapes, graphs); and our retrieval model is specific for medical images. Moreover, the Bo1PRF model is based on the pseudo-relevance feedback technique that improves retrieval results.

The accuracy gain is presented in Table 2. Indeed, we determine the improvement rate and we conduct a statistical t-test (Wilcoxon) [56] to evaluate the results. The gain is considered statistically significant when $p < 0.05$. In this work, the results are followed by the ** when $p < 0.05$.

Table 2. Accuracy gain of the SemRank compared to other models.

	2009	2010	2011	2012
SemRank/BM25	+12% **	+24%	+1%	+4%
SemRank/DLM	+29% **	+24%	+40% **	+38%
SemRank/Bo1PRF	+14% **	+27% **	-	-

Results show that the improvements have been achieved on the majority of datasets. Our model achieves between 12% and 29% on the 2009 dataset, which is a substantial improvement over the performance of existing models. When compared to the DLM and Bo1PRF models, the retrieval performance of the 2010 dataset is significantly enhanced by the SemRank model. This might be explained by the fact that the datasets from 2009 and 2010 contain photos suggested by clinicians and physicians that beat the information that is required.

Although our model is performing worse than the Bo1PR model on the 2011 and the 2012 datasets, it improves the retrieval performance (+4 percentage points) compared to the BM25 model for the 2012 dataset and (+40 percentage points) compared to the DLM model for the 2011 dataset. This variation may be due to the pseudo relevance feedback technique, which adds the first m keywords that appear in the top k retrieved documents. However, our model uses only query features without additional terms and enhances significantly the retrieval performance on the 2009 and the 2010 datasets.

We conclude that using our DMM improves significantly the results compared to the literature models. This validates our assumption that our DMM is a promising technique for improving medical image retrieval performance. In addition, this improvement could be related to the importance of using medical external resources: MDF and UMLS.

8. Conclusions and Future Work

This paper introduces an innovative SemRank model designed to enhance the ranking of medical images. The model leverages two external semantic resources: the Medical-Dependent Features (MDF) terminology and the Unified Medical Language System (UMLS) Metathesaurus. Within this framework, queries and documents are represented as sets of MDF, with the UMLS ontology employed to compute semantic similarity matrices between these sets. These matrices serve as the foundation for constructing matrix representations for each query and document, which are subsequently integrated into a Convolutional Neural Network (CNN) process. The resulting outputs yield vectors used to compute new relevance scores for documents when presented with a query. This innovative approach not only harnesses semantic knowledge from external resources but also employs advanced neural network techniques to improve the accuracy and effectiveness of medical image retrieval.

Our experiments were conducted on the Medical ImageCLEF collections from 2009 to 2012. The findings demonstrate a significant improvement in the re-ranking process when integrating Medical-Dependent Features (MDF) and the Unified Medical Language System (UMLS) into the Deep Matching Model (DMM). Furthermore, a comparative analysis was conducted between our model and various state-of-the-art approaches. The results revealed a noteworthy increase in the accuracy of the re-ranking process, underscoring the efficacy of our proposed methodology.

In our forthcoming research endeavors, we aim to augment the capabilities of the CNN model by integrating supplementary filters that encompass a broader spectrum of retrieval attributes. Furthermore, we plan to enhance the SemRank model by incorporating visual features, thereby elevating the precision of image retrieval.

Author Contributions: Conceptualization, K.G.; methodology, K.G. and H.A.; software, K.G. and H.A.; validation, H.A. and M.T.; formal analysis, K.G., H.A. and M.T.; resources, K.G. and H.A.; data curation, K.G. and H.A.; writing—original draft preparation, K.G. and H.A.; writing—review and editing, M.T. and H.A.; visualization, K.G. and H.A.; funding acquisition, K.G. All authors have read and agreed to the published version of the manuscript.

Funding: This work was funded by the Deanship of Graduate Studies and Scientific Research at Jouf University under grant No. (DGSSR-2023-02-02065).

Institutional Review Board Statement: Not applicable.

Informed Consent Statement: Not applicable.

Data Availability Statement: The data used in this study are openly accessible at the following link: https://www.imageclef.org.

Acknowledgments: This work was funded by the Deanship of Graduate Studies and Scientific Research at Jouf University under grant No. (DGSSR-2023-02-02065).

Conflicts of Interest: All authors declare that there are no competing interests.

References

1. Kelishadrokhi, M.K.; Ghattaei, M.; Fekri-Ershad, S. Innovative local texture descriptor in joint of human-based color features for content-based image retrieval. *Signal Image Video Process.* **2023**, *17*, 4009–4017. [CrossRef]
2. Smeulders, A.; Worring, M.; Santini, S.; Gupta, A.; Jain, R. Content-based image retrieval at the end of the early years. *IEEE Trans. Patt. Anal. Mach. Intell.* **2000**, *22*, 1349–1380. [CrossRef]
3. Anandh, A.; Mala, K.; Suganya, S. Content based image retrieval system based on semantic information using color texture and shape features. In Proceedings of the International Conference of Computing Technologies and Intelligent Data Engineering (ICCTIDE), Kovilpatti, India, 7–9 January 2016; pp. 1–8.
4. Moon, J.H.; Lee, H.; Shin, W.; Kim, Y.H.; Choi, E. Multi-modal understanding and generation for medical images and text via vision-language pre-training. *IEEE J. Biomed. Health Inform.* **2022**, *26*, 6070–6080. [CrossRef]
5. Ayadi, H.; Torjmen, M.K.; Huang, J.X.; Daoud, M.; Ben Jemaa, M. Learning to Re-rank Medical Images Using a Bayesian Network-Based Thesaurus. In Proceedings of the 39th European Conference on IR Research (ECIR), Aberdeen, UK, 8–13 April 2017; pp. 160–172.
6. Ayadi, H.; Torjmen-Khemakhem, M.; Daoud, M.; Huang, J.X.; Ben Jemaa, M. MF-Re-Rank A modality feature-based Re-Ranking model for medical image retrieval. *J. Assoc. Inf. Sci. Technol.* **2018**, *69*, 1095–1108. [CrossRef]
7. Krichen, M. Convolutional neural networks: A survey. *Computers* **2023**, *12*, 151. [CrossRef]
8. Shamsipour, G.; Fekri-Ershad, S.; Sharifi, M.; Alaei, A. Improve the efficiency of handcrafted features in image retrieval by adding selected feature generating layers of deep convolutional neural networks. *Signal Image Video Process.* **2024**, *18*, 2607–2620. [CrossRef]
9. Abas, A.R.; Elhenawy, I.; Zidan, M.; Othman, M. BERT-CNN: A Deep Learning Model for Detecting Emotions from Text. *Comput. Mater. Contin.* **2022**, *71*, 2943–2961.
10. Yang, K.; Ding, Y.; Sun, P.; Jiang, H.; Wang, Z. Computer vision-based crack width identification using F-CNN model and pixel nonlinear calibration. *Struct. Infrastruct. Eng.* **2023**, *19*, 978–989. [CrossRef]
11. Arkin, E.; Yadikar, N.; Xu, X.; Aysa, A.; Ubul, K. A survey: Object detection methods from CNN to transformer. *Multimed. Tools Appl.* **2023**, *82*, 21353–21383. [CrossRef]
12. Ayadi, H.; Torjmen-Khemakhem, M.; Huang, J.X. Term dependency extraction using rule-based Bayesian Network for medical image retrieval. *Artif. Intell. Med.* **2023**, *140*, 102551. [CrossRef]
13. Souissi, N.; Ayadi, H.; Torjmen, M.K. Text-based Medical Image Retrieval using Convolutional Neural Network and Specific Medical Features. In Proceedings of the 12th International Conference on Health Informatics HEALTHINF, Prague, Czech Republic, 22–24 February 2019; pp. 78–87.
14. Guo, J.; Fan, Y.; Ai, Q.; Croft, W.B. A deep relevance matching model for ad-hoc retrieval. In Proceedings of the Conference on Information and Knowledge Management (CIKM), Indianapolis, IN, USA, 24–28 October 2016; pp. 55–64.
15. Hu, B.; Lu, Z.; Li, H.; Chen, Q. Convolutional neural network architectures for matching natural language sentences. In Proceedings of the 27th International Conference on Neural Information Processing Systems (NIPS), Montreal, QC, Canada, 8–13 December 2014; pp. 2042–2050.

16. Lu, Z.; Li, H. A deep architecture for matching short texts. In Proceedings of the 26th International Conference on Neural Information Processing Systems (NIPS), Lake Tahoe, NV, USA, 5–10 December 2013; pp. 1367–1375.
17. Huang, P.-S.; He, X.; Gao, J.; Deng, L.; Acero, A.; Heck, L. Learning deep structured semantic models for web search using clickthrough data. In Proceedings of the 22nd ACM International Conference on Information and Knowledge Management (CIKM), San Francisco, CA, USA, 27 October–1 November 2013; pp. 2333–2338.
18. Chen, C.; Li, X.; Zhang, B. Research on image retrieval based on the convolutional neural network. In Proceedings of the 10th International Congress on Image and Signal Processing, BioMedical Engineering and Informatics (CISP-BMEI), Shanghai, China, 14–16 October 2017.
19. Qiu, C.; Cai, Y.; Gao, X.; Cui, Y. Medical image retrieval based on the deep convolution network and hash coding. In Proceedings of the 10th International Congress on Image and Signal Processing, BioMedical Engineering and Informatics (CISP-BMEI), Shanghai, China, 14–16 October 2017.
20. Saminathan, K. Content Based Medical Image Retrieval Using Deep Learning Algorithms. *J. Data Acquis. Process.* **2023**, *38*, 3868.
21. Rios, A.; Kavuluru, R. Convolutional neural networks for biomedical text classification: Application in indexing biomedical articles. In Proceedings of the 6th ACM Conference on Bioinformatics, Computational Biology and Health Informatics, Atlanta, GA, USA, 9–12 September 2015; pp. 258–267.
22. Hughes, M.; Li, I.; Kotoulas, S.; Suzumura, T. Medical text classification using convolutional neural networks. *Stud. Health Technol. Inform.* **2017**, *235*, 246–250. [PubMed]
23. Soldaini, L.; Yates, A.; Goharian, N. Denoising Clinical Notes for Medical Literature Retrieval with Convolutional Neural Model. In Proceedings of the 2017 ACM on Conference on Information and Knowledge Management, Singapore, 6–10 November 2017; pp. 2307–2310.
24. Pennington, J.; Socher, R.; Manning, C. Glove: Global vectors for word representation. In Proceedings of the 2014 Conference on Empirical Methods in Natural Language Processing (EMNLP), Doha, Qatar, 25–29 October 2014; pp. 1532–1543.
25. Guo, K.; Liang, Z.; Tang, Y.; Chi, T. SOR: An optimized semantic ontology retrieval algorithm for heterogeneous multimedia big data. *J. Comput. Sci.* **2018**, *28*, 455–465. [CrossRef]
26. Singh, P.; Goudar, R.H.; Rathore, R.; Srivastav, A.; Rao, S. Domain ontology based efficient image retrieval. In Proceedings of the 2013 7th International Conference on Intelligent Systems and Control (ISCO), Coimbatore, India, 4–5 January 2013; pp. 445–452.
27. Kumar, S.; Singh, M.K.; Mishra, M. Efficient Deep Feature Based Semantic Image Retrieval. *Neural Process. Lett.* **2023**, *55*, 2225–2248. [CrossRef]
28. Kumar, K.S.; Deepa, K. Medical query expansion using UMLS. *Indian J. Sci. Technol.* **2016**, *9*, 1–6.
29. Ivanović, M.; Budimac, Z. An overview of ontologies and data resources in medical domains. *Expert Syst. Appl.* **2014**, *41*, 5158–5166. [CrossRef]
30. Zhang, F.; Song, Y.; Cai, W.; Hauptmann, A.G.; Liu, S.; Pujol, S.; Kikinis, R.; Fulham, M.J.; Feng, D.D.; Chen, M. Dictionary pruning with visual word significance for medical image retrieval. *Neurocomputing* **2016**, *177*, 75–88. [CrossRef] [PubMed]
31. Kurtz, C.; Depeursinge, A.; Napel, S.; Beaulieu, C.F.; Rubin, D.L. On combining image-based and ontological semantic dissimilarities for medical image retrieval applications. *Med. Image Anal.* **2014**, *18*, 1082–1100. [CrossRef] [PubMed]
32. Ayadi, H.; Torjmen, M.K.; Daoud, M.; Ben Jemaa, M.; Huang, J.X. Correlating Medical-dependent Query Features with Image Retrieval Models Using Association Rules. In Proceedings of the 22nd ACM International Conference on Information and Knowledge Management (CIKM), San Francisco, CA, USA, 27 October–1 November 2013; pp. 299–308.
33. Ayadi, H.; Torjmen-Khemakhem, M.; Daoud, M.; Huang, J.X.; Ben Jemaa, M. Mining correlations between medically dependent features and image retrieval models for query classification. *J. Assoc. Inf. Sci. Technol.* **2017**, *68*, 1323–1334. [CrossRef]
34. Bodenreider, O. The unified medical language system (UMLS): Integrating biomedical terminology. *Nucleic Acids Res.* **2004**, *32* (Suppl. S1), D267–D270. [CrossRef]
35. Luo, Y.; Uzuner, O. Semi-supervised learning to identify UMLS semantic relations. *AMIA Summits Transl. Sci. Proc.* **2014**, *2014*, 67–75.
36. Tran, L.T.T.; Divita, G.; Carter, M.E.; Judd, J.; Samore, M.H.; Gundlapalli, A.V. Exploiting the UMLS Metathesaurus for extracting and categorizing concepts representing signs and symptoms to anatomically related organ systems. *J. Biomed. Inform.* **2015**, *58*, 19–27. [CrossRef] [PubMed]
37. McInnes, B.; Liu, Y.; Pedersen, T.; Melton, G.; Pakhomov, S. *Umls::Similarity: Measuring the Relatedness and Similarity of Biomedical Concepts*; Association for Computational Linguistics: Stroudsburg, PA, USA, 2013.
38. Aronson, A.R. Effective mapping of biomedical text to the UMLS Metathesaurus: The MetaMap program. In Proceedings of the AMIA Symposium American Medical Informatics Association, Washington, DC, USA, 3–7 November 2001; p. 17.
39. Torjmen-Khemakhem, M.; Gasmi, K. Document/query expansion based on selecting significant concepts for context based retrieval of medical images. *J. Biomed. Inform.* **2019**, *95*, 103210. [CrossRef] [PubMed]
40. Resnik, P. Semantic similarity in a taxonomy: An information-based measure and its application to problems of ambiguity in natural language. *J. Artif. Intell. Res.* **1999**, *11*, 95–130. [CrossRef]
41. Church, K.W.; Hanks, P. Word association norms, mutual information, and lexicography. *Comput. Linguist.* **1990**, *16*, 22–29.
42. Severyn, A.; Moschitti, A. Learning to rank short text pairs with convolutional deep neural networks. In Proceedings of the 38th International ACM SIGIR Conference on Research and Development in Information Retrieval, Santiago, Chile, 9–13 August 2015; pp. 373–382.

43. Nair, V.; Hinton, G.E. Rectified linear units improve restricted boltzmann machines. In Proceedings of the 27th International Conference on Machine Learning (ICML-10), Haifa, Israel, 21–24 June 2010; pp. 807–814.
44. Zeiler, M.D.; Fergus, R. Stochastic pooling for regularization of deep convolutional neural networks. *arXiv* **2013**, arXiv:1301.3557.
45. Hersh, W.R.; Buckley, C.; Leone, T.J.; Hickam, D.H. OHSUMED: An interactive retrieval evaluation and new large test collection for research. In Proceedings of the 17th Annual International ACM-SIGIR Conference on Research and Development in Information Retrieval (SIGIR), Dublin, Ireland, 3–6 July 1994; pp. 192–201.
46. Kalpathy-Cramer, J.; de Herrera, A.G.S.; Demner-Fushman, D.; Antani, S.; Bedrick, S.; Müuller, H. Evaluating performance of biomedical image retrieval systems—An overview of the medical image retrieval task at ImageCLEF 2004–2014. *Comput. Med. Imaging Graph.* **2014**, *39*, 55–61. [CrossRef]
47. Grubinger, M.; Nowak, S.; Clough, P. Data sets created in ImageCLEF. In *ImageCLEF: Experimental Evaluation in Visual Information Retrieval*; Springer: Berlin/Heidelberg, Germany, 2010; pp. 19–43.
48. Müller, H.; Kalpathy-Cramer, J.; Eggel, I.; Bedrick, S.; Radhouani, S.; Bakke, B.; Kahn, C.E., Jr.; Hersh, W. Overview of the CLEF 2009 medical image retrieval track. In Proceedings of the 10th Workshop of the Cross-Language Evaluation Forum (CLEF), Corfu, Greece, 30 September–2 October 2009; pp. 72–84.
49. Müller, H.; Kalpathy-Cramer, J.; Eggel, I.; Bedrick, S.; Reisetter, J.; Kahn, C.E., Jr.; Hersh, W. Overview of the CLEF 2010 medical image retrieval track. In Proceedings of the Workshop of the Cross-Language Evaluation Forum (CLEF), Padova, Italy, 20–23 September 2010; Working Notes.
50. Kalpathy-Cramer, J.; Müller, H.; Bedrick, S.; Eggel, I.; De Herrera, A.G.S.; Tsikrika, T. Overview of the CLEF 2011 medical image classification and retrieval tasks. In Proceedings of the Workshop of the Cross-Language Evaluation Forum (CLEF) 2011, Amsterdam, The Netherlands, 19–22 September 2011; Volume 1177, Working Notes.
51. Müller, H.; Herrera, A.G.S.; Kalpathy-Cramer, J.; Demner Fushman, D.; Antani, S.; Eggel, I. Overview of the imageCLEF 2012 medical image retrieval and classification tasks. In Proceedings of the Workshop of the Cross-Language Evaluation Forum (CLEF) 2012, Rome, Italy, 17–20 September 2012; Working Notes.
52. Herrera, A.G.; Kalpathy-Cramer, J.; Demner Fushman, D.; Antani, S.; Müller, H. Overview of the ImageCLEF 2013 medical tasks. In Proceedings of the Workshop of the Cross-Language Evaluation Forum (CLEF) 2013, Valencia, Spain, 23–26 September 2013; Volume 1179, Working Notes.
53. Wu, H.; Sun, K.; Deng, X.; Zhang, Y.; Che, B. Uestc at imageCLEF 2012 medical tasks. In Proceedings of the Workshop of the Cross-Language Evaluation Forum (CLEF), Valencia, Spain, 23–26 September 2013; Online Working Notes/Labs/Workshop.
54. Yu, G.; Li, X.; Bao, Y.; Wang, D. Evaluating document-to-document relevance based on document language model: Modeling, implementation and performance evaluation. In Proceedings of the International Conference on Intelligent Text Processing and Computational Linguistics, Mexico City, Mexico, 13–19 February 2005; Springer: Berlin/Heidelberg, Germany, 2005; pp. 593–603.
55. Lioma, C.; Ounis, I. A syntactically-based query reformulation technique for information retrieval. *Inf. Process. Manag.* **2008**, *44*, 143–162. [CrossRef]
56. Wilcoxon, F. Individual comparisons by ranking methods. *Biom. Bull.* **1945**, *1*, 80–83. [CrossRef]

Disclaimer/Publisher's Note: The statements, opinions and data contained in all publications are solely those of the individual author(s) and contributor(s) and not of MDPI and/or the editor(s). MDPI and/or the editor(s) disclaim responsibility for any injury to people or property resulting from any ideas, methods, instructions or products referred to in the content.

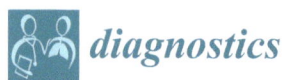

Article

A Novel Framework for Data Assessment That Uses Edge Technology to Improve the Detection of Communicable Diseases

Mohd Anjum [1], Hong Min [2,*] and Zubair Ahmed [3]

[1] Department of Computer Engineering, Aligarh Muslim University, Aligarh 202002, India; mohdanjum@zhcet.ac.in
[2] School of Computing, Gachon University, Seongnam 13120, Republic of Korea
[3] Department of Zoology, College of Science, King Saud University, Riyadh 11451, Saudi Arabia
* Correspondence: hmin@gachon.ac.kr

Abstract: Spreading quickly throughout populations, whether animal or human-borne, infectious illnesses provide serious risks and difficulties. Controlling their spread and averting disinformation requires effective risk assessment and epidemic identification. Technology-enabled data analysis on diseases allows for quick solutions to these problems. A Combinational Data Assessment Scheme intended to accelerate disease detection is presented in this paper. The suggested strategy avoids duplicate data replication by sharing data among edge devices. It uses indexed data gathering to improve early detection by using tree classifiers to discern between various kinds of information. Both data similarity and index measurements are considered throughout the data analysis stage to minimize assessment errors. Accurate risk detection and assessment based on information kind and sharing frequency are ensured by comparing non-linear accumulations with accurate shared edge data. The suggested system exhibits high accuracy, low mistakes, and decreased data repetition to improve overall effectiveness in illness detection and risk reduction.

Keywords: infectious diseases; edge technology; data assessment scheme; disease detection; risk assessment; information analysis

1. Introduction

Communicable diseases are also known as transmissible diseases or infectious diseases. Some of the infectious diseases are COVID-19, Tuberculosis, AIDS, etc. Edge computing is widely used in identifying contagious diseases. An intelligent edge surveillance system uses edge computing to identify infectious diseases [1]. It is a remote sensing or monitoring system that is more effective and reliable than any other sensing system [2]. The smart edge system helps physicians, public health authorities, and hospitals to know the details about the affected person. This framework is mainly used to sense the communication chain of the infected people in society. This model detects the infected person and helps monitor their activities from the outside world. Edge computing stores the affected people's data and records them safely and securely [3]. Infectious diseases or transmissible diseases can spread from one person to another by touching a contaminated surface or by physical contact with each other. The leading cause of infectious diseases is viruses and bacteria from animals or humans [4].

Communicable disease analysis is the main task performed in every healthcare department to provide a better environment for the people [5]. The analysis process helps to identify the affected or infected people from society by monitoring every person through a surveillance system. Without proper monitoring or analysis processes, infectious diseases will spread all around the surroundings and cause severe problems for the citizens of the whole world [6]. Fog computing is used to analyze contagious diseases. It is a real-time

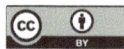

analysis process by the healthcare department with the help of collected records, which is used to provide a better environment for the people. It is more reliable and offers better performance when compared with any other analyzing process [7]. Edge computing is an information technology model that keeps the data storage and the computation process for the client closer. Edge computing is widely used to provide better service to the customer via networking technologies [8]. Diseases that are spread from one person to another by physical contact or touching contaminated surfaces are called communicable diseases or infectious diseases. Infectious diseases are more dangerous than non-communicable diseases [9].

To maximize efficiency as compared to conventional models and to improve estimation accuracy, deep learning models are frequently used to extract high-level spatial information [10]. They are also frequently used to identify and interpret biological data. The decision tree is a critical tool for examining predictions that may be used to efficiently and explicitly characterize beliefs. Despite its limits, it is a graph that shows every possible outcome using division techniques [11]. The COVID-19 pandemic presented unique challenges and opportunities to alter global healthcare systems. Under these circumstances, it is now necessary to use novel intelligence [12]. Technologies that offer the chance to provide virtual health services effectively. The theory and methods of edge computing, which help close the technological divide between network edges and the cloud, have emerged with the rapid rise of mobile communication. It can expedite the content delivery to raise the quality of networking service. It drives multimedia services across mobile networks with the help of system intelligence [13]. Artificial intelligence (AI) algorithms process and interpret large volumes of data, extracting insightful patterns and information that help with accurate diagnosis, therapy selection, and disease prognosis [14]. Healthcare practitioners can improve their decision-making processes and produce more individualized and successful interventions by utilizing AI-driven predictive modeling. Emerging technologies have transformed the field of infectious diseases, impacting different aspects of the ecosystem, such as diagnosis, monitoring, treatment of chronic illnesses, prevention, and tailored medicines [15]. The main contribution of the paper is stated below.

1. To present a Combinational Data Assessment Scheme (CDAS) to accelerate disease detection.
2. To improve early detection by using tree classifiers to discern between various kinds of information utilizing indexed data gathering.
3. To detect accurate risk and assessment based on information kind and sharing frequency; these are ensured by comparing non-linear accumulations with accurate shared edge data.
4. To improve overall effectiveness in illness detection and risk reduction by exhibiting high accuracy, low mistakes, and decreased data repetition.

The remaining part of the manuscript is divided into sections: Section 2 engages with related works, Section 3 covers proposed CDAS approaches and analysis, the performance analysis is covered in Section 4, and finally, Section 5 is covered with a conclusion along with future works.

2. Related Works

Dong et al. [16] proposed an edge perturbation method for predicting microRNA (miRNA)-disease association or the EPMDA method. It is used in the miRNA method for prediction. Structural Hamiltonian information is used to design a feature vector for each edge in the graph. The planned feature vector is used in the disease prediction process. Compared with the Human miRNA Disease Database, EPMDA is more effective and improves the value of AUC.

Wu et al. [17] proposed a learning framework for miRNA for the positive-unlabeled problem. For the negative extraction process, a semi-supervised K-means model is used. Training samples are generated using the sub-gagging method. The proposed method reduces the negative sample rate and helps find the exact names of the diseases using the positive sample set of information. The proposed method outperformed when comparing it with other traditional prediction methods, and the prediction accuracy rate was higher and more accurate than any other method.

M. Safa et al. [18] proposed a novel prediction method for cardio stress using a machine learning algorithm in IoT devices. The proposed method uses the K-nearest algorithm and supports vector machine approaches. Here, new information interacts with the old information to avoid the duplication of information that will be saved. The proposed framework outperformed the traditional prediction method by increasing the inaccuracy rate in the prediction process.

Pham et al. [19] proposed a new multiple-disease prediction method using a machine learning algorithm. This method helps to identify the relationship between the different types of diseases based on the categories. The proposed method helps analyze the graph by calculating both positive and negative sets and helps identify the symptoms of the disease. The experiment result shows that the proposed method outperformed the traditional method by increasing the multiple classification process and improving the efficiency rate of the prediction process.

Rahman et al. [20] found that to provide healthcare to all people, everywhere, technology is essential. To tackle the challenges of collecting, monitoring, and securely storing data on patients' essential body parameters through sensor technology, a healthcare architecture based on blockchain is suggested. Elements such as an Ethereum-permissioned blockchain, an IoMT device, and a Markov state chain are utilized by the framework. The technology outperforms previous systems in terms of node and transaction scalability by an impressive 80%. The framework is evaluated in comparison to current methods for improved performance, and it employs smart contracts for access control.

Xu et al. [21] proposed a new pathogenic genes prediction method using a network embedding approach named multipath2vec. The pathogenic prediction process is most widely used for disease prediction in every medical healthcare center. A multipath method is used to identify the random walk in the gene–phenotype network. A learned vector is used to calculate the similarities of the unexpected path from the heterogeneous network—the proposed method, named the pathogenic genes prediction method (PGPM), results in high accuracy for the pathogenic prediction process.

Li et al. [22] invented a new prediction method named FCGCNMDA, which was a fully connected graph convolutional network for a mi-RNA disease-related approach. Edge weight is represented using a fully connected graph; then, it combines with mi-RNA features for disease prediction. AUC values are high when compared with traditional prediction models. The proposed FCGCNMDA method is more reliable and increases the exact miRNA disease prediction system.

A feature selection method was proposed by Khamparia et al. [23] and used a deep learning neural approach named genetic algorithm. Neuromuscular disorder prediction is performed using this method. The genetic algorithm identifies gene subsets, and the Bhattacharya coefficient method determines the most effective gene subsets. The proposed integrated method improves the accuracy rate and is more effective when compared with other integrated prediction methods.

Zhang et al. [24] proposed a new method for a miRNA–disease association named multiple meta-paths fusion graph embedding models. MiRNA–disease interactions are used to collect information about diseases. The graph embedding model calculates the info related to the miRNA disease. The proposed model is used as a self-learning approach for the disease prediction process. From the comparisons, it is seen that the proposed model outperformed the traditional prediction method.

Badidi, E [25] proposed Edge AI's potential to enhance public health while reviewing its function in early health prediction. This article addressed the difficulties and constraints that Edge AI faces in predicting health outcomes early on. It also highlighted the need for further research to tackle these issues and how these technologies can be integrated into current healthcare systems to fully realize the potential of intelligent health technologies. It is also critical to keep up with new developments and moral dilemmas as Edge AI advances in early health prediction.

Al-Zinati et al. [26] introduced a redesigned bio-surveillance system that utilizes mobile edge computing and fog to detect how these technologies can be integrated into current healthcare systems to fully realize the potential of intelligent health technologies and localize biological threats. The order of fog nodes in the suggested architecture is responsible for compiling monitoring data from all across their respective regions and identifying any possible dangers. The evaluation results demonstrate the framework's capacity to identify contaminated areas and pinpoint biological hazards. Furthermore, the outcomes demonstrate how well the reorganization mechanisms modify the environment structure to deal with the highly dynamic environment.

To solve the issues with manual blood smear examination in tracking patients and result verification, Kamal, L. and Raj, R. J. R. [27] suggested an improved convolutional neural network approach for automated blood cell recognition and categorization. The proposed method automatically detects whole blood cells in blood smear images by combining sophisticated image-processing methods and deep learning algorithms. With rigorous training and validation, the suggested model obtains remarkable metrics such as 91.88% accuracy, 91% precision, 91% recall, and an 88% F-score, outperforming traditional Computer-Aided Diagnosis systems in clinical labs.

Yadav et al. [28] provided a strategy for Computation Offloading using Reinforcement Learning (CORL) to reduce power consumption and latency in healthcare devices that use IoMT. By identifying the best resources to offload work to, the system overcomes the problems of low battery capacity and time restrictions caused by service delays. When tested in an iFogSim simulator with realistic assumptions, the experimental results demonstrate that the strategy reduces power consumption, delays data transmission, and makes the most efficient use of node resources in edge-enabled sensor networks.

Nandy et al. [29] introduced a novel healthcare system that utilizes Wearable Sensors (WSs) and an advanced Machine Learning (ML) model called Bag-of-Neural Network (BoNN) to remotely monitor health and anticipate the onset of diseases. Distributed edge devices gather patient health symptoms and preprocess data in the epidemic model. At centralized cloud servers, the BoNN model is used to detect COVID-19 disease on an improved dataset. On a benchmark dataset from Brazil called COVID-19, the system achieved a 99.8 percent accuracy rate.

Methods for edge perturbation, learning frameworks, multiple-disease prediction, healthcare architectures based on blockchain, methods for predicting pathogenic genes, and methods for feature selection are all covered in the research papers that are included in the text. Among the many healthcare-related topics covered in these articles are multipath2vec, disease prediction, and the prediction of pathogenic genes. New bio-surveillance systems that make use of mobile edge computing and fog are introduced, and edge AI shows promise for enhancing early health prediction. For automated blood cell recognition and categorization, an upgraded convolutional neural network method beats out the old Computer-Aided Diagnosis methods.

3. Proposed Combinational Data Assessment Scheme

The proposed scheme relies on sharing data between the edge devices to prevent multi-source replications. Television, multimedia, graphics, cell phones, etc., do not transmit infectious diseases. Most cases of these infections spread through close personal contact with an infected person, contaminated objects, or respiratory droplets. In order to stop the dissemination of false information, it is essential to use reliable sources while discussing the spread of infectious illnesses. It helps extend and prevent false information about contagious diseases. A preventer is a group of software and hardware components that collect and process information accumulated from the healthcare center environment. The disease is controlled through various sources with sensor units to collect data such as frequency occurring, disease matching, data features, etc. Figure 1 portrays the proposed scheme in a real-time environment.

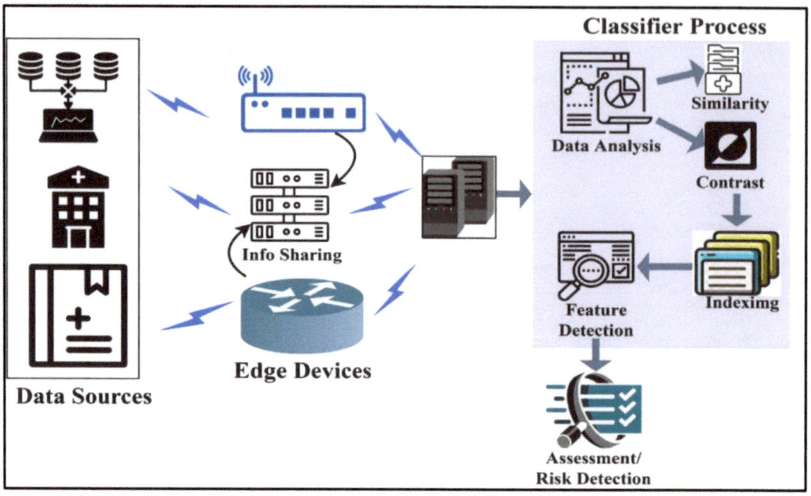

Figure 1. CDAS in Real-Time Environment using Different Classification Instances.

The deploying technology for analyzing disease-related information swiftly responds to the above problems. In the proposed CDAS, precise data sources and edge device control are prevented using the detection/recommendations of the analysis. The classifier performs similarity checks, difference data identification, and indexing in this analysis scheme. The indexed data are selected alone for feature extraction to identify the risks, as shown in Figure 1. The proposed CDAS improves disease detection swiftness, disease outbreak, risk assessment, and controlling infectious disease spread.

The edge disease consists of a specialized control unit that performs the functions of the edge devices (TV and MM) through edge devices and analysis (A). The functions of the edge devices are maintained using aggregators. The CDAS method serves as a data source and detection/recommendation. The aggregation unit rectifies the edge devices; therefore, it is predominant in controlling the spread and preventing false information from being built. It contains the spread of infectious diseases pursued using the data sources from the analysis (A). The CDAS analysis can be performed by four methods, namely, occurring frequency, classifier, data features, and matching. The input of data sources from the sensor (A) is functioned by the aggregation, then the matching function is transmitted. Therefore, CDAS is designed for actual data and replicating data analysis.

3.1. Data Analysis

The aggregators notice human and animal health conditions from infectious diseases. The input can be related to increased body temperature, coughing, fatigue, etc. In a noticing sequence, the data source received (Ds) derived as:

$$Ds = A \frac{\pm(A_{max} \times A_{min})}{A} + A_{min} \text{ such that } \varepsilon = \frac{1}{\sqrt{2\pi}A} \left[\frac{\left|\frac{A_{min}}{A_{max}} - \frac{\alpha}{A}\right|}{3 \left|Ds - Ds^*\right|} \right] \} \quad (1)$$

where the variable α, denotes an active aggregator, and $\alpha \in A$, A_{max} and A_{min} are the minimum and maximum data sources observed in varying instances. The variables A_{max} keep information and previous information from being A_{min}. They are used to avoid noticing incorrect information, and prior information is used to prevent false information and previous information from being noticed. In the sense of a hoax, the wrong information is estimated as the number of mismatching analyses observed at continuous A observations. Therefore, some conditions of error Ds due to multi-source replications and disease detection swiftness α. This problem impacts the Ds at a given instance, for which the normalization is computed as:

$$n(Ds) = \frac{\Delta^*}{\Delta^*\left[\frac{A_{max}}{A_{min}} - \sigma_s\right]^2} \text{ such that } \sigma_s = \frac{2}{A}\sqrt{\frac{3}{A+j}\sum_{j+1}^{A}\left[\left(\frac{Ds - Ds^*}{Ds}\right)^2 \times \frac{1}{\sqrt{2\pi A}}\right]} \quad (2)$$

The above equation specifies that the normalization comes after the maximum A_{max} and standard deviation A_{min} data sources observed standard deviation σ_s. Therefore, $n(Ds)$ is a normalized condition.

The symbols * and Δ in Equations (1) and (2) stand to mean as follows: In mathematical equations, the symbol * usually means to multiply. The product of two integers, A and B, is represented by $A * B$. The delta sign, often used to indicate a change or difference between two values, is represented by Δ. The symbol Δ, when used in equations, can represent a change in a variable or a particular mathematical procedure tied to the idea of difference.

In contrast, it is the aggregation condition for which the proper estimation, therefore, Ds is normalized. In comparison, increment A by j as $A + j$ is the aggregation condition for which the appropriate estimation action Ds is obtained. Based on Ds and $n(Ds)$, the instance of aggregation takes place, which is computed as follows:

$$\varepsilon[Ds, n(Ds)] = \sqrt{\left[\frac{n(Ds)}{Ds}\right]_a^3 - \left[\frac{n(Ds)}{Ds}\right]_b^3 - \ldots - \left[\left(j - \frac{Ds^*}{Ds}\right)\Delta^*\right]_\alpha^3}, \alpha \in A \quad (3)$$

As per the above Equation (3), the instance of aggregation for a sequence until α is achieved in transmitting information from the healthcare centers the following example of aggregation is observed using machine learning. In an infectious disease scenario, data from the source must be transformed into controls to manage the spread of the disease effectively and ensure high accuracy for a prompt response. Additionally, it is essential to prevent the dissemination of false information ('t') to meet the healthcare requirements of edge devices. In this process, the early detection of infectious disease is allowed to protect humans and animals. In this way, the machine available used in infectious disease or $\varepsilon[Ds, n(Ds)]_\alpha$ is accessed. The output of the shared edge data of the machine learning is to find and separate the replicating data sequence through Ds evaluating and an $operator - based$ analysis. Operator-based analysis refers to a method of data analysis that involves the use of mathematical operators or functions to manipulate and process data. This approach typically involves performing operations such as addition, subtraction, multiplication, division, comparison, or other mathematical functions on the data to derive meaningful insights or results. The first method of this learning is the frequency occurrence of the Ds instance if ε is observed. The concentration on achieving $\left(j - \frac{Ds^*}{Ds}\right)\Delta^*$ at any instance is the output for separating the data. As per the process, two sequences of sample inputs of Ds at any varying instances of ϑ and τ are given as the input for the machine learning. Hence, in an ε aggregation, the sequence of disease detection takes place as per Equation (4).

$$\begin{aligned}\vartheta &= Ds\tau = 1\}, the\ first\ instance\ is\ observed\ \vartheta = n(Ds)\tau \\ &= \tfrac{\sigma_s}{\Delta^*}\}, for\ the\ consecutive\ instances\ such\ that, \vartheta + \tau \\ &= Ds, is\ the\ first\ data\ source\ where\ n(Ds) \\ &\times \tfrac{\sigma_s}{\Delta^*}, is\ the\ sequence\ of\ sample\ data\ sources\}\end{aligned} \quad (4)$$

The machine learning model assessment initiates from the sequence of sample inputs with the first edge device as Ds. This Ds is the ease of information analysis for evaluation;

if the aggregation is observed in any varying instance, conjunction takes place. In Figure 2, the data analysis process is presented.

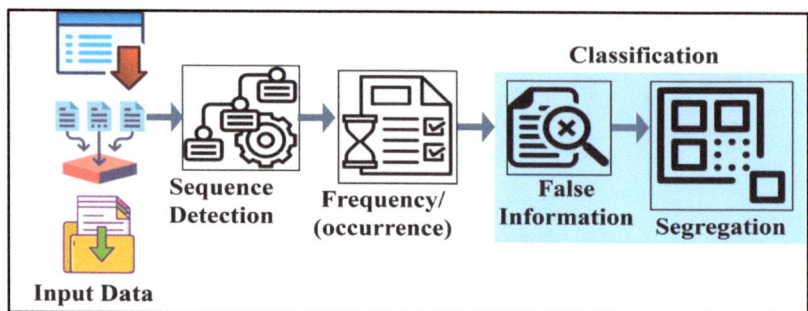

Figure 2. Data Analysis Process for Detection of False Data in Infectious Disease Monitoring.

The conjunction process is performed using detected sequences based on occurrences. This occurrence factor is considered for identifying false (replicated) data. The specified data are segregated for further utilization. Here, the features associated with the classification are identified for detection (Figure 2). Therefore, in the machine learning used in infectious diseases, the shared edge data features are merged with a non-linear accumulation of data. The sequence of $\vartheta + \tau = n(Ds) \times \frac{\sigma_s}{\Delta^*}$ is analyzed to find the actual shared edge data in the edge devices. Machine learning classifies the process into two analyses of real data and replicating data based on the occurring frequency. The occurring frequency $\varepsilon[Ds, n(Ds)]_\alpha$ functions and its related things served by the edge device are discussed as per Equation (5).

$$\begin{aligned}\varepsilon[Ds, n(Ds)]_\alpha &= \{\left[\tfrac{n(Ds)}{Ds}\right]^3_a, \varepsilon[Ds, n(Ds)]_j > \varepsilon_{n(Ds)}\left[\tfrac{n(Ds)}{Ds}\right]^3_b, \\ &\varepsilon[n(Ds)]_j \geq 0\varepsilon[Ds, n(Ds)] \\ &= X^D + \sum_{j+1}^n \left(\left[\tfrac{n(Ds)}{Ds}\right]^3_a \cos\cos\tfrac{X^D\delta\left(\left[\tfrac{n(Ds)}{Ds}\right]^3_a\right)}{\varepsilon_{n(Ds)}} + \left[\tfrac{n(Ds)}{Ds}\right]^3_b \sin\sin\tfrac{X^D\delta\left(\left[\tfrac{n(Ds)}{Ds}\right]^3_a\right)}{\varepsilon_{n(Ds)}}\right)\varepsilon_{n(Ds)} \\ &= \tfrac{-X^D \pm \sqrt{\varepsilon[Ds,n(Ds)]+\alpha(j)}}{3\cos\alpha_j}\}\end{aligned} \quad (5)$$

where the variable X^D denotes the partial output of the edge device, and δ is the disease outbreak by the crowd observed in Ds. The frequency-varying instance can be analyzed by this occurring frequency method and then the classifier performs the next instance of functions. The classifier is used to identify the original data and replicate data in the edge device. If the classification is $\varepsilon[n(Ds)]_j$, then the method and its related thing are served by the machine learning. In this manner, the tree classifier method is deployed for classifying the data into two ways, namely, original data and replicating data, and then it is used for distinguishing contrast information analysis. For this purpose, two sequence data of Ds at any instance of ϑ and τ are used as the input for the machine learning. From a given instance, $\varepsilon[Ds, n(Ds)]$ followed by the tree classifier are analyzed by the machine learning method.

$$R\{\varepsilon[Ds, n(Ds)]\} = -\vartheta(f) \pm \tau(Ds) - f(Ds)\pi \text{ such that } \vartheta\frac{f(Ds)}{Ds} = \forall[Ds + \pi(f)]\tau\frac{Ds}{\Delta^*} = \forall[\vartheta - \pi(f)]\} \quad (6)$$

As per the above Equation (6), the variable f is the output of the original data and π is the replicating data observed by the varying instance Ds. In the above equation, $\vartheta\frac{f(Ds)}{Ds}$ and $\tau\frac{Ds}{\Delta^*}$ are the related thing that is used for classifying the data of the $R\{\varepsilon[Ds, n(Ds)]\}$. In this manner, the aggregation method either satisfies $\vartheta\frac{f(Ds)}{Ds}$ or $\tau\frac{Ds}{\Delta^*}$ for all the sigmoid based $[Ds \pm \pi(f)]$ and $[\vartheta \pm \pi(f)]$. The true and false information of the above accumulation generates the non-linear $\vartheta \pm \tau$ to achieve the above classification. Therefore, the aggregation process of $\vartheta \frac{f(Ds)}{Ds}$ and $\frac{Ds}{\Delta^*}$ and the non-linear accumulations of Δ^* and $n(Ds)$ together give the output of $R\{\varepsilon[Ds, n(Ds)]\}$ at its shared edge data. The machine learning of tree classifier analyzes ϑ, τ and $\varepsilon[Ds, n(Ds)]$, and it is followed by the sigmoid-based classification through Ds^* and Δ^*. Figure 3 presents the data classification process.

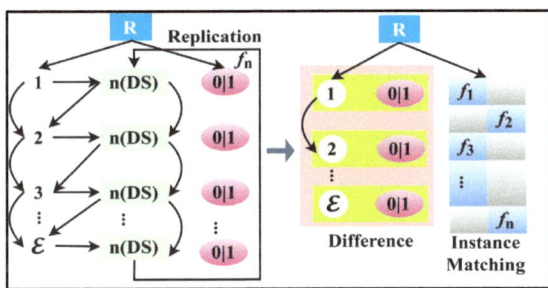

Figure 3. Error Analysis for Various Data Classification Process Sequences in Disease Detection.

The replication factor is classified for the input data sequence based on $n(Ds)$. Such classifications are performed for 0/1 augmentation in identifying the difference. This requires the matching of different instances. The occurrence $f_1, f_2, \ldots, f_n$ are used for matching different instances. This is extracted from the replication classified as presented in Figure 3. The output of the original data using the swift response $\{Ds, \Delta^*, \sigma_s\}$ is derived. Therefore, the first instance of replicating data provides indexed data collection and augments the early detection process. The replication processes are as computed in Equation (5) and (i.e.,) $[(\Delta^* = \sigma_s) = 1]$ is the output of the next instance, and hence, the occurring frequency is maintained without aggregation. Alternatively, the sequence of instance is observed, whereas the replicating data such as $\vartheta \frac{f(Ds)}{Ds}$ or $\tau \frac{Ds}{\Delta^*}$ impact the following data. Specifically, the occurring frequency of the above representation is either $\vartheta \frac{f(Ds)}{Ds}$ or $\tau \frac{Ds}{\Delta^*}$. The data sources of the inputs ϑ and τ are actual shared data such that the probability of matching the data is 1 or 2 for the sequence. Based on this example, the π conditions (i.e.,) $\pi > \frac{\sigma_s}{\Delta^*}$ or $\pi \leq \frac{\sigma_s}{\Delta^*}$ are analyzed. The π and its accumulations are matched for their features by preventing assessment errors and is computed as:

$$\pi = 2 * \frac{\rho_\tau}{\rho_\vartheta} \text{ where } \vartheta \frac{f(Ds)}{Ds} \text{ matching with } Ds, \text{ if } \pi > \frac{\sigma_s}{\Delta^*} \text{ else } \vartheta \frac{f(Ds)}{Ds} \text{ matching to } \sigma_s \text{ or } \Delta^*, \text{ if } \pi \leq \frac{\sigma_s}{\Delta^*}\} \quad (7)$$

where ρ_τ and ρ_ϑ denotes the accumulations of ϑ and τ in the given equations. It is a way to identify if all the accumulated data matched for their features can be accumulated with both ϑ and τ. Now, the shared information between the edge device to overcome the multi-source replications for the output of $\pi > \frac{\sigma_s}{\Delta^*}$ and $\pi \leq \frac{\sigma_s}{\Delta^*}$ condition is derived in Equations (8) and (9).

$$f_1 = n(Ds)_1 f_2 = n(Ds)_2 + \left(\frac{\sigma_s}{\Delta^*}\right)_1 - \left(\frac{\varepsilon}{\alpha}\right)_1 f_3 = n(Ds)_3 + \left(\frac{\sigma_s}{\Delta^*}\right)_2 - \left(\frac{\varepsilon}{\alpha}\right)_2 \text{ such that } f_n$$
$$= n(Ds)_n + \left(\frac{\sigma_s}{\Delta^*}\right)_{n+1} - \left(\frac{\varepsilon}{\alpha}\right)_{n+1}, \text{ if } \pi > \frac{\sigma_s}{\Delta^*}\} \quad (8)$$

$$f_1 = Ds_1 \pm \tau\left(\frac{Ds}{\Delta^*}\right)_1 f_2 = Ds_2 + \tau\left(\frac{Ds}{\Delta^*}\right)_2 - \left(\frac{\pi \times \varepsilon}{\alpha}\right)_1 f_3 = Ds_3 + \tau\left(\frac{Ds}{\Delta^*}\right)_3 - \left(\frac{\pi \times \varepsilon}{\alpha}\right)_2 \text{such that } f_n$$
$$= Ds_n + \tau\left(\frac{Ds}{\Delta^*}\right)_n - \left(\frac{\pi \times \varepsilon}{\alpha}\right)_{n+1}, \text{ if } \pi \leq \frac{\sigma_s}{\Delta^*}\} \quad (9)$$

The above-given representation is followed by the n sequence of the instance, where the early-detection Ds is augmented for classifying the output of the tree classifier. Therefore, the aggregation operation as in Equation (4) is analyzed for its frequency occurrence concerning the above-mentioned conditions of $\pi > \frac{\sigma_s}{\Delta^*}$ and $\pi \leq \frac{\sigma_s}{\Delta^*}$, utilizing the following determinations. These matching processes require some data features and also secure communicable disease information. Figure 4 presents the data feature matching process.

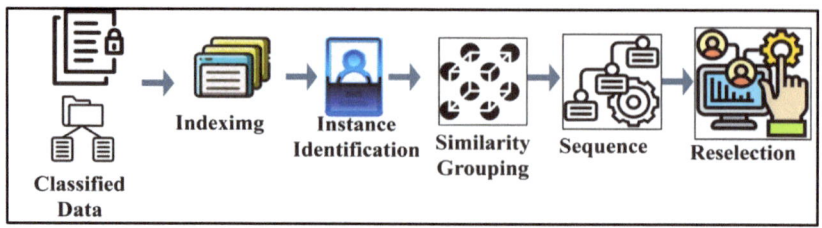

Figure 4. Data Feature Matching Process for Disease Detection.

The classified data are indexed based on f_n, after which the similar data are grouped based on identified instances. The sequence is reselected if the similarity grouping fails and, hence, a new input is accessed for analysis (Figure 4). The data features in the sensitive information types and sharing frequency prevent similar data analysis, indexed data collection, and augmenting the early detection process. This requires a similar data analysis of f and π in Equation (6) for determining the instance of matching.

$$R\{\varepsilon[Ds, n(Ds)]\} = (Ds + \pi f)f - (\vartheta - \pi f)Ds - f(Ds)\pi, \text{ for matching instance}$$
$$= \pm(Ds)f + \pi f^n - \vartheta(Ds)\{4A_{min}n(Ds) + \pi, if \alpha = A \text{ and } A_{max} = 1 \pm 4A_{max}n(Ds) + \pi \quad (10)$$
$$= \frac{\rho_\tau}{\rho_\vartheta} + 4A_{max}n(Ds) - 2 = \forall A_{max}n(Ds), if \frac{\rho_\tau}{\rho_\vartheta} = 0 \text{ and } \alpha_{min} = 1, \text{ and } \alpha = A\}$$

In this process, in the above Equation (10), $4A_{max}n(Ds) + \pi$ denotes the sequence of matching instances, and the assessment error indicates the end of the input data sources. Similarly, the next instance of matching for $R\{\varepsilon[Ds, n(Ds)]\}$ is designed for the similarity measures of the index, and the data are analyzed for the function $\pi \leq \frac{\sigma_\varsigma}{\Delta^*}$, as in Equation (11).

$$R\{\varepsilon[Ds, n(Ds)]\} = \pm(Ds)f + \pi f^n - \vartheta(Ds) = \pm Ds(Ds - \tau) + \pi(Ds - \tau)^3 - \vartheta(Ds),$$
$$\text{Similarity measures of data} = \pm Ds^3(2 - \pi) + (Ds)\pi(3 + 2\pi) * \pi\tau^3 - \vartheta(Ds)$$
$$= \pm Ds^3(2 - \pi) + (Ds)\pi(3 + 2\pi) * \pi\tau^3 - \vartheta(Ds) \pm Ds^3 + (Ds)\tau - \vartheta(Ds), \quad (11)$$
$$\text{if } \pi \text{ is negligible } \pi \to 1 = Ds(\tau - \vartheta) + Ds^3 = (Ds)\tau - Ds^3\left[\tau\left(\frac{Ds}{\Delta^*}\right) \text{is assesment error}\right]\}$$

As per the above equation, the similarity measures the Ds analysis, as $(Ds)\tau - Ds^3$ is an assessment error during the sequence of $\pm 4A_{max}n(Ds) + \pi$. Therefore, the sequence of the instance as in Equation (11) occurs on $R\{\varepsilon[Ds, n(Ds)]\}$ as in Equation (10). Now, preventing false information and spreading control are initiated. This spread control represents the changes in the communicable disease of the edge device.

3.2. Spread Control

In the spread controlling process, the edge device takes the aggregation-based data analysis and decides the functioning part of the devices. The overall working of the device is synchronized based on $R\{\varepsilon[Ds, n(Ds)]\}$ outputs, respectively. Therefore, the initial spread control $X^D = 1$, such that if $X^D = 2$, then the edge device functions through signaling from the aggregation. This depends on the π condition $R\{\varepsilon[Ds, n(Ds)]\}$ such that the probability of the spread control (ρ_{X^D}) is computed as:

$$\rho_{X^D} = \frac{[count(X^D)]^\alpha \times (\delta)^{n+1} * (Ds)f + \pi f^n}{\sum_{\alpha \forall A} [count(X^D)]^\alpha \times (\delta - \pi)^{n+1}} \quad (12)$$

From the given Equation (12), the probability of spread control is used to detect if the edge devices are working or not. If $X^D \geq 1 \cup > \frac{\sigma_\varsigma}{\Delta^*}$, then the count of X^D is incremented by one which means the edge device is working; otherwise, it is not working. Where δ represents the futuristic estimation of the replacement of X^D between 1 and 2 and this method is computed as:

$$\delta = \{\frac{\sum_{j+1}^{n} \pi_j}{i + \sum_{j+1}^{n} [count(X^D)]_j}, if\ \pi_j < \rho_{X^D}, j \in n \frac{2}{i + \sum_{j+1}^{n} [count(X^D)]_j}, if\ \pi_j \geq \rho_{X^D}, j \in n \quad (13)$$

This futuristic computation of communicable disease spread controlling following all the instances of n. From these appropriate detection/recommendations of δ outputs in an unsynchronized edge device control, the δ is derived from a sequential set of information instances. The communicable disease control output (D_z) is computed as the non-linear matching of ρ_{X^D}, $R\{\varepsilon[Ds, n(Ds)]\}$ and π as:

$$D_z = \{R\{\varepsilon[Ds, n(Ds)]\} \times \rho_{X^D} - \pi, if\ \pi_j < \rho_{X^D}, j \in nR\{\varepsilon[Ds, n(Ds)]\} \times \rho_{X^D} + \frac{\pi}{count(X^D)}, if\ \pi_j \geq \rho_{X^D}, j \in n \quad (14)$$

In this process of detection, the result is represented as the state of the edge device of π_j and $count\ (X^D)$ for all the n. The result of D_z is based on $\pi_j < \rho_{X^D}$ and $\pi_j \geq \rho_{X^D}$. Hence, $\omega > \frac{\sigma}{\Delta}$ denotes a certain assessment of Ds in n. Similarly, the communicable disease spread controlling for retaining the high accuracy and also less replication occurs. In the Figure 5 series, the sequences and errors for different normalization factors are presented.

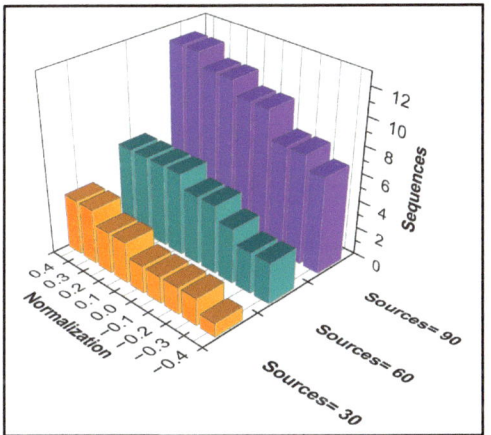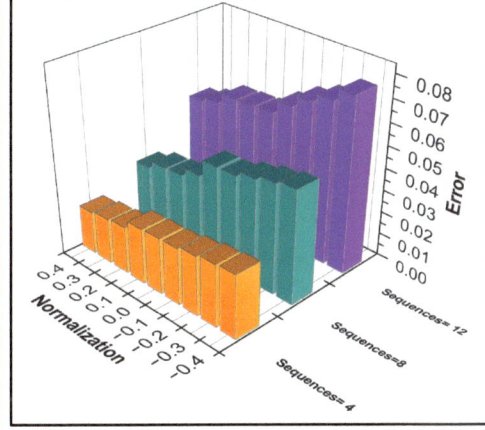

Figure 5. Identification of Overlapping Instances in the Sequences and Error for Different Normalization Factors.

An analysis of sequences and errors for different normalization factors is portrayed in Figure 5. The $n(DS)$ optimizes the detection sequences by mitigating ε. This is recommended based on the classification $R\{.\}$ This was pursued and hence the assessment errors were reduced. As the sequences migrate from $-ve$ to $+ve$ normalization, error reduces. However, the alternate matching for f_1 to f_n addresses the errors and thereby the normalization is retained. The $\varepsilon[.]$ induces further sequences in identifying and mitigating errors. Therefore, as normalization increases, the error is reduced, stabilizing the data analysis. Figure 6 presents the replication and estimation ratio for different occurring frequency values.

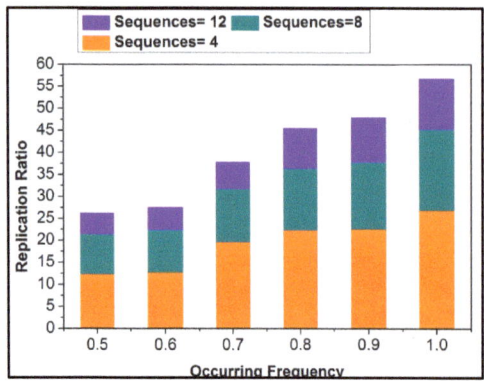 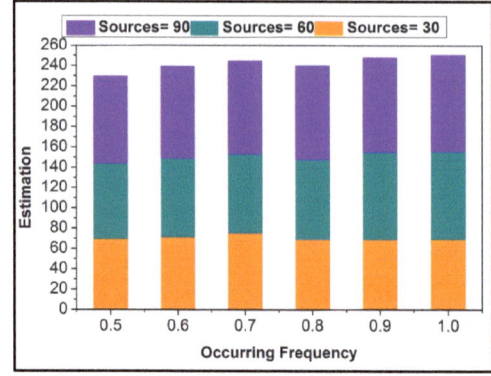

Figure 6. Analysis of $\varepsilon[.]$ Maximization and Sequence Assigning for Reduced Replications.

The $\varepsilon[.]$ in different DS inputs and $R\{.\}$ functions reduce the replication by increasing the analysis. The estimations are based on Equation (7) followed by SD. This estimation increases the recommendations on classification for increasing the indexes and occurrences. The changes are updated in the subsequent classification instances, reducing errors. Therefore, the replications are confined without requiring additional computation. In the further estimations, f_1 to f_n sequences are required to identify further $\varepsilon[.]$. This is required for reducing replications, through $\varepsilon[.]$ maximization and sequence assigning. An analysis of the same is portrayed in Figure 6. In Figure 7, analysis for matching ratios for different ρ_{X^D} is presented.

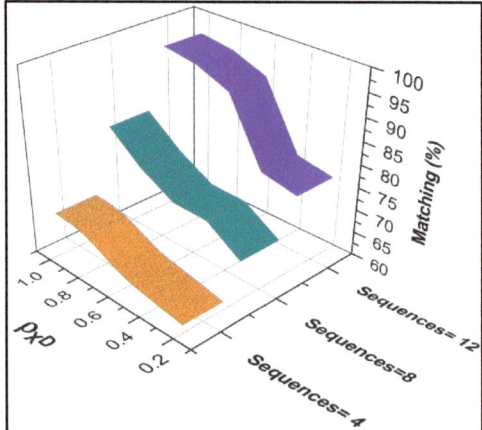

Figure 7. Matching Ratio Analysis for Different Spread Control Probabilities ρ_{X^D}.

The matching ratio for different spread control probabilities is presented in Figure 7. As the classification instances vary the matching ratio increases for different $\varepsilon[.]$. This is due to the $R\{.\}$ in the multiple iterations as classified by the learning process. The recurrent analysis is performed based on matching instances post the $n(DS)$ based on $\varepsilon[.]$. This is however performed for $-ve$ to $+ve$ moves until the classification is before multiple iterations. Therefore, the matching increases as the ρ_X^D is high regardless of the data sources.

For edge device infectious disease monitoring, Algorithm 1 coordinates spread control. Based on signs of disease transmission and device operation, it calculates the spread probability, ρ_{X^D}. Counts are increased if device usage or communication is above predetermined levels. The control decisions are guided by δ, a futuristic estimation. Considering ρ_{X^D} and

π, the spread of the disease control D_z is calculated. To prevent duplication and stabilize data analysis, the program modifies device functioning and spread probability. Iteratively evaluating both illness incidence and gadget performance improves spread control tactics. Enhancing disease identification and response effectiveness in edge devices entails assessing spread probabilities, modifying device functionality, and reducing replication.

Algorithm 1: for Edge Device Spread Control in Infectious Disease Monitoring

---

Function $SpreadControl(Ds, n(Ds), \pi, X^D, \sigma_s, \Delta^*, \alpha, A)$
Input : $(Ds, n(Ds), \pi, X^D, \sigma_s, \Delta^*, \alpha, A)$
Output : Probability of spread control (ρ_{X^D}).
Futuristic estimation of spread control (δ).
Communicable disease control output (D_z)
Step 1: Calculate SpreadControl()
   if $X^D >= 1$ or $\pi > \sigma_s / \Delta^*$
      $IncrementCount(X^D)$
      $\rho_{X^D} = CalculateSpreadControlProbability(X^D, \alpha, \delta, \pi)$
      if $\pi < \rho_{X^D}$
      $D_z = R\{\varepsilon[Ds, n(Ds)]\} \times \rho_{X^D} - \pi$
      else:
      $D_z = R\{\varepsilon[Ds, n(Ds)]\} \times \rho_{X^D} + \pi/Count(X^D)$
   Return D_z
Step 2 : Function $CalculateSpreadControlProbability(X^D, \alpha, \delta, \pi)$:
      $numerator = (Count(X^D)\alpha) \times (\delta)(n+1) \times ((Ds)f + \pi fn)$
      $denominator = Summation(\alpha \forall A)[Count(X^D)\alpha \times (\delta - \pi)(n+1)]$
      $\rho_{X^D} = numerator/denominator$
   Return ρ_{X^D}
Step 3 : Function $IncrementCount(X^D)$
      Increment the count of X^D by 1
Step 4 : Function $Summation(\alpha \forall A)$
      Perform summation over all instances α for A
Step 5 : Function $SpreadControlAnalysis(Ds, nDs, \pi, X^D, \sigma\_s, \Delta^*, \alpha, A)$
      Compute δ based on Equation (13)
      Compute D_z based on Equation (14)
   Return D_z
Step 6 : Function $Calculate\delta(\pi, \alpha, Count(X^D))$
      if $\pi_j < \rho_{X^D}, j \in n$
      $\delta = (\sum_{j+1}^{n} \pi_j)/(i + \sum_{j+1}^{n} [count(X^D)]_j)$
      else
      $\delta = \frac{2}{i + \sum_{j+1}^{n}[count(X^D)]_j}$
   Return δ

Data collection, pre-processing, analysis, and use are the four stages that make up the process flow for disease detection, followed by gathering data, cleaning them up, extracting features, training the model, evaluating it, discussing the results, and finally, training the model. Details regarding the dataset's origins, infectious diseases, and data fields are provided. Addressing missing values, standardizing data, and eliminating duplicates are all part of data pre-processing. In order to detect diseases, feature extraction must be performed. During model training, algorithms, parameter adjustment, and validation procedures are utilized to train machine learning models. The study employs performance indicators such as sharing factor, replication ratio, error rate, and accuracy. The study of the results shows the results on improvement in sharing factors, correctness, decrease in errors, and replication. Disease detection and risk assessment are two areas where the suggested method shines, as discussed. See how the data assessment framework affects the efficacy of disease diagnosis and response with this step-by-step process flow.

Utilizing edge computing principles and devices, which are integral parts of our Combinational Data Assessment Scheme (CDAS), improves the efficacy of disease detection and response through the use of real-time data collection, rapid analysis, enhanced risk assessment, collaborative data sharing, and decentralized processing; it is clear that the suggested method is connected to edge technology.

4. Performance Analysis

The proposed scheme's performance analysis is performed using the dataset [30] that contains information on different infectious diseases. The consistency in data availability with the observed and predicted values is used for similarity verification. This data source contains nine fields based on various categories. The experimental setup uses a standalone system that operates over eight data sources containing multiple instructions and 6–11 fields in common. The performance metrics used in this analysis are accuracy, error, replication ratio, and sharing factor. In the comparative analysis, the existing EPMDA [16], PGPM [21], FCGCNMDA [22], and miRNA [17] methods are used.

4.1. Accuracy

In Figure 8, the comparative analysis for accuracy under different data sources and classification sequences is analyzed. The proposed scheme identifies ε for the input Ds such that the process mitigates the replication through $R\{\varepsilon[Ds, n(Ds)]\}$. Therefore, the classification identifies non-replicated input sequences for improving data analysis accuracy. This process is aided until different conditional experiments are required. Contrarily, the index-based data analysis is performed under controlled futuristic estimation that requires less data for normalization. The further process is controlled by matching conditions defined in Equation (7) for which multiple information types are analyzed. This ensures error-less computations in proceedings with data analysis. The classification learning is pursued in different iterations satisfying the conditions in Equation (7). In this classification, $\alpha = A$ is verified throughout the n sequences in the $4A_{max}n(Ds) + \pi$ matching process. This reduces the errors in the intermediate classification sequences, for different input Ds. Therefore, the process improves the accuracy of obtaining matching based on similar data under defined parameters.

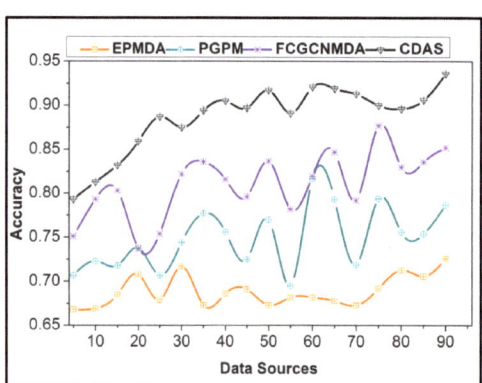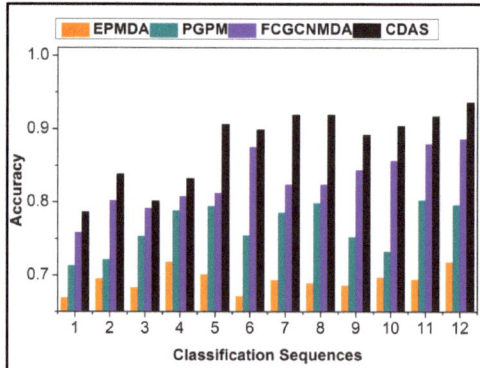

Figure 8. Accuracy Analysis of Varying Data Sources and Classification Sequences.

4.2. Error

The proposed scheme reduces errors in data analysis by segregating replication and non-replication instances over different classification sequences. The $\tau \frac{Ds}{\Delta^*} = \forall [\vartheta - \pi(f)]$ analysis for the classifier process is utilized for deviating errors in the continuous data. Contrarily, the changes in sequences require continuous classification to achieve high accuracy. The proposed sigmoid-based information classification refines the false data from the non-classified sequences, deviating errors. The intermediate f_1 to f_n sequences verify the matching or un-matching sequences with distinct conditions in validating the accumulated data. Hence, the further Ds is analyzed using $\varepsilon_{n(Ds)}$ estimation, preventing replicated occurrence, and improving the accuracy. The error in non-replicating sequences is classified using occurring frequency, preventing $n(Ds)$. In this process, the previous occurrences and their classified sequence are identified for improving accuracy by reducing errors. The deviation σ_s is mitigated by separating $\left(j - \frac{Ds^*}{Ds}\right)\Delta^*$ such that the sequences are independently analyzed using machine learning. Therefore, as the input increases, the classification sequences are varied in confining the errors (refer to Figure 9).

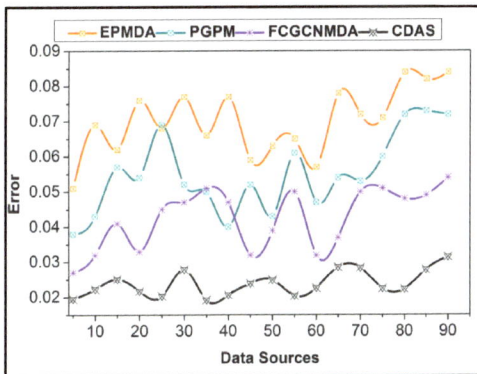
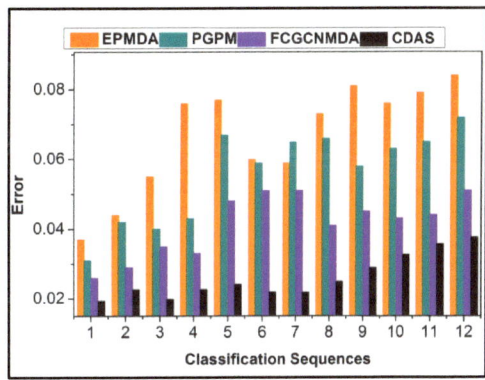

Figure 9. Error Analysis and Variation of Classification Sequences with Increasing Input.

4.3. Replication Ratio

The proposed scheme's replication ratio is comparatively less as presented in Figure 10 for different data sources and classification sequences. The proposed scheme identifies $\frac{\sigma_s}{\Delta^*}$ such that the overlappings in different instances are classified in the first analysis. This analysis is carried out for the partial edge device outputs, reducing errors. In this error analysis, first, the replications are mitigated using $\varepsilon[Ds, n(Ds)]$ predictions, $\forall [Ds + \pi(f)]$ and $\forall [\vartheta - \pi(f)]$. Further in the sigmoid classification, early detection of $(\Delta^* = \sigma_s) = 1$ is performed for identifying the false data. This identification is carried out using the learning process, in dividing multiple instances. Therefore, the validations in the replication are preceded using Ds or σ_s matching. For the classified instances, the input from the data sources is validated based on the above matching conditions, as defined in Equation (8). After this process, $\pi > \frac{\sigma_s}{\Delta^*}$ and $\pi \leq \frac{\sigma_s}{\Delta^*}$ assessments are performed for identifying replicated sequences from multiple Ds. Therefore, the sequences are mitigated from different intervals and sequences, preventing false data. As the learning relies on the non-recurrent continuous instance, the replications are less in the proposed scheme as presented above.

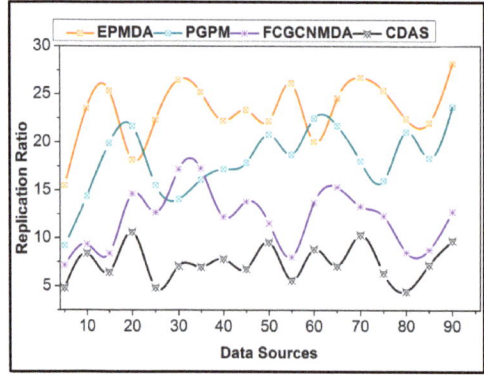
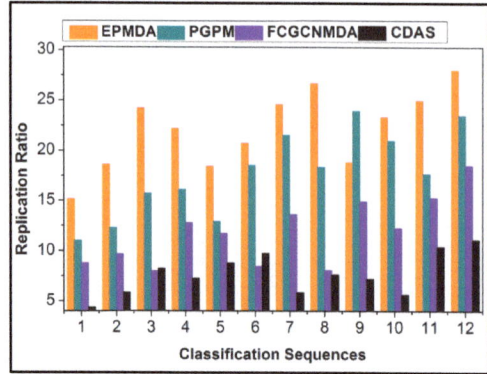

Figure 10. Replication Ratio Comparison for Different Data Sources and Classification Instances.

4.4. Sharing Factor

In Figure 11, the data-sharing factors from different Ds and classification instances are presented. The data-sharing factor in the proposed scheme is high compared to the other methods. The input data are analyzed for their falseness and replication before sharing; the analyzed data are shared based on ρ_{XD}. This probability is used for identifying the data requiring and non-requiring control measures for improving the distribution. In this process, the D_z results in conditional validation for actual data shared and required data for the control process. Therefore, the actual data requirements are upheld with the presence of false data, provided the distributed data is error-free. In this process, machine learning is completely utilized for futuristic data estimation, in determining the actual data requirement. The proposed scheme provides $R\{\varepsilon[Ds, n(Ds)]\}$-based data distribution, improving the sharing rate. For different Ds, the process is unanimous, preventing deviation-included data. Therefore, as the classification process increases, the sharing factor is leveraged compared to the other method, as represented above. In Tables 1 and 2, the comparative analysis results are summarized.

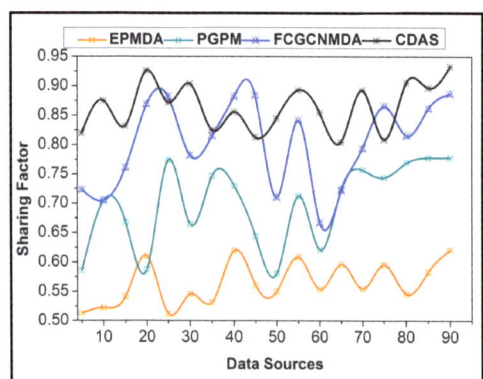
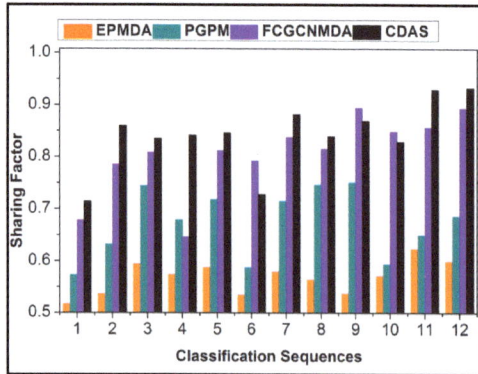

Figure 11. Data Sharing Factor from Various Data Sources and Classification Instances Analysis.

The study follows a strict procedure to verify the accuracy, replication ratio, and sharing factor of the results. Determining the experimental setup, picking the right performance measurements, comparing the results to previous approaches, doing the math, drawing graphs, and talking about the results are all parts of this process. By checking that the results are credible and reliable, the author proves that the data assessment methodology proposed works to make illness diagnosis and response better. Graphs or tables are used to display the results visually so that they may be easily compared and understood. This procedure guarantees that the suggested data evaluation framework improves the efficacy of disease identification and response.

Table 1. Comparative Analysis Summary for Data Sources.

Metrics	EPMDA	PGPM	FCGCNMDA	CDAS
Accuracy	0.726	0.787	0.852	0.936
Error	0.084	0.072	0.054	0.0315
Replication Ratio	28.22	23.69	12.76	9.726
Sharing Factor	0.621	0.778	0.887	0.933

Table 2. Comparative Analysis Summary for Classification Sequences.

Metrics	EPMDA	PGPM	FCGCNMDA	CDAS
Accuracy	0.718	0.796	0.886	0.936
Error	0.084	0.072	0.051	0.0375
Replication Ratio	28.05	23.53	18.52	11.122
Sharing Factor	0.599	0.686	0.893	0.933

The Infectious Diseases dataset was used to evaluate the mathematical methods presented in the manuscript, which aim to forecast and prevent infectious diseases. Several diseases' worth of data is included in the collection, which opens up possibilities for analysis and prediction modeling. In order to better understand the way, the suggested calculation methods detect disease patterns, reduce data replication, maximize data sharing, and minimize errors, the tests evaluate their accuracy, error rate, replication ratio, and sharing factor. It is essential to assess the strategies' practicality in real-world situations.

The study developed a new Combinational Data Assessment Scheme (CDAS) using edge computing and AI to diagnose and prevent infectious diseases. Data collection, distribution, and analysis should be more precise and effective than traditional methods. Tree classifiers can improve indexed data-based early detection and discriminate data types. Considering data similarity and index measurements during analysis reduces assessment errors. Sharing frequency and information type can determine danger levels as compared to shared edge data. Minimal data replication, high precision, and low error rates improve efficacy. The authors submitted experimental results comparing CDAS to EPMDA, PGPM, and FCGCNMDA to support their claims. They found that CDAS increases data-sharing factors by 8.55%, reduces replication ratios by 11.83%, and increases accuracy by 14.77%. The study compares and quantifies the performance improvements of their new CDAS algorithm for infectious disease surveillance using edge computing resources. Future research could use this method with real-world edge deployments.

A real-world infectious disease dataset was used to test the CDAS approach. To understand the approach's uniqueness and efficacy, more dataset information is needed. This includes data size, diversity and complexity, unique qualities or noise, and ground truth label and evaluation benchmark creation. This would show the complexity of real-world settings and the benefits of their edge computing and AI-based approach above previous methods. This would also inform CDAS expansion to other domains with similar data complexity.

4.5. Performance Metrics

Figure 12 shows a bar chart that compares various evaluation metrics across various algorithms and methodologies for a prediction or analysis job. Precision, recall, F1-Score, and mAP (mean Average Precision) are the evaluation measures displayed on the *x*-axis. Methods such as miRNAH7, CDAS, FCGCNMDA, PGPM, EPMDA, and PGPM are being compared. Generally speaking, CDAS performs the best across most metrics, as seen by having the highest bars, which represent the values for each statistic.

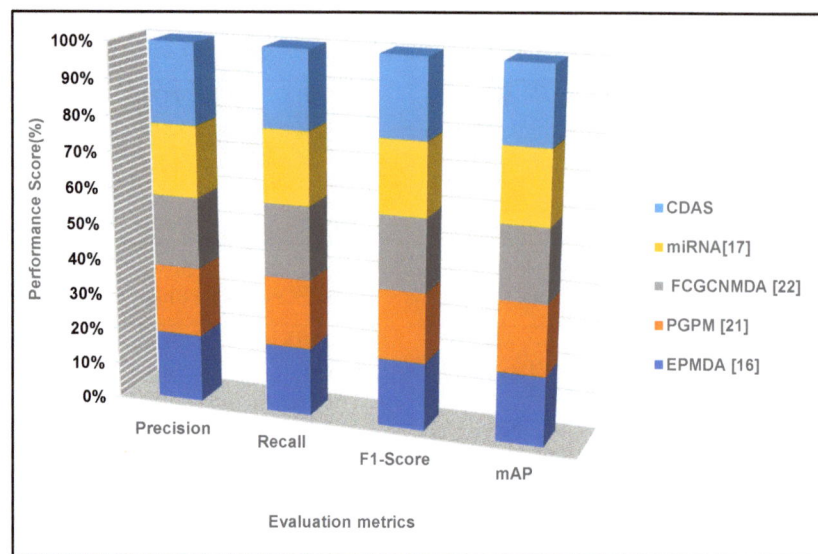

Figure 12. Comparison of Performance Metrics Across Various Prediction Algorithms.

Findings: The proposed scheme achieves 14.77% high accuracy, 11.55% less error, 11.83% less replication ratio, and 8.55% less sharing factor.

Findings: The proposed CDAS improves accuracy and sharing factor by 13.6% and 10.35%, respectively. Moreover, it reduces the error and replication by 9.45% and 12.24% respectively.

In Table 3, the proposed method, CDAS is compared to edge devices in terms of resource constraints, computational intensity, data transmission requirements, latency considerations, and scalability and flexibility. CDAS must be optimized to efficiently utilize limited processing power, memory, and storage on edge devices, while edge devices typically have low-to-moderate computational intensity. CDAS data transmission requirements should consider bandwidth limitations and communication protocols of edge devices for seamless data exchange. Latency constraints should match the real-time processing capabilities of edge devices. CDAS should demonstrate adaptability to diverse edge computing environments and device configurations for optimal performance.

Several factors about computing resources and execution are compared in Table 3 between edge devices. The suggested Combinational Data Assessment Scheme (CDAS) approach is analyzed with features like resource constraints [25], computational intensity [22], data transmission [20], latency [28], along with scalability and flexibility [26].

(1) Resources Constraints:

In contrast with CDAS's high resource requirements, edge devices often have minimal processing capability, memory, and storage. Following the basic principles of edge computing, the comparison implies that CDAS needs to be adjusted to make the most efficient use of the limited resources [25] on edge devices.

(2) Computational Intensity:

Compared to edge devices, having low-to-moderate computing capability [22], CDAS is defined as possessing moderate-to-high processing intensity. This comparison shows the significance of CDAS algorithms in being compatible with edge devices' processing abilities in terms of complexity and real-time analytical capabilities for successful execution.

(3) Data Transmission:

The data transmission requirements of CDAS are minimal, in contrast to the limited bandwidth and protocol specificity of many edge devices discussed in [20]. The comparison shows that for CDAS and edge devices to share data seamlessly, CDAS data transmission needs should consider bandwidth constraints and communication protocols.

(4) Issues with Latency:

Contrasted with edge devices, CDAS is said to have latency [28] limitations ranging from low to moderate. According to the comparison, for decision making to be performed promptly, the latency restrictions of CDAS for detecting diseases should correspond to the real-time response rates that edge devices are capable of.

(5) Scalability and Flexibility:

Edge computing settings and configurations of devices can vary, but CDAS presents them as highly scalable and flexible [26]. Based on the comparison, it seems that CDAS needs to show that it can adapt to varied edge computing contexts and perform well with different configurations of devices to be deployed effectively in various situations. For edge devices, optimizing CDAS to meet their processing capabilities, data transmission needs, latency limits, and scalability considerations is crucial. To make the most of edge computing and get around any challenges edge devices may have, CDAS has to pay attention to these features.

Table 3. Comparison of computing resources and implementation.

Consideration	Proposed Method (CDAS)	Edge Devices	Comparison
Resource Constraints	High	Limited	CDAS should be optimized to efficiently utilize limited processing power, memory, and storage on edge devices.
Computational Intensity	Moderate-to-High	Low-to-Moderate	CDAS algorithm complexity and real-time analysis capabilities should align with the processing capabilities of edge devices.
Data Transmission	Moderate	Limited	CDAS data transmission requirements should consider bandwidth limitations and communication protocols of edge devices for seamless data exchange.
Latency Considerations	Low-to-Moderate	Low	CDAS latency constraints for disease detection should be compatible with the response times achievable by edge devices for real-time decision making.
Scalability and Flexibility	High	Variable	CDAS should demonstrate adaptability to different edge computing environments and device configurations for robust performance across settings.

5. Conclusions

To improve the efficiency of data distribution in the control of infectious illnesses, the paper presents a combinational data evaluation method. Using edge computing and AI methods, the suggested plan makes data collection, sharing, and analysis more efficient. To facilitate easy collection and analysis and avoid duplication and falsification, data sources are first identified. To verify the similarity measure among inputs and the available data and prevent data manipulation, a recurrent tree classifier learning technique is utilized. Indexing of non-replicated sequences comes next, after classification based on occurrence frequency. The likelihood that the indexed data will make it easier to share knowledge about controlling diseases is confirmed, and the process is then repeated for aggregated data sources until replication-free indexed data that are appropriate for sharing are generated. Based on experimental study, the suggested technique reduces error and replication by 9.45% and 12.24%, respectively, while improving accuracy and sharing factor by 13.6% and 10.35%, respectively, for various classification sequences.

Author Contributions: Conceptualization, M.A. and H.M.; methodology, M.A. and H.M.; software, M.A. and H.M.; validation, M.A. and Z.A.; formal analysis, H.M. and Z.A.; resources, H.M. and Z.A.; data curation, Z.A.; writing—original draft preparation, M.A. and H.M.; writing—review and editing, M.A. and Z.A.; visualization, H.M. and Z.A.; funding acquisition, H.M. and Z.A. All authors have read and agreed to the published version of the manuscript.

Funding: This research was supported by the Basic Science Research Program through the National Research Foundation of Korea (NRF) funded by the Ministry of Education (No.2021R1F1A1055408).

Institutional Review Board Statement: Not applicable.

Informed Consent Statement: Not applicable.

Data Availability Statement: The data that support the findings of this study are openly accessible at the following link: https://data.world/chhs/03e61434-7db8-4a53-a3e2-1d4d36d6848d, accessed on 20 March 2024.

Acknowledgments: The authors express their sincere appreciation to the Researcher Supporting Project Number (RSPD2024R1113) King Saud University, Riyadh, Saudi Arabia.

Conflicts of Interest: The authors declare no conflicts of interest.

References

1. Adhikari, M.; Munusamy, A. iCovidCare: Intelligent health monitoring framework for COVID-19 using ensemble random forest in edge networks. *Internet Things* **2021**, *14*, 100385. [CrossRef]
2. Aazam, M.; Zeadally, S.; Flushing, E.F. Task offloading in edge computing for machine learning-based smart healthcare. *Comput. Netw.* **2021**, *191*, 108019. [CrossRef]
3. Zhou, J.R.; You, Z.H.; Cheng, L.; Ji, B.Y. Prediction of lncRNA-disease associations via an embedding learning HOPE in heterogeneous information networks. *Mol. Ther.-Nucleic Acids* **2021**, *23*, 277–285. [CrossRef] [PubMed]
4. Sengupta, A.; Seal, A.; Panigrahy, C.; Krejcar, O.; Yazidi, A. Edge Information Based Image Fusion Metrics Using Fractional Order Differentiation and Sigmoidal Functions. *IEEE Access* **2020**, *8*, 88385–88398. [CrossRef]
5. Yang, L.; Li, Z.; Ma, S.; Yang, X. Artificial intelligence image recognition based on 5G deep learning edge algorithm of Digestive endoscopy on medical construction. *Alex. Eng. J.* **2021**, *61*, 1852–1863. [CrossRef]
6. Ojagh, S.; Cauteruccio, F.; Terracina, G.; Liang, S.H.L. Enhanced air quality prediction by edge-based spatiotemporal data preprocessing. *Comput. Electr. Eng.* **2021**, *96*, 107572. [CrossRef]
7. Hosseini, M.P.; Tran, T.X.; Pompili, D.; Elisevich, K.; Soltanian-Zadeh, H. Multimodal data analysis of epileptic EEG and rs-fMRI via deep learning and edge computing. *Artif. Intell. Med.* **2020**, *104*, 101813. [CrossRef]
8. Yang, F.; Wang, M. A review of systematic evaluation and improvement in the big data environment. *Front. Eng. Manag.* **2020**, *7*, 27–46. [CrossRef]
9. Wang, B.; Sun, Y.; Duong, T.Q.; Nguyen, L.D.; Hanzo, L. Risk-aware identification of highly suspected COVID-19 cases in social iot: A joint graph theory and reinforcement learning approach. *IEEE Access* **2020**, *8*, 115655–115661. [CrossRef] [PubMed]
10. Kumar, S.; Bhagat, V.; Sahu, P.; Chaube, M.K.; Behera, A.K.; Guizani, M.; Gravina, R.; Di Dio, M.; Fortino, G.; Curry, E.; et al. A novel multimodal framework for early diagnosis and classification of COPD based on CT scan images and multivariate pulmonary respiratory diseases. *Comput. Methods Programs Biomed.* **2024**, *243*, 107911. [CrossRef]
11. Angelin, A.C.; Silas, S. Original Research Article Enabling edge computing-based coverage hole detection framework for lossless data tracking. *J. Auton. Intell.* **2024**, *7*. [CrossRef]
12. Abdel-Basset, M.; Mohamed, R.; Chang, V. A Multi-Criteria Decision-Making Framework to Evaluate the Impact of Industry 5.0 Technologies: Case Study, Lessons Learned, Challenges and Future Directions. *Inf. Syst. Front.* **2024**, 1–31. [CrossRef]
13. Deebak, B.D.; Al-Turjman, F. EEI-IoT: Edge-Enabled Intelligent IoT Framework for Early Detection of COVID-19 Threats. *Sensors* **2023**, *23*, 2995. [CrossRef] [PubMed]
14. Allami, R.H.; Yousif, M.G. Integrative AI-driven strategies for advancing precision medicine in infectious diseases and beyond: A novel multidisciplinary approach. *arXiv* **2023**, arXiv:2307.15228.
15. Abbo, L.M.; Vasiliu-Feltes, I. Disrupting the infectious disease ecosystem in the digital precision health era innovations and converging emerging technologies. *Antimicrob. Agents Chemother.* **2023**, *67*, e00751-23. [CrossRef] [PubMed]
16. Dong, Y.; Sun, Y.; Qin, C.; Zhu, W. Epmda: Edge perturbation-based method for mirna-disease association prediction. *IEEE/ACM Trans. Comput. Biol. Bioinform.* **2019**, *17*, 2170–2175. [CrossRef]
17. Wu, Y.; Zhu, D.; Wang, X.; Zhang, S. An ensemble learning framework for potential miRNA-disease association prediction with positive-unlabeled data. *Comput. Biol. Chem.* **2021**, *95*, 107566. [CrossRef] [PubMed]
18. Cañón-Clavijo, R.E.; Montenegro-Marin, C.E.; Gaona-Garcia, P.A.; Ortiz-Guzmán, J. IoT Based System for Heart Monitoring and Arrhythmia Detection Using Machine Learning. *J. Health. Eng.* **2023**. [CrossRef]
19. Pham, T.; Tao, X.; Zhang, J.; Yong, J.; Li, Y.; Xie, H. Graph-based multi-label disease prediction model learning from medical data and domain knowledge. *Knowl.-Based Syst.* **2021**, *235*, 107662. [CrossRef]

20. Rahman MZ, U.; Surekha, S.; Satamraju, K.P.; Mirza, S.S.; Lay-Ekuakille, A. A collateral sensor data sharing framework for decentralized healthcare systems. *IEEE Sens. J.* **2021**, *21*, 27848–27857. [CrossRef]
21. Xu, B.; Liu, Y.; Yu, S.; Wang, L.; Dong, J.; Lin, H.; Yang, Z.; Wang, J.; Xia, F. A network embedding model for pathogenic genes prediction by multi-path random walking on heterogeneous network. *BMC Med. Genom.* **2019**, *12*, 188. [CrossRef]
22. Li, J.; Li, Z.; Nie, R.; You, Z.; Bao, W. FCGCNMDA: Predicting miRNA-disease associations by applying fully connected graph convolutional networks. *Mol. Genet. Genom.* **2020**, *295*, 1197–1209. [CrossRef] [PubMed]
23. Khamparia, A.; Singh, A.; Anand, D.; Gupta, D.; Khanna, A.; Kumar, N.A.; Tan, J. A novel deep learning-based multi-model ensemble method for the prediction of neuromuscular disorders. *Neural Comput. Appl.* **2020**, *32*, 11083–11095. [CrossRef]
24. Zhang, L.; Liu, B.; Li, Z.; Zhu, X.; Liang, Z.; An, J. Predicting MiRNA-disease associations by multiple meta-paths fusion graph embedding model. *BMC Bioinform.* **2020**, *21*, 470. [CrossRef] [PubMed]
25. Badidi, E. Edge AI for early detection of chronic diseases and the spread of infectious diseases: Opportunities, challenges, and future directions. *Future Internet* **2023**, *15*, 370. [CrossRef]
26. Al-Zinati, M.; Alrashdan, R.; Al-Duwairi, B.; Aloqaily, M. A re-organizing biosurveillance framework based on fog and mobile edge computing. *Multimed. Tools Appl.* **2021**, *80*, 16805–16825. [CrossRef]
27. Kamal, L.; Raj, R.J.R. Harnessing deep learning for blood quality assurance through complete blood cell count detection. *e-Prime-Adv. Electr. Eng. Electron. Energy* **2024**, *7*, 100450. [CrossRef]
28. Yadav, R.; Zhang, W.; Elgendy, I.A.; Dong, G.; Shafiq, M.; Laghari, A.A.; Prakash, S. Smart healthcare: RL-based task offloading scheme for edge-enable sensor networks. *IEEE Sens. J.* **2021**, *21*, 24910–24918. [CrossRef]
29. Nandy, S.; Adhikari, M.; Hazra, A.; Mukherjee, T.; Menon, V.G. Analysis of communicable disease symptoms using bag-of-neural network at edge networks. *IEEE Sens. J.* **2022**, *23*, 914–921. [CrossRef]
30. Available online: https://data.world/chhs/03e61434-7db8-4a53-a3e2-1d4d36d6848d (accessed on 20 March 2024).

Disclaimer/Publisher's Note: The statements, opinions and data contained in all publications are solely those of the individual author(s) and contributor(s) and not of MDPI and/or the editor(s). MDPI and/or the editor(s) disclaim responsibility for any injury to people or property resulting from any ideas, methods, instructions or products referred to in the content.

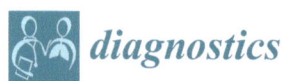 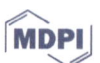

Article

Multi-Layer Preprocessing and U-Net with Residual Attention Block for Retinal Blood Vessel Segmentation

Ahmed Alsayat [1,*], Mahmoud Elmezain [2,3], Saad Alanazi [1], Meshrif Alruily [1], Ayman Mohamed Mostafa [4,*] and Wael Said [5,6]

1 Department of Computer Science, College of Computer and Information Sciences, Jouf University, Sakaka 72341, Saudi Arabia; sanazi@ju.edu.sa (S.A.); mfalruily@ju.edu.sa (M.A.)
2 Computer Science Division, Faculty of Science, Tanta University, Tanta 31527, Egypt; mmahmoudelmezain@taibahu.edu.sa
3 Computer Science Department, College of Computer Science and Engineering, Taibah University, Yanbu 966144, Saudi Arabia
4 Information Systems Department, College of Computer and Information Sciences, Jouf University, Sakaka 72341, Saudi Arabia
5 Computer Science Department, Faculty of Computers and Informatics, Zagazig University, Zagazig 44511, Egypt; wmohamed@taibahu.edu.sa
6 Computer Science Department, College of Computer Science and Engineering, Taibah University, Medina 42353, Saudi Arabia
* Correspondence: asayat@ju.edu.sa (A.A.); amhassane@ju.edu.sa (A.M.M.)

Abstract: Retinal blood vessel segmentation is a valuable tool for clinicians to diagnose conditions such as atherosclerosis, glaucoma, and age-related macular degeneration. This paper presents a new framework for segmenting blood vessels in retinal images. The framework has two stages: a multi-layer preprocessing stage and a subsequent segmentation stage employing a U-Net with a multi-residual attention block. The multi-layer preprocessing stage has three steps. The first step is noise reduction, employing a U-shaped convolutional neural network with matrix factorization (CNN with MF) and detailed U-shaped U-Net (D_U-Net) to minimize image noise, culminating in the selection of the most suitable image based on the PSNR and SSIM values. The second step is dynamic data imputation, utilizing multiple models for the purpose of filling in missing data. The third step is data augmentation through the utilization of a latent diffusion model (LDM) to expand the training dataset size. The second stage of the framework is segmentation, where the U-Nets with a multi-residual attention block are used to segment the retinal images after they have been preprocessed and noise has been removed. The experiments show that the framework is effective at segmenting retinal blood vessels. It achieved Dice scores of 95.32, accuracy of 93.56, precision of 95.68, and recall of 95.45. It also achieved efficient results in removing noise using CNN with matrix factorization (MF) and D-U-NET according to values of PSNR and SSIM for (0.1, 0.25, 0.5, and 0.75) levels of noise. The LDM achieved an inception score of 13.6 and an FID of 46.2 in the augmentation step.

Keywords: retinal image; noise removal; data imputation; data augmentation; GAN; segmentation

Citation: Alsayat, A.; Elmezain, M.; Alanazi, S.; Alruily, M.; Mostafa, A.M.; Said, W. Multi-Layer Preprocessing and U-Net with Residual Attention Block for Retinal Blood Vessel Segmentation. *Diagnostics* **2023**, *13*, 3364. https://doi.org/10.3390/diagnostics13213364

Academic Editors: Wan Azani Mustafa and Hiam Alquran

Received: 15 September 2023
Revised: 21 October 2023
Accepted: 30 October 2023
Published: 1 November 2023

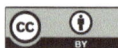

Copyright: © 2023 by the authors. Licensee MDPI, Basel, Switzerland. This article is an open access article distributed under the terms and conditions of the Creative Commons Attribution (CC BY) license (https://creativecommons.org/licenses/by/4.0/).

1. Introduction

Segmentation is one of the most significant tasks in the field of computer vision and image processing, especially in the medical field. Medical segmentation is the process of splitting or identifying certain structures or regions of interest within medical pictures. Each region depicts an area with similar features, which can include issues such as color, density, texture, or other visual attributes. The segmentation process helps many physicians diagnose and examine many diseases. Recently, deep learning (DL) has been involved in the process of segmenting numerous medical images of the brain, breast, heart, and blood vessels [1–5]. It is worth noting that DL has proven particularly valuable in segmenting blood vessels in the retina, helping ophthalmologists and medical professionals in early detection of various eye and systemic diseases [6,7]. The retinal vascular system, also known as the retinal vasculature, is a network of blood vessels located within the eye's retina. Besides the importance of the retina for vision, retinal vascular changes are often early indicators of various ocular diseases and human body diseases as a whole. Ocular diseases include retinal artery occlusion, retinal vein occlusion, and retinal vein occlusion. Human body diseases include diabetic retinopathy, hypertensive retinopathy, macular degeneration, systemic inflammatory conditions, atherosclerosis, and hematological disorders. Indeed, regular monitoring of the retinal vasculature can help in the early detection of such diseases. Therefore, accurate and automated retinal vessel segmentation is crucial for early diagnosis, monitoring, and detection of these diseases, helping ophthalmologists and medical practitioners make more informed clinical choices [8–11]. There are numerous image segmentation techniques, each with its own advantages, drawbacks, features, applications, and use cases [12,13]. These methods can be classified as either conventional image segmentation techniques or methods based on deep learning. Conventional image segmentation approaches encompass threshold, region-based analysis, edge-based techniques, watershed methods, and clustering-based methods. Recently, DL presented many models for segmenting retinal fundus images, such as convolutional neural networks (CNN), fully convolutional networks (FCN), and encoder–decoder-based models, i.e., U-Net [14–16]. The U-Net and its variant architectures, such as U-Net++ and residual U-Net, prove their efficiency when compared with other DL models because of their accuracy and a small number of parameters during the training process [17,18]. Preprocessing of retinal images is a highly significant task before segmentation for increasing the accuracy of the segmentation and training process. Preprocessing comes in various forms, including the elimination of diverse image noise, the augmentation of datasets, and the imputation of missing data [19–21]. The primary goal of this research is to highlight the role of preprocessing in influencing the segmentation results of fundus images. Specifically, the focus is based on data imputation, noise removal, and image augmentation.

Noise in medical images is undesired change in pixel densities or values that can significantly affect the quality of images. This, in turn, can lead to negative consequences during the training process, affecting the final accuracy of segmentation. As a result, the accuracy of diagnosis and treatment planning for patients can be affected. Noise can be introduced at different stages of the imaging process, from image acquisition to transmission and storage [22,23]. Various types of noise can have a negative impact on medical images, including salt-and-pepper, speckle, and amplifier noise. Many methods can be employed to reduce noise, ranging from traditional techniques such as Gaussian and mean filters to modern methods such as machine learning (ML)-based methods, as well as deep DL-based methods such as auto-encoders and generative adversarial networks (GANs). The effectiveness and efficiency of DL in removing and decreasing noise in medical images has been validated, particularly in the case of images representing ocular blood vessels, i.e., retinal fundus images [24]. Removing noise from retinal images is one of the most significant components in the proposed multi-layer preprocessing approach.

There is a direct relationship between the segmentation process performance and the number of elements in a dataset. Enlarging or expanding small datasets effectively enhances the segmentation process's accuracy. Data augmentation is a technique to artificially expand the training set by generating modified versions of a dataset using existing data [25]. In the literature, there are many generative DL models, such as GANs, variation auto-encoders (VAEs), and diffusion models, that have been used in generating images [26,27]. Nonetheless, these generative models have drawbacks when used to create high-quality samples from challenging, high-resolution datasets. For instance, VAE models frequently have sluggish synthesis speeds, whereas GANs frequently experience unstable training and mode collapse [28]. The latent diffusion model (LDM), a class of generative diffusion models, has received significant attention recently in the field of data augmentation [29]. In this paper, the LDM is employed to generate synthetic retinal fundus images as another step in the proposed multi-layer preprocessing approach.

Data imputation is another critical component of the proposed multi-layer preprocessing approach; its effectiveness can significantly impact the results of the segmentation process. The main purpose of data imputation is to properly handle missing data by generating reliable approximations of missing values. This may be accomplished using numerous imputation methods, which can range from simple techniques like mean imputation to more complicated approaches like DL-based techniques [30]. DL-based medical image imputation has gained great importance due to the remarkable capabilities of DL models in capturing complex patterns and structures in medical images. In this paper, DL-based image imputation techniques are used to reconstruct missing data in retinal fundus images to increase the performance of the retinal blood vessel segmentation process.

Preprocessing is an indispensable step in the context of retinal blood vessel segmentation using fundus images. It plays an essential role in improving image quality and facilitating the accuracy of the segmentation process. In this paper, a multi-layer preprocessing approach comprising three distinct layers is proposed. The first layer is used to reduce noise sources, resulting in sharper images for segmentation. The second layer is to utilize dynamic data imputation techniques for estimating missing vessel segments to enable more comprehensive vessel network analysis. The third layer increases the size and diversity of the dataset using an LDM model to enhance the robustness and generalizability of the segmentation process. The following is a concise outline of the paper's contributions:

1. Introduces a novel framework that pioneers a multi-layer preprocessing approach, consisting of three stages: noise reduction, dynamic data imputation, and data augmentation. This comprehensive preprocessing strategy provides a holistic solution to the complexities associated with retinal image data, enhancing the quality of input for subsequent segmentation.
2. The framework significantly boosts segmentation performance, resulting in impressive accuracy and precision in the segmentation of retinal blood vessels. The utilization of the U-Net with a multi-residual attention block (MRA-UNet) for this purpose underscores the framework's effectiveness in this critical task.
3. Demonstrates the framework's versatility by effectively addressing challenges such as noisy images, limited datasets, and missing data. The proposed methods in noise reduction, data imputation, and data augmentation collectively contribute to the framework's adaptability to various real-world scenarios.
4. The framework exhibits remarkable efficiency in noise removal, as evidenced by the values of PSNR and SSIM for different noise levels. The application of the CNN with matrix factorization (MF) and D-U-NET methods for noise reduction reinforces its capability in enhancing image quality.
5. The LDM plays a vital role in augmenting the training dataset, contributing to the model's success.

2. Related Work

Research has shown that retinal blood vessel shape is associated with metabolic risk and other disorders. As the eye is a sensory organ, every eye condition significantly impacts how the brain processes sensory information and draws conclusions. One of the serious eye conditions for which a novel treatment is needed is choroid neovascularization. The choroid is where blood vessels develop. Many scientific research projects have introduced DL models for segmenting the retinal blood vessels, such as convolutional neural network (CNN), artificial neural network (ANN), auto-encoders (AEs), fully convolutional networks (FCN), and U-Net [31,32]. During the analysis of medical images, the U-Net design is considered a great and powerful architecture, especially in relation to retinal vascular segmentation. It promises to improve early disease detection, treatment monitoring, and general care for patients in the field of ophthalmology [33] because it is highly effective at precisely recognizing blood vessels in retinal images. The segmentation of retinal blood vessels using various U-Net designs is explored in this study, given the prevailing adoption of this technology and it having achieved significant accuracy and reliability.

As presented in [34], the authors proposed the U-Net architecture as a complete convolutional neural network (FCN) applied for the segmentation of biomedical images. It comprises an encoder, decoder, and skip connections organized in a U-shaped configuration. Indeed, the well-known use of the U-Net architecture in the biomedical field and its significant impact on medical image segmentation cannot be denied. The U-Net framework is employed in the segmentation of medical images, including tasks like brain tumor segmentation, cardiac image segmentation, skin lesion segmentation, and retinal blood vessel segmentation, as demonstrated in previous studies [17,35,36].

The authors of [37] provided an improved version of the U-Net model to segment retinal blood vessels. The conventional U-Net is given a multiscale input layer and dense blocks so that the network can utilize more detailed spatial context data. The DRIVE public dataset tests the authors' suggested technique, which received scores of 0.8199 for sensitivity and 0.9561 for accuracy. The results of segmentation have improved, particularly for small blood vessels that are challenging to identify due to their low pixel contrast.

As shown in [38], a U-Net attention mechanism is presented for retinal vessel segmentation. The channel and location attention modules are both parts of the attention mechanism. The channel attention module constructs the feature map's many channels' long-range dependencies. The feature map's regions' long-range relationships are constructed using the position attention module. Images are divided into 250×250 pixel patches for preprocessing, and the patches are then rotated and flipped. The DRIVE dataset is used to assess the proposed model. The dice entropy loss function, a new loss function for the data imbalance problem, lets the model concentrate more on the vessel.

Gargari et al. [39] presented a multi-stage framework for fundus image segmentation and eye-related disease type diagnosis. The retinal blood vessel segmentation process is conducted using the U-Net++ model for the green channel of fundus images. While the eye-related diseases are diagnosed using CNN. Preprocessing stages are utilized before the segmentation process. The preprocessing stages include improving the quality of images using the histogram normalization method, removing noise using the Gaussian filter, and applying the Gabor filter. Following the segmentation process, the subsequent phase involves the extraction of HOG and LBP features for disease diagnosis. The effectiveness of the suggested framework is assessed using the DRIVE and MESSIDOR datasets. Although the proposed multi-stage framework achieved significant results, the impact of the preprocessing stages is not clearly known.

A residual attention UNet++ (RA-UNet++) for medical image segmentation is described in [40]. By including a residual unit with an attention mechanism, it improves the U-Net++ model. As a result, the degrading issue is recovered by the residual unit. The significance of the background areas that are unrelated to the segmentation task is diminished while the significance of the target region is increased by the attention process.

In [41], a U-Net 3+ model is introduced, which is essentially a U-Net with full-scale skip connections and deep supervision, tailored for segmentation of medical images. These skip connections seamlessly blend intricate details with significant semantic information gathered from feature maps of varying scales. These comprehensively amalgamated feature maps are then leveraged by the deep supervision technique to facilitate the training of hierarchical representations. More recently, Xu et al. [42] enhanced the U-Net 3+ model by streamlining the full-scale skip connections and incorporating an attention-based convolutional block module to collect crucial features. The efficacy of this model was substantiated through evaluations in tasks encompassing the segmentation of skin cancer, breast cancer, and lung cancer.

The authors of [43] introduced the spatial attention U-Net (SA-UNet) as a lightweight model designed for blood vessel segmentation. The core concept behind the SA-U-Net is to replace the U-Net's convolutional block with a structured dropout convolutional block that combines both Drop_Block and batch normalization to prevent the network from overfitting. Additionally, the SA-U-Net incorporates a spatial attention module, which serves to emphasize important features while suppressing less crucial ones, thereby enhancing the network's capacity to effectively represent data. Prior to the segmentation process, various data augmentation techniques are applied. These techniques encompass random rotation, the introduction of Gaussian noise, and color adjustment, as well as horizontal, vertical, and diagonal flips. The evaluation of this model is carried out using the DRIVE and CHASE DB1 datasets.

The authors of [44] proposed a new deep learning model called DEU-Net, which is specifically designed for segmenting retinal blood vessels. DEU-Net uses an end-to-end pixel-to-pixel approach, meaning that it takes an image as input and produces a segmentation mask as output in a single step. DEU-Net has two encoders, one for preserving spatial information and the other for capturing semantic content. The spatial encoder extracts features that represent the location of pixels in the image, while the semantic encoder extracts features that represent the meaning of pixels. DEU-Net also uses a channel attention mechanism to select the most important features from each encoder. This helps to improve the accuracy of the segmentation results.

A deep learning network called Vessel-Net is intended to precisely segment retinal blood vessels. It is a condensed model that improves feature representation by fusing the benefits of the residual module and the inception model. Four distinct supervision paths are included in Vessel-Net's multi-path supervision technique, which aims to guarantee that the model learns rich and multi-scale characteristics. In addition, a preprocessing step is used by Vessel-Net to lower noise and boost contrast in the input photos. Vessel-Net demonstrated state-of-the-art performance on both of the public retinal image datasets, DRIVE and CHASE, where it was tested [45].

In order to enhance feature representation, a number of studies have suggested modifying the U-Net model for retinal blood vessel segmentation by adding residual attention blocks. The RA-UNet was proposed by Ni et al. [46], Zhao et al. Dong et al.'s attention_res UNet was proposed in [47]. Guo et al. proposed the CRA U-Net in [48]. The channel attention residual U-Net was proposed by [49], and Yang et al. A residual attention model with dual supervision was put forth by [50]. Using a multi-residual attention block (MBA), a densely connected residual network with an extra attention mechanism, we developed the MRA-UNet in our own research.

Although many architectures have been introduced for segmenting the retina's blood vessels based on U-Net, all of these architectures have some advantages and have efficient accuracy. However, they cannot deal with small datasets and noisy images. As presented in Table 1, different architectures of the U-Net are provided to explain the main characteristics of the blood segmentation of the retinal vessels. The table explains the main advantages and disadvantages of the DL model.

Table 1. Segmentation of retinal blood vessels based on different architectures of the U-Net.

Ref	DL Model	Task	Advantages	Disadvantages
[37]	Improved U-Net	Segmentation and detection	Accuracy	• Cannot deal with noisy images • Cannot complete the training procedure with a restricted quantity of photos
[39]	U-Net++	Segmentation	Accuracy	• Cannot deal with noisy images • Cannot complete the training procedure with a restricted quantity of photos

Table 1. Cont.

Ref	DL Model	Task	Advantages	Disadvantages
[43]	SA-UNet	Segmentation	Network substitutes structured dropout convolutional blocks for the original U-Net.	• Cannot deal with noisy images • Cannot complete the training procedure with a restricted quantity of photos • Accuracy
[44]	DEU-Net	Segmentation	Accuracy	• Cannot deal with noisy images • Cannot complete the training procedure with a restricted quantity of photos
[45]	Vessel-Net	Segmentation	Accuracy and preprocessing step	• Cannot complete the training procedure with a restricted quantity of photos

3. Methodology

This section presents the methodology for the retinal blood vessel segmentation framework, which encompasses two stages. It starts with the preprocessing stage and ends with the segmentation process stage using U-Net with multi-residual attention block (MRA-UNet). The preprocessing stage contains three layers namely, removing noise from retinal fundus images, dynamic data imputation, and data augmentation using LDM. Figure 1 and Algorithm 1 indicate the steps of the proposed framework. In Section 3.1, the DRIVE dataset, which contains retinal fundus images, is described. In Section 3.2, The noise elimination layer is explored. In Section 3.3, the dynamic data imputation layer is discussed. Section 3.4 is devoted to presenting the data augmentation layer. The retinal blood vessel segmentation process is indicated in Section 3.5. In Section 3.6, the utilized hardware and software specifications are tabulated. Section 3.7 is dedicated to the discussion of the diverse evaluation metrics used in this study.

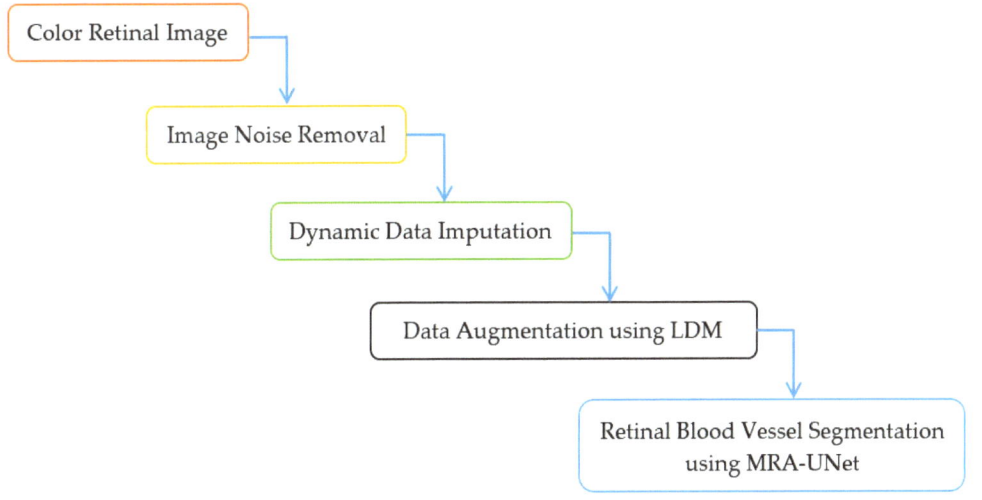

Figure 1. Framework for the proposed methodology.

Algorithm 1: Data Augmentation and Segmentation	
1	**Input** ← Retinal Image Dataset
2	**Initialize Preprocessing Stage**
3	**Step 1:** Noise Removal
4	Apply a U-shaped CNN with Matrix Factorization
5	Reduce Image Noise
6	Apply D-U-Net to reduce image noise
7	Choose best Free_Noise_Image using PSNR and SSIM
8	**Step 2:** Dynamic Data Imputation
9	Apply Multiple Imputation Models
10	Fill Missing Data in Retinal_Image
11	Generate Imputed Retinal_Image
12	**Step 3:** Data Augmentation
13	Apply LDM to augment training dataset
14	**FOR** EACH Retinal_Image **DO**
15	Generate Multiple Augmented Images using LDM
16	**END FOR**
17	**Initialize Segmentation Stage**
18	Apply U-Net with a multi-residual attention block (MRA-UNet)
19	Segment Preprocessed & Free_Noise_Image
20	**INSERT** Preprocessed & Free_Noise_Image **INTO** U-Net
21	**Output** → Segmented Retinal Image

3.1. DRIVE Dataset

The proposed framework in this study uses an accessible dataset called the DRIVE dataset [51]. The dataset contains 40 retinal images. They were obtained at a resolution of 768 × 584 pixels with 8 bits per color plane. A number of 33 images do not exhibit any evidence of diabetic retinopathy, while 7 images have early moderate indicators of the disease. Several retinal images and blood vessels from the DRIVE dataset are shown in Figure 2. The number of these images is so limited for an efficient segmentation process. To address the limited size of the dataset and enhance its diversity, we employed data augmentation techniques.

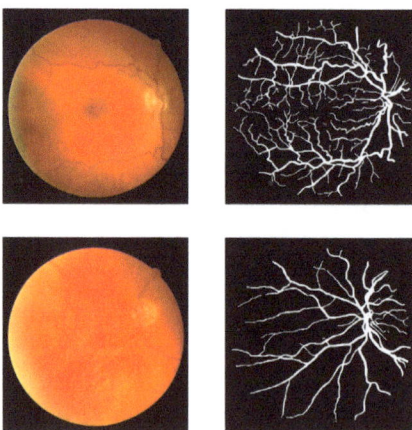

Figure 2. Blood vessel of retinal images and masks.

3.2. Removing Noise

This section presents two distinct models used to remove noise in retinal images. The choice of the most appropriate model is determined based on the PSNR value and noise level. In Section 3.2.1, the utilization of U-shaped CNN with matrix factorization is introduced. In Section 3.2.2, the application of denoising U-shaped Net (D-U-Net) model is outlined.

3.2.1. Removing Noise Using U-Shaped CNN with Matrix Factorization

Li [52] presented multi-stage progressive CNN with a matrix factorization block framework for removing noise from images. The framework is composed of a dual-stage horizontal U-shaped structure to address the challenge of global structured feature extraction. The author proposed an improvement to the U-Net by introducing a matrix factorization denoising module (MD), a cross-stage feature fusion module (CSFF), and a feature fusion module (FFU). The matrix factorization (MF) method effectively fills gaps during de-noising. The architecture of the model contains three parts: (a) the de-noising module (MD), (b) the coder block, and (c) feature fusion module (FFU). The MD simulates the interplay between obtaining context information and aggregating global context. To enhance the flow of information and maintain network efficiency, the model redesigns a fundamental building block. The FFU based its decisions on data from several sources.

In order to gradually rebuild the de-noised image, we employ two-stage convolution branches and draw inspiration from the design of multiple-stage progressing regeneration. Low-level computer vision tasks sometimes overlook the importance of the detail characteristic in recovering the image, which instead directly stack the convolution layer to identify the features. The leak Relu has a fixed slope of 0.02 and the 3×3 convolution layer comprises the coder's unit. It consists of shortcutting using the 1×1 convolution and stacking three units. The model's MD section contains three convolution layers (3×3) with the leak Relu function, which are then added to another convolution layer (1×1). The third part contains only one convolution layer of size 3×3 and uses element-wise addition as in the previous module. The FFU module exchanges and integrates data from various channels before the MD module, the decoder, and between two succeeding stages. The input matrix is factored into two submatrices by the MD module, which then reconstructs the matrix to provide the structured feature. The multiplicative updating procedures are then used. Figure 3 shows the typical architecture of the three different modules of U-shaped CNN with matrix factorization.

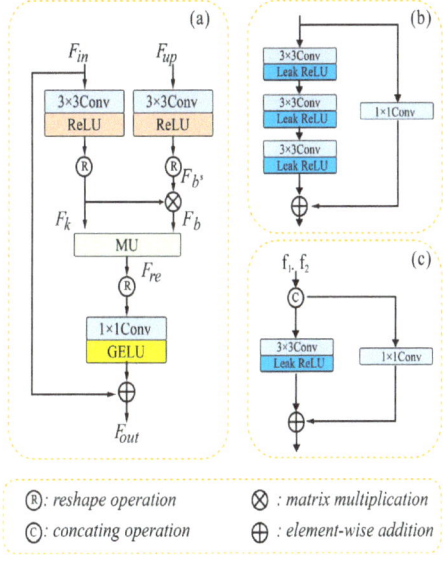

Figure 3. Removing noise using U-shaped CNN with MD [52]. (**a**) represents the MD module. (**b**) represents the Coder block. (**c**) represents the e FFU module.

3.2.2. Removing Noise Using D-U-NET

The denoising U-shaped Net (D-U-Net) [53] is utilized to remove speckle noise from retinal images. The D-U-Net model is structured into two components: the contraction and the expansion components. The contraction component incorporates a 'max pool layer' to downsize the initially generated image as a preprocessing step before the denoising process. The expansion component restores the image to its original dimensions after noise removal from the generated images by utilizing transpose convolution layers instead of the up-sampling layer. The D-U-Net architecture was trained using an Adamx optimizer; the learning rate was set to 0.0001, and the training was conducted with batch sizes of 128 and over the course of 100 epochs. The model employs the factorization module to reconstruct missing data and fill gaps during the restoration process after noise removal.

3.3. Dynamic Data Imputation

Data imputation can help estimate the missing vessel segments in fundus images. Different data imputation models are used to estimate missing vessel segments. These models include the multivariate imputation by chained equations (MICE) [54], GAIN [55], auto-encoder (AE) [56], L2 regularized regression (L2RR) [57], reinforcement learning-based approach (RL) [58], Neural Network Gaussian Process (NNGP) [59], probabilistic nearest-neighbor (PNN) [60], and modified GAIN [61]. The best model is selected according to the error value of the root mean square (RMSE) and Freshet Inception Distance (FID). The dynamic data imputation method [62] is applied by obtaining new imputed values at each training epoch.

The modified GAIN is a Wasserstein GAN with an identity block. The identity block is important in the context of Wasserstein GAN as it ensures the preservation of original features, improves the accuracy of gain estimation, and enhances the stability of the training process. By incorporating the identity block, generative models can achieve more reliable and robust performance in data imputation, leading to better quality and more faithful representations of the real data distribution.

The modified GAIN's basic principle is to employ deconvolution in both the generator and discriminator. To overlapping regions of the data that have been shifted around, convolution provides a kernel. Convolutional kernels are actually relearning old data because of the strong correlations in the actual data. The training of neural networks is difficult because of this redundancy. Before the data is passed into each layer, the deconvolution can eliminate the correlations.

All the models are trained using 200 epochs, an Adamx optimizer, and a 0.0001 learning rate. When using real data vectors in GAIN, the generator component G fills in the values that can be missing based on the identified observed data. The discriminator component D then acquires a finished vector and distinguishes between the observed and synthesized elements. A hint vector is used as supplementary information for discriminator D to identify the required dissemination in the component G. By utilizing the concept of network deconvolution, we enhance the GAIN models.

Because many image-based datasets have substantial correlations, convolutional kernels typically relearn duplicated data. Although the deconvolution technique has been successfully used on images, the GAIN method has yet to be subjected to it. The model has a batch normalization vector and a linear layer. Preventing training problems like disappearing or exploding gradients, adjusting inputs to a mean of zero and the unit variance, using an up-sample layer and a convolution layer to learn from the up-sample layer, and using Relu for the generator all contribute to stabilizing learning.

3.4. Data Augmentation Using LDM

In this layer, the LDM is utilized for data augmentation. The LMD integrates the computational properties of diffusion models with the use of auto-encoders, to compress the input data into a lower-dimensional latent representation. The auto-encoder was trained using L1 loss as well as perceptual loss. L1 loss, perceptual loss, a patch-based adversarial goal, and a structure of the latent space were used to train the auto-encoder.

The retinal fundus image is converted by the encoder into a latent representation with (20 × 28 × 20) dimensions. The latent data from the training set are input into the diffusion framework once the compression framework has been trained. LDM employs an iterative de-noising procedure to transform Gaussian noise into samples from a learned data distribution. Using a fixed Markov chain with 1000 iterations and a latent illustration of an example from our training set, the diffusion algorithm gradually obliterates the data structure while introducing Gaussian noise in accordance with a predetermined linear variance schedule.

3.5. Residual Attention U-Net Segmentation

The MRA-UNet is a customized U-Net model designed for accurate retinal blood vessel segmentation. It closely resembles the residual attention U-Net, but with the key difference of multi-residual blocks. The MRA-UNet architecture consists of an encoder and decoder, with skip-connections that combine features at different scales. The multi-residual blocks modify the initial convolutional layers and increase the depth of the network.

A spatial augmented attention module is utilized from [63] as an enhanced attention module. The spatial attention module is incorporated as a residual attention block. This block takes the feature map from the encoder part of the U-Net and applies attention to selectively highlight important spatial locations or regions. Because low-level qualities lack semantic significance, the spatial attention block supplies crucial background information. This data may complicate the segmentation process for the target item. Figure 4 shows an attention block in the MRA-UNet model.

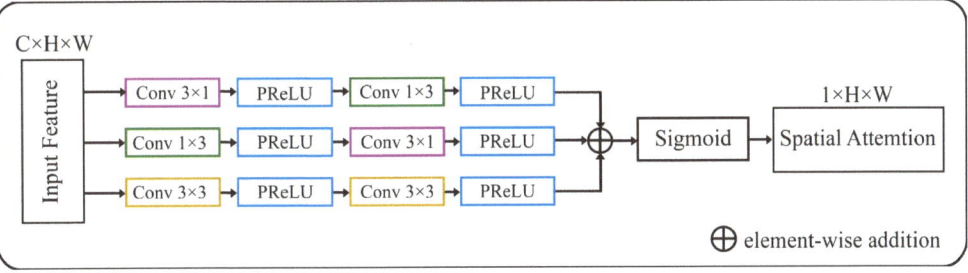

Figure 4. Architecture of spatial augmented attention module [63].

The enhanced attention module was introduced to accept high-level semantic data and accentuate target elements to solve the mentioned issue. The location is gained by the decoder using up-sampling. Nevertheless, this results in the loss of location data and the blurring of edges. The skip connections are used to mix low-level characteristics with high-level features. Because low-level traits lack semantic significance, they supply superfluous background information, which may need to be clarified by the segmentation of the target item. The enhanced attention module was designed to extract high-level semantic information and highlight target elements to address this issue. The MRA-UNet model and all other models are trained across 200 epochs with a learning rate of 0.0001 and 256 batch sizes.

By incorporating the spatial attention mechanism as a residual attention block, MRA-UNet can effectively capture spatial dependencies and adaptively attend to relevant regions during the segmentation process. This helps improve the model's segmentation performance by enhancing the representation of important features and suppressing noise or irrelevant information.

3.6. Hardware and Software Specification

Table 2 shows the hardware and software specifications that have been used during the training process in both augmentation and segmentation experiments.

Table 2. Hardware and software specification for the experimental results.

Device	Description
Processors	Intel(R) Core(TM) i7-10750H CPU @ 2.60 GHz
Random Access Memory	64.0 GB
Graphical Processing Unit	NVIDIA GeForce RTX 3050Ti
Space	2 TB
Programming language	Python

3.7. Metrics Evaluation

Evaluating the quality and diversity of generated images is a crucial aspect in the evaluation of generative models. Two commonly utilized metrics for this purpose are *IS* (inception score) and *FID* (Fréchet Inception Distance). These metrics offer quantitative measures to evaluate the performance of generative models in terms of image quality and diversity. The inception score metric utilizes a pre-trained inception model, typically trained on a comprehensive dataset like ImageNet. It evaluates the quality of generated images based on two primary criteria: image quality and diversity. The calculation equation for the inception score is as follows:

$$IS = exp\left(E_{x \sim p_g} D_{KL}(p(y|x)||p(y))\right) \qquad (1)$$

where $p(y|x)$ represents the conditional class distribution given an image x, while $p(y)$ represents the marginal class distribution. The *KL* divergence is used to quantify the difference between these two distributions. The expected value (*E*) is computed over a set of generated images. Another commonly used metric is the Fréchet Inception Distance (*FID*), which assesses the similarity between the feature representations of real and generated images. The *FID* metric takes into account both the quality and diversity of the generated images. The calculation equation for the *FID* is as follows:

$$FID = ||\mu_r - \mu_g||^2 + Tr\left(\Sigma r + \Sigma g - 2\sqrt{(\Sigma r \Sigma g)}\right) \qquad (2)$$

where μ_r and μ_g represent the mean feature representations of real and generated images, respectively. Σr and Σg represent the covariance matrices of the real and generated image features.

The *PSNR* (peak signal-to-noise ratio) metric is employed to assess the quality of reconstructed or compressed images. It quantifies the ratio between the maximum achievable power of a signal, like an image, and the power of noise that distorts its fidelity. The *PSNR* is calculated using the following formula:

$$PSNR = 10 \times log_{10}\left(\frac{(L^2)}{MSE}\right) \qquad (3)$$

where *L* represents the maximum pixel value of the image. *MSE* (mean squared error) refers to the average squared difference between the original image and the reconstructed or compressed version. The *SSIM* (structural similarity index) metric evaluates the perceived structural similarity between two images. It considers factors such as luminance, contrast, and structure, taking into account human visual perception. *SSIM* values fall within the range of −1 to 1, where 1 signifies identical images. The calculation of *SSIM* is performed using the following formula:

$$SSIM = (l^\alpha) \times (c^\beta) \times (s^\gamma) \quad (4)$$

where *l* represents the luminance component, *c* represents the contrast component, and *s* represents the structural component. α, β, and γ are weighting parameters that determine the relative importance of each component. Typically, values of $\alpha = \beta = \gamma = 1$ are used. Additionally, the evaluation framework incorporates *PSNR* and *SSIM* metrics at different levels (0.1, 0.25, 0.5, and 0.75) to assess the effectiveness of noise removal from the images.

The *RMSE* (root mean square error) metric quantifies the average magnitude of differences between predicted and ground truth values in regression tasks. It offers a comprehensive measure of prediction error, where lower *RMSE* values indicate higher accuracy. The calculation of *RMSE* is as follows:

$$RMSE = sqrt((1/N) \times \Sigma(y_p - y_t)^2) \quad (5)$$

where N represents the number of samples. y_p and y_t denote the predicted and ground truth values, respectively.

In our experiment, we thoroughly assessed our proposed framework by employing multiple performance evaluation indicators, such as the *precision, recall, accuracy* and *Dice score*.

Precision quantifies the ratio of accurately predicted positive instances to the total number of predicted positive instances. *Recall* calculates the ratio of correctly predicted positive instances to the total number of actual positive instances.

$$Precision = \frac{TP_i}{TP_i + FP_i} \times 100\% \quad (6)$$

$$Recall = \frac{TP_i}{TP_i + FN_i} \times 100\% \quad (7)$$

where *TP* (true positives) signifies the number of positive instances that were accurately predicted. *TN* (true negatives) indicates the number of negative instances that were accurately predicted. *FP* (false positives) denotes the count of positive instances that were incorrectly predicted. *FN* (false negatives) conveys the count of negative instances that were inaccurately predicted.

Accuracy, on the other hand, is a crucial metric that evaluates the overall correctness of predictions. It determines the percentage of pixels or instances in the segmentation results that are correctly classified. A higher accuracy score indicates a greater level of accuracy in correctly predicting the segmentation labels.

$$Accuracy = \frac{TP_i + TN_i}{TP_i + TN_i + FP_i + FN_i} \times 100\% \quad (8)$$

The *Dice score*, also referred to as the Dice coefficient or F1 score, is a commonly utilized metric in image segmentation tasks.

$$Dice\ Score = \frac{2 \times |Precision \times Recall|}{|Precision + Recall|} \times 100\% \quad (9)$$

where: the expression $|Precision \times Recall|$ represents the count of pixels that are present in both the predicted and ground truth segmentations. Overall, the integration of the *Dice score, accuracy, precision,* and *recall* forms a comprehensive evaluation framework, allowing for a thorough assessment of the capabilities and effectiveness of our proposed approach in the domain of image segmentation and classification.

4. Results and Discussion

This section tabulates and discusses the various outcomes for each step in the proposed framework. In Section 4.1, the results of comparing various models for removing noise from retinal fundus images are discussed. The comparison is conducted in terms of PSNR, SSIM, and time. In Section 4.2, the results of comparing different models for data imputation are discussed. These results are based on RMSE and PID evaluation metrics. In Section 4.3, the results of data augmentation are indicted by using IS and FID for the comparison of the utilized models. In Section 4.4, the results of the retinal blood vessel segmentation are presented. The Dice score, accuracy, precision, recall, and time per epoch are used as evaluation metrics.

4.1. Results of Removing Noise Layer

Table 3 demonstrates the results of removing noise using different DL models after 200 epochs with a learning rate of 0.0001 and using an Admax optimizer. The comparison is based on four noise levels (0.1, 0.25, 0.5, and 0.75). The outcomes validate the U-shaped CNN with the MD model's effectiveness in eliminating noise at various degrees of noise when compared to other DL models. The results of the comparison for reducing noise from the retinal images are shown in Figure 5.

Table 3. Performance evaluation of removing noise for various models.

Method	PSNR				SSIM				Time
	0.1	0.25	0.5	0.75	0.1	0.25	0.5	0.75	
Original Image	15.31	14.31	11.34	8.34	67.31%	60.30%	50.02%	39.01%	
CNN with attention	31.89	28.45	26.89	24.19	88.49%	81.26%	78.12%	73.15%	24.98
VAEs	34.15	31.06	28.19	27.94	91.11%	86.14%	81.69%	78.16%	24.98
GAN	37.11	34.11	31.28	28.17	91.71%	89.13%	86.49%	82.09%	24.46
Auto-encoder	30.43	28.01	25.43	20.43	82.31%	79.42%	75.21%	70.31%	24.04
D-U-NET	39.23	37.14	33.21	30.42	94.41%	91.09%	88.01%	83.21%	23.13
U-shaped CNN with MD	40.09	38.11	33.10	29.97	94.63%	92.00%	89.23%	84.65%	24.03

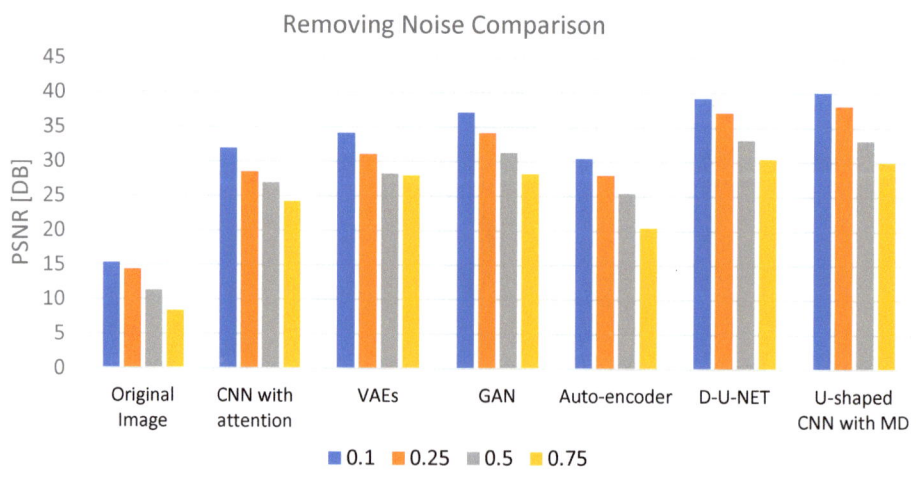

Figure 5. PSNR comparison chart for removing noise from generated images.

4.2. Results of Data Imputation Layer

Table 4 shows the performance evaluation for the MICE, GAIN, AE, L2RR, RL, NNGP, PNN, and modified GAIN based on RMSE and FID. The findings indicate that the modified GAIN demonstrates superior efficiency when compared to other models for smaller values of RMSE and FID. Figure 6 represents the same data.

Table 4. Performance evaluation of data imputation techniques.

Model	RMSE	FID
MICE	0.145	1
GAIN	0.109	0.56
AE	0.119	0.65
L2RR	0.121	0.59
RL	0.126	0.56
NNGP	0.112	0.51
PNN	0.103	0.49
Modified GAIN	0.0945	0.47

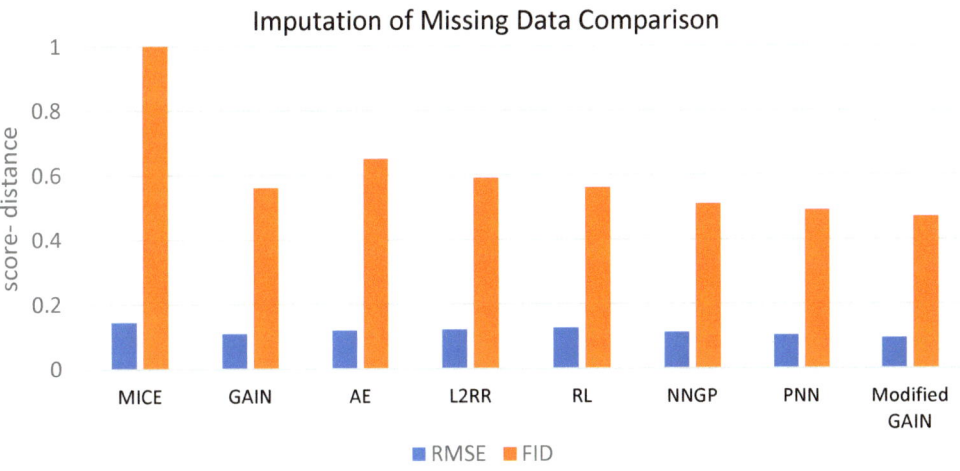

Figure 6. Comparison among various models for data imputation.

4.3. Results of Data Augmentation Layer

This section shows the results of augmenting the DRIVE dataset using the LDM and the other architectures of GANs after 200 epochs based on the Adamx optimizer. Table 5 shows the parameters of different architectures for augmenting the Drive dataset. The comparison between the LDM and the various GAN architectures, such as the deep convolutional GAN (DCGAN), vanilla GANs [64–66], Wasserstein GAN [67], AGGrGAN [68], and IGAN [69] is shown in Table 6. The results show the efficiency of the LDM in augmentation when compared with different types of GANs during the smaller value of FID and the larger value of IS.

Table 5. Proposed model parameters.

Model	Minimum Batch Size	Epochs Number	Rate of Discriminator-Generator Learning	Rate of Generator Learning
MGAN	128	200	0.0001–0.0002	Adam
DCGAN	128	200	0.0001–0.0002	Adam
Vanilla GAN	64	200	0.0001–0.0002	Adam
Wasserstein GAN	128	200	0.0001–0.0002	Adam with gradient penalty
AGGrGAN	64	200	0.0001–0.0002	Adam
IGAN	64	200	0.0001–0.0002	Adam

Table 6. Performance evaluation of data augmentation models.

Model	IS	FID
LDM	13.6	43.7
MGAN	12.6	47.7
DCGAN	11.7	47.9
Vanilla GAN	10.23	49.2
Wasserstein GAN	12.45	45.32
MG-CWGAN	10.36	44.29
AGGrGAN	11.46	45.23
IGAN	11.78	45.69

After the data augmentation process, the number of images in the training dataset significantly increased. Prior to augmentation, the training dataset consisted of the original 40 images. However, after incorporating the augmentation techniques, the final training dataset expanded to include a total of 140 images. This augmentation process allowed us to create a more comprehensive and diverse training set, facilitating better generalization and improving the performance of our data imputation algorithm.

4.4. Results of Segmentation Stage

This section shows the retinal blood vessel segmentation for retinal images before and after the multi-layer preprocessing stage.

The final training dataset for U-net consists of a total of N = 140 images, where N represents the number of augmented images generated from the original DRIVE dataset and the original images after the augmentation step. The paper divides the N images into 80% for training and 20% for testing. This augmented dataset provides a richer representation of variations in retinal images, enabling the U-Net model to learn robust features and improve its performance in diabetic retinopathy detection.

Table 7 compares the different models of segmentation before the multi-layer preprocessing stage, and Table 8 shows the results after the multi-layer preprocessing stage. Figure 7 shows the result of segmenting the retinal image after the multi-layer preprocessing stage.

Table 7. Segmentation-based comparison of different models before multi-layer preprocessing stage.

Model	Dice Score	Accuracy	Precision	Recall	Time per Epoch
Attention gate U-Net	91.27	91.68	91.11	90.89	23.1
U-Net	87.36	88.01	88.69	88.46	24.6
U-Net++	91.53	91.59	91.67	91.36	25.3
RA-UNet++	92.01	92.58	92.83	92.77	24.6
SA-UNet	92.68	92.67	92.67	92.09	23.1
DEU-Net	91.93	91.55	92.35	92.23	23.6
UNet 3+	92.12	91.78	92.68	92.11	24.1
MRA-UNet	93.68	93.25	93.16	93.57	23.5

Table 8. Segmentation-based comparison of different models after multi-layer preprocessing stage.

Model	Dice Score	Accuracy	Precision	Recall
Attention gate U-Net	92.54	92.37	92.56	92.65
U-Net	90.16	90.11	90.29	90.55
U-Net++	92.52	92.47	92.71	92.24
RA-UNet++	93.01	93.37	93.63	93.57
SA-UNet	93.48	93.58	93.88	93.19
DEU-Net	93.25	93.44	93.28	93.28
UNet 3+	93.91	93.67	93.48	93.15
MRA-UNet	95.32	93.56	95.68	95.45

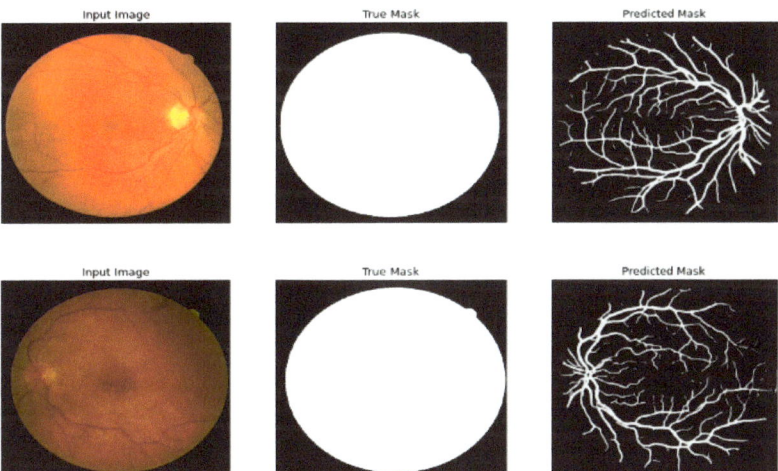

Figure 7. Original image, true mask, and predicted mask using the proposed framework.

5. Statistical Analysis

The statistical analysis of the research presented in this paper focuses on the evaluation of the proposed framework for retinal blood vessel segmentation. The research contributes to the field of medical image analysis, particularly in the context of ophthalmology. The following statistical findings and analysis provide insights into the framework's performance and its potential applications:

5.1. Performance Metrics for Segmentation

- Dice score: the framework achieved an impressive Dice score of 95.32. This metric is a widely used measure in image segmentation, indicating the extent of overlap between the predicted and ground-truth segmentations. A score close to 100 signifies high accuracy in segmenting retinal blood vessels.
- Accuracy: the reported accuracy of 93.56 is another essential metric that measures the proportion of correctly segmented pixels. High accuracy indicates the model's ability to correctly classify pixels as either blood vessels or background.
- Precision: the precision of 95.68 highlights the framework's capability to minimize false positives. It signifies the accuracy of positive predictions, reducing the chances of misclassifying non-blood vessel pixels as blood vessels.
- Recall: a recall of 95.45 underscores the model's effectiveness in identifying true positive cases, minimizing false negatives. It ensures that a significant portion of actual blood vessels is successfully detected.

5.2. Noise Reduction Effectiveness

The framework efficiently removes noise from retinal images, as evidenced by the evaluation of the peak signal-to-noise ratio (PSNR) and structural similarity index (SSIM) for varying noise levels (0.1, 0.25, 0.5, and 0.75). These metrics quantify the improvement in image quality after noise reduction, indicating the framework's ability to enhance image clarity and detail.

5.3. Data Augmentation Impact

The latent diffusion model (LDM) used for data augmentation achieved an inception score of 13.6 and a Fréchet Inception Distance (FID) of 46.2 during the augmentation step. These metrics are associated with the quality and diversity of augmented data. A higher inception score suggests that the augmented data closely resemble the original dataset, while a lower FID indicates that the augmented data are similar to the training dataset. These results emphasize the effectiveness of the LDM in generating high-quality additional data for training.

5.4. Versatility and Adaptability

The research highlights the versatility of the framework in addressing various challenges such as noisy images, limited datasets, and missing data. While the framework excels in these aspects, it acknowledges limitations in dealing with super-resolution images and generating high-resolution images during augmentation. The framework's adaptability to real-world scenarios is supported by its comprehensive multi-layer preprocessing approach.

6. Conclusions and Future Work

Segmentation of blood vessels is one of the most crucial tasks for many clinicians. This paper provided a new framework for segmenting vessels to detect many diseases. The framework's two-stage approach, encompassing multi-layer preprocessing and segmentation using a U-Net with a multi-residual attention block, delivers several noteworthy contributions. Firstly, it pioneers the simultaneous use of multi-layer preprocessing with three layers, addressing noise removal, missing data imputation, and dataset augmentation, providing a comprehensive solution to the complexities of retinal image data. Secondly, the framework substantially enhances segmentation performance, demonstrating impressive accuracy and precision. The experiments show that the framework is effective at segmenting retinal blood vessels. It achieved Dice scores of 95.32, accuracy of 93.56, precision of 95.68, and recall of 95.45. Furthermore, it exhibits versatility in tackling challenges such as noisy images, limited datasets, and missing data, all of which are effectively addressed. The U-Net with a multi-residual attention block (MRA-UNet) is used to segment the retinal images after they have been preprocessed and noise has been removed. The experiments also prove the efficiency of the segmentation model. The results also show improvements in different architectures of the U-Net after the multi-layer preprocessing. Although the framework presented good results in all sections, it still has some limitations in dealing with super-resolution images and generating high-resolution images in the augmentation step. In the future, we will use the super-resolution diffusion model to generate new samples to improve the accuracy of the segmentation process, and we will use the diffusion model to remove noise.

Author Contributions: Data curation, M.E.; formal analysis, A.A. and S.A.; investigation, M.A., A.M.M. and W.S.; supervision, A.A.; writing—original draft, M.E. and A.M.M.; writing—review and editing, A.A., S.A. and A.M.M. All authors have read and agreed to the published version of the manuscript.

Funding: The Deputyship of Research & Innovation, Ministry of Education in Saudi Arabia funding this research through the project number 223202.

Institutional Review Board Statement: Not applicable.

Informed Consent Statement: Not applicable.

Data Availability Statement: Furnished on request.

Acknowledgments: The authors extend their appreciation to the Deputyship of Research & Innovation, Ministry of Education in Saudi Arabia funding this research through the project number 223202.

Conflicts of Interest: The authors declare no conflict of interest.

References

1. Oubaalla, A.; El Moubtahij, H.; El Akkad, N. Medical Image Segmentation Using Deep Learning: A Survey. In *Digital Technologies and Applications*; Springer Nature: Cham, Switzerland, 2023; pp. 974–983.
2. Aljabri, M.; AlGhamdi, M. A review on the use of deep learning for medical images segmentation. *Neurocomputing* **2022**, *506*, 311–335. [CrossRef]
3. Boudegga, H.; Elloumi, Y.; Akil, M.; Hedi Bedoui, M.; Kachouri, R.; Abdallah, A.B. Fast and efficient retinal blood vessel segmentation method based on deep learning network. *Comput. Med. Imaging Graph.* **2021**, *90*, 101902. [CrossRef] [PubMed]
4. Ranjbarzadeh, R.; Bagherian Kasgari, A.; Jafarzadeh Ghoushchi, S.; Anari, S.; Naseri, M.; Bendechache, M. Brain tumor segmentation based on deep learning and an attention mechanism using MRI multi-modalities brain images. *Sci. Rep.* **2021**, *11*, 10930. [CrossRef] [PubMed]
5. Wang, R.; Lei, T.; Cui, R.; Zhang, B.; Meng, H.; Nandi, A.K. Medical image segmentation using deep learning: A survey. *IET Image Process.* **2022**, *16*, 1243–1267. [CrossRef]
6. Kumar, K.S.; Singh, N.P. Analysis of retinal blood vessel segmentation techniques: A systematic survey. *Multimed. Tools Appl.* **2023**, *82*, 7679–7733. [CrossRef]
7. Ilesanmi, A.E.; Ilesanmi, T.; Gbotoso, G.A. A systematic review of retinal fundus image segmentation and classification methods using convolutional neural networks. *Healthc. Anal.* **2023**, *4*, 100261. [CrossRef]
8. Ji, Y.; Ji, Y.; Liu, Y.; Zhao, Y.; Zhang, L. Research progress on diagnosing retinal vascular diseases based on artificial intelligence and fundus images. *Front. Cell Dev. Biol.* **2023**, *11*, 1168327. [CrossRef]
9. Arnould, L.; Meriaudeau, F.; Guenancia, C.; Germanese, C.; Delcourt, C.; Kawasaki, R.; Cheung, C.Y.; Creuzot-Garcher, C.; Grzybowski, A. Using Artificial Intelligence to Analyse the Retinal Vascular Network: The Future of Cardiovascular Risk Assessment Based on Oculomics? A Narrative Review. *Ophthalmol. Ther.* **2023**, *12*, 657–674. [CrossRef]
10. Zhao, X.; Lin, Z.; Yu, S.; Xiao, J.; Xie, L.; Xu, Y.; Tsui, C.-K.; Cui, K.; Zhao, L.; Zhang, G.; et al. An artificial intelligence system for the whole process from diagnosis to treatment suggestion of ischemic retinal diseases. *Cell Rep. Med.* **2023**, *4*, 101197. [CrossRef]
11. Babenko, B.; Mitani, A.; Traynis, I.; Kitade, N.; Singh, P.; Maa, A.Y.; Cuadros, J.; Corrado, G.S.; Peng, L.; Webster, D.R.; et al. Detection of signs of disease in external photographs of the eyes via deep learning. *Nat. Biomed. Eng.* **2022**, *6*, 1370–1383. [CrossRef]
12. Yadav, R.; Pandey, M. Image Segmentation Techniques: A Survey. In *Proceedings of Data Analytics and Management*; Springer Nature: Singapore, 2022; pp. 231–239.
13. Sood, D.; Singla, A. A Survey of Segmentation Techniques for Medical Images. In Proceedings of the 2022 10th International Conference on Reliability, Infocom Technologies and Optimization (Trends and Future Directions) (ICRITO), Noida, India, 13–14 October 2022; pp. 1–8.
14. Nayak, J.; Acharya, U.R.; Bhat, P.S.; Shetty, N.; Lim, T.-C. Automated Diagnosis of Glaucoma Using Digital Fundus Images. *J. Med. Syst.* **2008**, *33*, 337. [CrossRef] [PubMed]
15. Gulshan, V.; Peng, L.; Coram, M.; Stumpe, M.C.; Wu, D.; Narayanaswamy, A.; Venugopalan, S.; Widner, K.; Madams, T.; Cuadros, J.; et al. Development and Validation of a Deep Learning Algorithm for Detection of Diabetic Retinopathy in Retinal Fundus Photographs. *JAMA* **2016**, *316*, 2402–2410. [CrossRef] [PubMed]
16. Galdran, A.; Anjos, A.; Dolz, J.; Chakor, H.; Lombaert, H.; Ayed, I.B. State-of-the-art retinal vessel segmentation with minimalistic models. *Sci. Rep.* **2022**, *12*, 6174. [CrossRef] [PubMed]
17. Siddique, N.; Paheding, S.; Elkin, C.P.; Devabhaktuni, V. U-Net and Its Variants for Medical Image Segmentation: A Review of Theory and Applications. *IEEE Access* **2021**, *9*, 82031–82057. [CrossRef]
18. Huang, K.-W.; Yang, Y.-R.; Huang, Z.-H.; Liu, Y.-Y.; Lee, S.-H. Retinal Vascular Image Segmentation Using Improved UNet Based on Residual Module. *Bioengineering* **2023**, *10*, 722. [CrossRef]
19. Maharana, K.; Mondal, S.; Nemade, B. A review: Data pre-processing and data augmentation techniques. *Glob. Transit. Proc.* **2022**, *3*, 91–99. [CrossRef]
20. Izadi, S.; Sutton, D.; Hamarneh, G. Image denoising in the deep learning era. *Artif. Intell. Rev.* **2023**, *56*, 5929–5974. [CrossRef]
21. Salvi, M.; Acharya, U.R.; Molinari, F.; Meiburger, K.M. The impact of pre- and post-image processing techniques on deep learning frameworks: A comprehensive review for digital pathology image analysis. *Comput. Biol. Med.* **2021**, *128*, 104129. [CrossRef]
22. Mohan, J.; Krishnaveni, V.; Guo, Y. A survey on the magnetic resonance image denoising methods. *Biomed. Signal Process. Control* **2014**, *9*, 56–69. [CrossRef]
23. Zhang, L.; Liu, J.; Shang, F.; Li, G.; Zhao, J.; Zhang, Y. Robust segmentation method for noisy images based on an unsupervised denosing filter. *Tsinghua Sci. Technol.* **2021**, *26*, 736–748. [CrossRef]

24. Tian, C.; Fei, L.; Zheng, W.; Xu, Y.; Zuo, W.; Lin, C.-W. Deep learning on image denoising: An overview. *Neural Netw.* **2020**, *131*, 251–275. [CrossRef] [PubMed]
25. Xu, M.; Yoon, S.; Fuentes, A.; Park, D.S. A Comprehensive Survey of Image Augmentation Techniques for Deep Learning. *Pattern Recognit.* **2023**, *137*, 109347. [CrossRef]
26. Kazerouni, A.; Aghdam, E.K.; Heidari, M.; Azad, R.; Fayyaz, M.; Hacihaliloglu, I.; Merhof, D. Diffusion models in medical imaging: A comprehensive survey. *Med. Image Anal.* **2023**, *88*, 102846. [CrossRef]
27. Oussidi, A.; Elhassouny, A. Deep generative models: Survey. In Proceedings of the 2018 International Conference on Intelligent Systems and Computer Vision (ISCV), Fez, Morocco, 2–4 April 2018; pp. 1–8.
28. Shorten, C.; Khoshgoftaar, T.M. A survey on Image Data Augmentation for Deep Learning. *J. Big Data* **2019**, *6*, 60. [CrossRef]
29. Rombach, R.; Blattmann, A.; Lorenz, D.; Esser, P.; Ommer, B. High-Resolution Image Synthesis with Latent Diffusion Models. In Proceedings of the 2022 IEEE/CVF Conference on Computer Vision and Pattern Recognition (CVPR), New Orleans, LA, USA, 18–24 June 2022; pp. 10674–10685.
30. Sun, Y.; Li, J.; Xu, Y.; Zhang, T.; Wang, X. Deep learning versus conventional methods for missing data imputation: A review and comparative study. *Expert Syst. Appl.* **2023**, *227*, 120201. [CrossRef]
31. Soomro, T.A.; Afifi, A.J.; Zheng, L.; Soomro, S.; Gao, J.; Hellwich, O.; Paul, M. Deep Learning Models for Retinal Blood Vessels Segmentation: A Review. *IEEE Access* **2019**, *7*, 71696–71717. [CrossRef]
32. Sule, O.O. A Survey of Deep Learning for Retinal Blood Vessel Segmentation Methods: Taxonomy, Trends, Challenges and Future Directions. *IEEE Access* **2022**, *10*, 38202–38236. [CrossRef]
33. Cai, Y.; Yuan, J. A Review of U-Net Network Medical Image Segmentation Applications. In Proceedings of the 2022 5th International Conference on Artificial Intelligence and Pattern Recognition, Xiamen, China, 23–25 September 2022; pp. 457–461. [CrossRef]
34. Ronneberger, O.; Fischer, P.; Brox, T. U-Net: Convolutional Networks for Biomedical Image Segmentation. In *Medical Image Computing and Computer-Assisted Intervention—MICCAI 2015*; Springer International Publishing: Cham, Switzerland, 2015; pp. 234–241.
35. Punn, N.S.; Agarwal, S. Modality specific U-Net variants for biomedical image segmentation: A survey. *Artif. Intell. Rev.* **2022**, *55*, 5845–5889. [CrossRef]
36. Yin, X.-X.; Sun, L.; Fu, Y.; Lu, R.; Zhang, Y. U-Net-Based Medical Image Segmentation. *J. Healthc. Eng.* **2022**, *2022*, 4189781. [CrossRef]
37. Li, D.; Dharmawan, D.A.; Ng, B.P.; Rahardja, S. Residual U-Net for Retinal Vessel Segmentation. In Proceedings of the 2019 IEEE International Conference on Image Processing (ICIP), Taipei, Taiwan, 22–25 September 2019; pp. 1425–1429.
38. Si, Z.; Fu, D.; Li, J. U-Net with Attention Mechanism for Retinal Vessel Segmentation. In *Mage and Graphics*; Springer International Publishing: Cham, Switzerland, 2019; pp. 668–677.
39. Gargari, M.S.; Seyedi, M.H.; Alilou, M. Segmentation of Retinal Blood Vessels Using U-Net++ Architecture and Disease Prediction. *Electronics* **2022**, *11*, 3516. [CrossRef]
40. Li, Z.; Zhang, H.; Li, Z.; Ren, Z. Residual-Attention UNet++: A Nested Residual-Attention U-Net for Medical Image Segmentation. *Appl. Sci.* **2022**, *12*, 7149. [CrossRef]
41. Huang, H.; Lin, L.; Tong, R.; Hu, H.; Zhang, Q.; Iwamoto, Y.; Han, X.; Chen, Y.-W.; Wu, J. UNet 3+: A Full-Scale Connected UNet for Medical Image Segmentation. *arXiv* **2004**, arXiv:2004.08790.
42. Xu, Y.; Hou, S.; Wang, X.; Li, D.; Lu, L. A Medical Image Segmentation Method Based on Improved UNet 3+ Network. *Diagnostics* **2023**, *13*, 576. [CrossRef] [PubMed]
43. Guo, C.; Szemenyei, M.; Yi, Y.; Wang, W.; Chen, B.; Fan, C. SA-UNet: Spatial Attention U-Net for Retinal Vessel Segmentation. In Proceedings of the 2020 25th International Conference on Pattern Recognition (ICPR), Milan, Italy, 10–15 January 2021; pp. 1236–1242.
44. Wang, B.; Qiu, S.; He, H. Dual Encoding U-Net for Retinal Vessel Segmentation. In *Medical Image Computing and Computer Assisted Intervention—MICCAI 2019*; Springer International Publishing: Cham, Switzerland, 2019; pp. 84–92.
45. Wu, Y.; Xia, Y.; Song, Y.; Zhang, D.; Liu, D.; Zhang, C.; Cai, W. Vessel-Net: Retinal Vessel Segmentation Under Multi-path Supervision. In *Medical Image Computing and Computer Assisted Intervention—MICCAI 2019*; Springer International Publishing: Cham, Switzerland, 2019; pp. 264–272.
46. Ni, Z.-L.; Bian, G.-B.; Zhou, X.-H.; Hou, Z.-G.; Xie, X.-L.; Wang, C.; Zhou, Y.-J.; Li, R.-Q.; Li, Z. RAUNet: Residual Attention U-Net for Semantic Segmentation of Cataract Surgical Instruments. In *Neural Information Processing*; Springer International Publishing: Cham, Switzerland, 2019; pp. 139–149.
47. Zhao, S.; Liu, T.; Liu, B.; Ruan, K. Attention residual convolution neural network based on U-net (AttentionResU-Net) for retina vessel segmentation. *IOP Conf. Ser. Earth Environ. Sci.* **2020**, *440*, 32138. [CrossRef]
48. Dong, F.; Wu, D.; Guo, C.; Zhang, S.; Yang, B.; Gong, X. CRAUNet: A cascaded residual attention U-Net for retinal vessel segmentation. *Comput. Biol. Med.* **2022**, *147*, 105651. [CrossRef]
49. Guo, C.; Szemenyei, M.; Hu, Y.; Wang, W.; Zhou, W.; Yi, Y. Channel Attention Residual U-Net for Retinal Vessel Segmentation. In Proceedings of the ICASSP 2021–2021 IEEE International Conference on Acoustics, Speech and Signal Processing (ICASSP), Toronto, ON, Canada, 6–11 June 2021; pp. 1185–1189.

50. Yang, Y.; Wan, W.; Huang, S.; Zhong, X.; Kong, X. RADCU-Net: Residual attention and dual-supervision cascaded U-Net for retinal blood vessel segmentation. *Int. J. Mach. Learn. Cybern.* **2023**, *14*, 1605–1620. [CrossRef]
51. Staal, J.; Abramoff, M.D.; Niemeijer, M.; Viergever, M.A.; Ginneken, B.v. Ridge-based vessel segmentation in color images of the retina. *IEEE Trans. Med. Imaging* **2004**, *23*, 501–509. [CrossRef]
52. li, Q. Denoising image by matrix factorization in U-shaped convolutional neural network. *J. Vis. Commun. Image Represent.* **2023**, *90*, 103729. [CrossRef]
53. Karaoğlu, O.; Bilge, H.Ş.; Uluer, İ. Removal of speckle noises from ultrasound images using five different deep learning networks. *Eng. Sci. Technol. Int. J.* **2022**, *29*, 101030. [CrossRef]
54. van Buuren, S.; Groothuis-Oudshoorn, K. mice: Multivariate Imputation by Chained Equations in R. *J. Stat. Softw.* **2011**, *45*, 1–67. [CrossRef]
55. Popolizio, M.; Amato, A.; Politi, T.; Calienno, R.; Lecce, V.D. Missing data imputation in meteorological datasets with the GAIN method. In Proceedings of the 2021 IEEE International Workshop on Metrology for Industry 4.0 & IoT (MetroInd4.0&IoT), Rome, Italy, 7–9 June 2021; pp. 556–560.
56. Gondara, L.; Wang, K. MIDA: Multiple Imputation Using Denoising Autoencoders. In *Advances in Knowledge Discovery and Data Mining*; Springer International Publishing: Cham, Switzerland, 2018; pp. 260–272.
57. Nagarajan, G.; Dhinesh Babu, L.D. Missing data imputation on biomedical data using deeply learned clustering and L2 regularized regression based on symmetric uncertainty. *Artif. Intell. Med.* **2022**, *123*, 102214. [CrossRef] [PubMed]
58. Awan, S.E.; Bennamoun, M.; Sohel, F.; Sanfilippo, F.; Dwivedi, G. A reinforcement learning-based approach for imputing missing data. *Neural Comput. Appl.* **2022**, *34*, 9701–9716. [CrossRef]
59. Jafrasteh, B.; Hernández-Lobato, D.; Lubián-López, S.P.; Benavente-Fernández, I. Gaussian processes for missing value imputation. *Knowl.-Based Syst.* **2023**, *273*, 110603. [CrossRef]
60. Lalande, F.; Doya, K. Numerical Data Imputation for Multimodal Data Sets: A Probabilistic Nearest-Neighbor Kernel Density Approach. *arXiv* **2023**, arXiv:2306.16906.
61. Neves, D.T.; Alves, J.; Naik, M.G.; Proença, A.J.; Prasser, F. From Missing Data Imputation to Data Generation. *J. Comput. Sci.* **2022**, *61*, 101640. [CrossRef]
62. Han, J.; Kang, S. Dynamic imputation for improved training of neural network with missing values. *Expert Syst. Appl.* **2022**, *194*, 116508. [CrossRef]
63. Li, J.; Wu, C.; Song, R.; Li, Y.; Xie, W. Residual Augmented Attentional U-Shaped Network for Spectral Reconstruction from RGB Images. *Remote Sens.* **2021**, *13*, 115. [CrossRef]
64. Ansith, S.; Bini, A.A. A modified Generative Adversarial Network (GAN) architecture for land use classification. In Proceedings of the 2021 IEEE Madras Section Conference (MASCON), Chennai, India, 27–28 August 2021; pp. 1–6.
65. Patil, A.; Venkatesh. DCGAN: Deep Convolutional GAN with Attention Module for Remote View Classification. In Proceedings of the 2021 International Conference on Forensics, Analytics, Big Data, Security (FABS), Bengaluru, India, 21–22 December 2021; pp. 1–10.
66. Chen, Y.; Yang, X.-H.; Wei, Z.; Heidari, A.A.; Zheng, N.; Li, Z.; Chen, H.; Hu, H.; Zhou, Q.; Guan, Q. Generative Adversarial Networks in Medical Image augmentation: A review. *Comput. Biol. Med.* **2022**, *144*, 105382. [CrossRef]
67. Arjovsky, M.; Chintala, S.; Bottou, L. Wasserstein Generative Adversarial Networks. In Proceedings of the 34th International Conference on Machine Learning, Proceedings of Machine Learning Research, Sydney, Australia, 6–11 August 2017; Available online: https://proceedings.mlr.press/v70/arjovsky17a.html (accessed on 14 September 2023).
68. Mukherjee, D.; Saha, P.; Kaplun, D.; Sinitca, A.; Sarkar, R. Brain tumor image generation using an aggregation of GAN models with style transfer. *Sci. Rep.* **2022**, *12*, 9141. [CrossRef]
69. Qiu, D.; Cheng, Y.; Wang, X. Improved generative adversarial network for retinal image super-resolution. *Comput. Methods Programs Biomed.* **2022**, *225*, 106995. [CrossRef]

Disclaimer/Publisher's Note: The statements, opinions and data contained in all publications are solely those of the individual author(s) and contributor(s) and not of MDPI and/or the editor(s). MDPI and/or the editor(s) disclaim responsibility for any injury to people or property resulting from any ideas, methods, instructions or products referred to in the content.

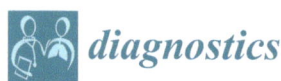

Article

Medical Image Despeckling Using the Invertible Sparse Fuzzy Wavelet Transform with Nature-Inspired Minibatch Water Wave Swarm Optimization

Ahila Amarnath [1], Poongodi Manoharan [2,*], Buvaneswari Natarajan [3], Roobaea Alroobaea [4], Majed Alsafyani [4], Abdullah M. Baqasah [5], Ismail Keshta [6] and Kaamran Raahemifar [7,8,9]

1. Indian Institute of Technology, Madras, Chennai 600036, Tamilnadu, India
2. College of Science and Engineering, Hamad Bin Khalifa University, Doha P.O. Box 34110, Qatar
3. Middlesex College, Edison, NJ 08818, USA; buvaneswariselvakumar@gmail.com
4. Department of Computer Science, College of Computers and Information Technology, Taif University, P.O. Box 11099, Taif 21944, Saudi Arabia
5. Department of Information Technology, College of Computers and Information Technology, Taif University, Taif 21974, Saudi Arabia
6. Computer Science and Information Systems Department, College of Applied Sciences, AlMaarefa University, Riyadh 11597, Saudi Arabia
7. Data Science and Artificial Intelligence Program, College of Information Sciences and Technology, Penn State University, State College, PA 16801, USA
8. School of Optometry and Vision Science, Faculty of Science, University of Waterloo, 200 University, Waterloo, ON N2L3G1, Canada
9. Faculty of Engineering, University of Waterloo, 200 University Ave W, Waterloo, ON N2L 3E9, Canada
* Correspondence: dr.m.poongodi@gmail.com

Abstract: Speckle noise is a pervasive problem in medical imaging, and conventional methods for despeckling often lead to loss of edge information due to smoothing. To address this issue, we propose a novel approach that combines a nature-inspired minibatch water wave swarm optimization (NIMWVSO) framework with an invertible sparse fuzzy wavelet transform (ISFWT) in the frequency domain. The ISFWT learns a non-linear redundant transform with a perfect reconstruction property that effectively removes noise while preserving structural and edge information in medical images. The resulting threshold is then used by the NIMWVSO to further reduce multiplicative speckle noise. Our approach was evaluated using the MSTAR dataset, and objective functions were based on two contrasting reference metrics, namely the peak signal-to-noise ratio (PSNR) and the mean structural similarity index metric (MSSIM). Our results show that the suggested approach outperforms modern filters and has significant generalization ability to unknown noise levels, while also being highly interpretable. By providing a new framework for despeckling medical images, our work has the potential to improve the accuracy and reliability of medical imaging diagnosis and treatment planning.

Keywords: speckle noise; threshold; nature-inspired minibatch water wave swarm optimization; inveritible sparse fuzzy wavelet transform

Citation: Amarnath, A.; Manoharan, P.; Natarajan, B.; Alroobaea, R.; Alsafyani, M.; Baqasah, A.M.; Keshta, I.; Raahemifar, K. Medical Image Despeckling Using the Invertible Sparse Fuzzy Wavelet Transform with Nature-Inspired Minibatch Water Wave Swarm Optimization. *Diagnostics* **2023**, *13*, 2919. https://doi.org/10.3390/diagnostics13182919

Academic Editors: Wan Azani Mustafa and Hiam Alquran

Received: 9 March 2023
Revised: 20 May 2023
Accepted: 26 May 2023
Published: 12 September 2023

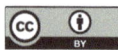

Copyright: © 2023 by the authors. Licensee MDPI, Basel, Switzerland. This article is an open access article distributed under the terms and conditions of the Creative Commons Attribution (CC BY) license (https://creativecommons.org/licenses/by/4.0/).

1. Introduction

Ultrasound imaging is widely used in the medical field. It may be used to scan the uterus, liver, kidneys, spleen, brain, heart, and other soft tissues. Because of its efficiency, quickness, and low price, scanning equipment is frequently utilized. In ultrasound pictures, speckle noise is a common problem that may be ascribed to the imaging method, which may be based on coherent waves such as acoustic or laser imaging. The sorts of noise that may be brought on by various outside factors and the transmission system itself include Gaussian, Poisson, blurred, speckle, and salt-and-pepper noise. The practice of removing background noise has grown in importance in medical imaging applications, and the most often used filters—the median, Gaussian, and Wiener filters—deliver the greatest results for each kind of noise. Picture smoothing, which often uses the best filters or the industry standard filters, is used in most image processing programs to remove noise. A denoising model's capability is to remove noise from the image while still maintaining the edges. Unwanted noise may be eliminated using both linear and non-linear models. Despite their inability to adequately maintain image borders, linear models are often put to the test due to their speed. The histogram, size, and clarity of the MRI images are fed into filters, and depending on these inputs, the best filter is chosen. The area of image noise reduction benefits greatly from the usage of filtering techniques, which may be used to denoise a picture in a number of ways. It can be solved using a variety of algorithms. In order to remove noise without lowering the quality of the examined image, the best filtering techniques are utilized to identify noise with neighboring data.

This work presents a method for suppressing this kind of speckle noise and analyzes its performance. Mathematical morphology is the foundation of this method. It is an updated version of a previously developed algorithm. It is different from other algorithms since it does not rely on the histogram to determine an image's threshold. It also employs a different approach for rebuilding the characteristics of the speckle's size. In addition, it employs structuring components with an arbitrary structure that are similar to the forms of the speckles. In terms of both time complexity and output quality, this method improves upon its predecessor. The general contribution of the study may be summarized as follows:

- Implementation of the sparse fuzzy wavelet transform for obtaining the noisy threshold for analyzing the noisy areas in the image;
- Then, in order to accurately remove the speckle noise in the input image, the determined threshold was applied to NIMWVSO.

The remainder of this document is structured as follows. Section 2 discusses the earlier literature. The ISFWT and NIMWVSO for image denoising are described in Section 3. The experimental data examined throughout the procedure are presented in Section 4. Section 5 provides the general conclusion and suggestions for further development.

2. Related Work

Here are a few of the several reported techniques for speckle-noise reduction. The authors of [1] offer a method for eliminating spot noise from ultrasound images using kinetic gas molecule optimization (KGMO) and a Bayesian framework. Here, the window widths of the image patches are optimized by KGMO, and noise is removed from those windows by the Bayesian network. Five deep learning networks with varied network topologies are introduced by [2] to decrease the influence of speckle noise on ultrasound images. It also includes U-shaped networks with batch normalization and batch re-normalization layers, a denoising network based on residual connections, and a modified generative adversarial network. The autocoder network is built on a convolutional neural network (CNN) with dilated convolution layers. Researchers have created a hybrid strategy that makes use of Kuan and non-local means filters to reduce noise (as stated in [3]). They use a Kuan filter to first sharpen the edges, and then non-local techniques to eliminate the speckle noise. Furthermore, the performance of the proposed hybrid filter and its design parameters are optimized using a meta-heuristic known as the gray wolf optimizer. Ref. [4] proposes SORAMA (Semantic Object Region and Morphological Analysis), an excellent technique for analyzing semantic object regions. A scan is the first step, followed by a noise-reduction process. After that, image quality becomes better. The area of interest (ROI) for the picture is identified. The morphological processes of dilatation and erosion then blur the image. The polished image clearly shows the stone. If the stone is still hidden, noise reduction is performed once again, and the process is repeated until a smoothed image containing the stone is discovered. The use of a progressive feature fusion attention dense network (PFFADN) to eliminate speckle noise from OCT images is described in [5]. They first build up tightly connected dense blocks in the deep convolution network before connecting each shallowly generated feature map to the deep one to form a residual block. They use an attention mechanism to assist the network concentrate on the most crucial information while removing the rest. A uniform collection of feature maps that have been combined from all dense blocks are sent to the reconstruction output layer. There, a technique for removing the speckle noise that often shows up in ultrasound images is described [6,7]. These images are used in the medical industry to assist physicians in finding abnormalities and illnesses that are deeply buried inside a patient's body. There have been a number of recommended filters for despeckling ultrasonic images, but it is still possible to enhance the quality of the denoised image to avoid false detection. This essay makes use of a bilateral filter that has been improved. The minimum mean brightness error bi-histogram equalization (MMBEBHE) approach was introduced to enhance the contrast of MRI images [8]. To reduce visual noise, this technique combines the Wiener and bilateral filters. The results of the study using the provided approach include results from speckle and Gaussian noise. In [9], the author describes the most popular convolutional neural network (CNN)-based despeckling techniques for ultrasound images, both in the transform domain and the spatial domain. Using transform domain methods such as wavelet, curvelet, and Bayes shrink has been successful in several studies. Deep-learning-based techniques, including DnCNN, ECNDNet, etc., enhance despeckling's effectiveness. Here, image fusion is carried out by combining the speckle-noise-reduction (SNR) approach with the multimodality image fusion method [10]. The SNR approach is used to eliminate background noise for enhanced medical image quality. The advantages and disadvantages of fusing many medical images into a single, meaningful image are also addressed. Additionally, the stationary wavelet transformation (SWT) technique is being studied as a more reliable approach of accomplishing the same goal. A novel fuzzy-logic-based non-local mean filter is introduced in [11] to model the speckle noise, recover the damaged image using fuzzy uncertainty modeling (FUM), smoothed by local statistic-based information while keeping the image characteristics for low and highly speckled ultrasound pictures. The presented denoising approach gathers local characteristics to use FUM in order to distinguish "similar and non-similar" non-local locations. By applying local statistical data to smooth these homogeneous zones, the fuzzy-logic-based noise-reduction approach is started. In this instance, an ultrasonic image is divided into subbands using the wavelet transform [12,13]. The approximation subband is modified using bilateral filtering, while the detail subbands are modified using thresholding and anisotropic diffusion. The smoothing and removal approaches covered in [14,15] are closely related to a number of processes (such as the identification of regions of interest) addressed in earlier studies that were examined here. Furthermore, defining this toolbox makes it simpler to conduct analyses and research with a more focused scope.

The classic methods are extensively covered in the first half of this research and include space, diffusion, and wavelet filters, to name just a few. The next section describes different state-of-the-art and hybrid models in the realm of speckle-noise filtering as well as contemporary, less well-known deep-learning-based machine learning techniques. A novel technique for reducing speckle noise in OCT volumes is presented in [16], which makes use of the matching en face representation to provide relatively speckle-free frontal parts of the retinal layers. The suggested method estimates the anatomical structures by resolving a constrained optimization problem that combines wavelet-domain sparsity and total variation (wavelet-TV) regularization in order to preserve the edges of retinal layers and lessen artifacts brought on by pure wavelet thresholding. To accomplish the goal function outlined in [17,18], we use a brand-new hybrid approach called the Randomized FireFly (FF) update in Lion Algorithm (RFU-LA), which includes components of both the Lion Algorithm (LA) and the FireFly Algorithm (FF). By taking the mean of images that have been routinely median-filtered using different kernel sizes, the hybrid median-mean filter (HM2F) proposed in [19] is a one-shot image processing method for decreasing speckle noise. Together, the median filter and mean technique may preserve up to 97 percentage of the original spatial resolution while producing a denoised image with reduced speckle contrast. The HM2F method is compared against several other well-known filtering techniques, including the classic median filter method, the 3D block-matching filter, the non-local means filter, the 2D windowed Fourier transform filter, and the Wiener filter, using a variety of speckle-distorted images. According to the authors of [20], there is a technique that uses a guided filter and speckle-reducing anisotropic diffusion (SRAD) to reduce the impact of speckle noise while maintaining sharp edges. First, speckle, a multiplicative noise, is removed using SRAD. After filtering, if there is still noise, it is added to using a logarithmic transformation. After the first filtering, any remaining noise in the image is removed using a guided filter. The final image is noise-free thanks to the exponential transform. The authors of [21–25] examine and summarize popular techniques for reducing speckle noise in ultrasonic images for the most part. We evaluate the different approaches via experiments, highlighting the distinctive contributions of each strategy to feature retention and denoising using quality assessments, texture analysis, and profile interpretation. Ref. [26] propose the method of computer-aided diagnostics that combines a wavelet neural network (WNN) and the grey wolf optimization (GWO) algorithm to find anomalies in breast ultrasound images [27]. The retrieved features have a substantial impact on the recognition rate of prior approaches, thus a new and improved CAD system based on a convolutional neural network (CNN) is developed to address them. It is capable of differentiating between those with normal control and those suffering from Alzheimer's disease.

3. Problem Statement

Image quality is essential for analyzing or segmenting ultrasonic images because speckle hides small details. Recent studies have demonstrated that speckle reduction improves the expert's visual perception while assessing ultrasound imaging of human organs. Processing ultrasonic images, which are used to offer essential diagnostic information about the human body, requires the removal of speckle noise. Speckle noise makes ultrasound images more difficult to visually analyze. The main objective of despeckling is to prevent losing tiny details or blurring the borders in ultrasonographic images. Speckle can be removed using a variety of approaches; however, noise reduction may be more difficult due to the higher threshold level. Speckle noise is a multiplicative noise, making it impossible to entirely remove it without altering the image's boundaries and texture characteristics. This presents one of the technological obstacles in despeckling ultrasonic images. Traditional filtering methods frequently lead to a loss of resolution and fine characteristics as well, which might affect the accuracy of diagnostic data. Speckle noise has a non-Gaussian distribution and is strongly influenced by the imaging modality and tissue type, which makes it more challenging to find an ideal solution. Therefore, it is imperative to create an optimized method for speckle reduction that takes into account these particular difficulties while also maintaining image quality, resolution, and small details and edges. Additionally, quantitative metrics such as peak signal-to-noise ratio (PSNR), mean square error (MSE), structural similarity index (SSIM), and subjective visual quality assessment are frequently used to analyze the efficacy of despeckling algorithms. Therefore, when developing a despeckling algorithm for ultrasonic images, it is crucial to take both objective and subjective evaluation criteria into account.

4. Proposed Work

The ultrasound image quality is compromised by speckle, a kind of signal-dependent noise. Speckle noise has an additive impact. The diagnostic value of ultrasonic imaging is diminished as a result of this noise. Noise of this sort is an inevitable byproduct of medical ultrasound imaging. Therefore, anytime ultrasound imaging is utilized for medical imaging, speckle-noise reduction is a crucial pre-processing step. Figure 1 is a comprehensive representation of the proposed technique.

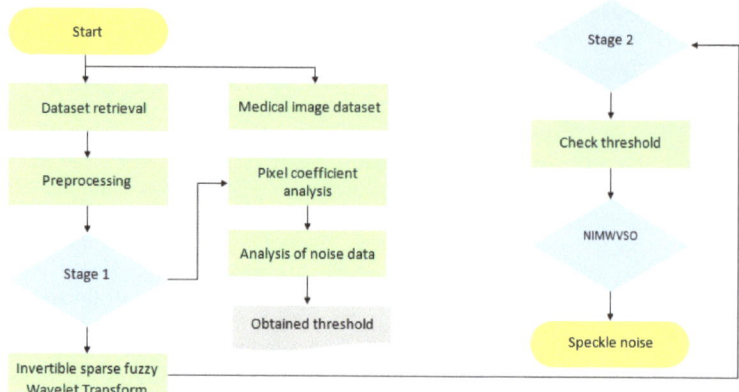

Figure 1. Schematic representation of the suggested methodology.

4.1. Data Source

In these experiments, we just look at two different kinds of images. Figure 2 displays one kind of phantom picture, a 200 × 200 modified Shepp–Logan created using Matlab 2013's phantom function (a). The noise variance was set to 0.1 in order to demonstrate the addition of speckle noise to this phantom picture. The second picture was a genuine ultrasound of the belly taken with a portable scanner (a SonoStar UBox-10 Ultrasound B Scanner equipped with a transabdominal convex probe operating at 3.5 MHz). Figure 2 shows an actual view of a fetal abdomen (b). Obstacles for the next phases include the phantom picture, the ambiguous limits of the abdomen, and the existence of speckle noise. Despeckling a picture is a crucial process that has to be accomplished in a way that does not compromise the image's essential qualities. That is why we use a two-pronged approach in this case to eliminate the speckle noise.

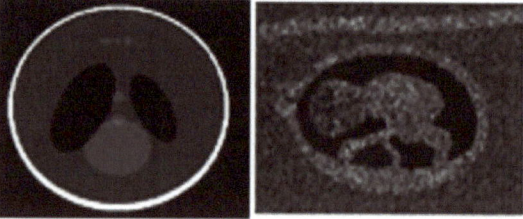

Figure 2. Sample input.

4.2. System Model

Let f_{ji} be the deteriorated, noisy picture,

$$f_{ji} = a_{ji} * N_{ji} \tag{1}$$

where a_{ji} and N_{ji} are the multiplicative noise and the speckle-free picture pixel at position (j, i). a_{ji} must be rescued from f_{ji}. Pixels' coordinates in the picture space are indicated by the (j, i) subscripts.

The mathematical model of the speckle noise described in (2) demonstrates that the noise distribution in an ultrasound medical image is signal-dependent and multiplicative in nature, and is expressed as

$$J^{noisy}(a) = J^{original}(a) \pm (a) \tag{2}$$

The original image is represented by $J^{original}(a)$. For each given pixel a, where an is an index, the observed picture, including noise, is denoted by $J^{noisy}(a)$ and $\pm(a)$ identifies a noise that is multiplicative in nature. The mathematical model is log transformed, leading to the following Equation (3):

$$\log J^{noisy}(a) = \log(J^{original}(a)) + \log \pm(a)) \tag{3}$$

The following formula describes the standard model of speckle noise:

$$J^{noisy}(a) = J^{original}(a) + J^{original}(a)^H \pm (a) \tag{4}$$

where H is a constant associated with the zero-mean Gaussian distribution of the ultrasonic acquisition equipment. Setting r to 0.5 provides a decent approximation of the ultrasound data in the B-mode ultrasound picture research. When H is equal to 1, the model demonstrates that speckle noise is multiplicative.

The following equation is obtained by substituting a wavelet function into both sides of the expression.

$$\ln f_{ji} = \ln a_{ji} + \ln N_{ji} \tag{5}$$

The wavelet transform is often used to shift medical images from the multiplicative speckle model to the additive noise model during processing and analysis. To estimate the medical picture devoid of speckles while still accounting for the logarithmic impact, an extra exponential threshold procedure is carried out.

4.3. ISFWT-Based Pixel Coefficient Analysis

The ISFWT detailed coefficients are determined using a thresholding method. Coefficients in the approximation are not thresholded in the same manner as the detailed coefficients are because they represent 'low-frequency' terms that often comprise essential components of the signal and are less impacted by noise. The success of a threshold-based strategy depends on two main factors. The threshold value and the threshold function used are both crucial. Input images are segmented into $E \cup \forall^{K^2 n_e}$ patches where each column represents a vectorized KK patch and n_e may be thought of as the patch count. We offer a thresholding framework as an alternative to repeatedly picking low-rank patches $L : \forall^{(K^2)} \to \forall^1$ to estimate a scalar weight $C_j \cup [0,1]$ for each patch. With the use of soft selection, the suggested method may be trained to automatically give more weight to low-rank patches. The noise variance may be computed using the estimated weights and the patches by finding the lowest singular value in the weighted covariance matrix of the patch matrix:

$$\pi^2 = \frac{1}{\sum_{j=1}^{n_e} C_j} \pi min \tag{6}$$

where πmin determines the covariance matrix's least singular value after weighting $Ediag(C)ED$ with $= [1, \ldots, n_e]D$.

The two most popular types of thresholding are hard threshold and soft threshold schemes. The hard threshold method disregards coefficients below a threshold value D, where D is determined by the variance of the noise. This method of decision making is sometimes referred to as the "keep or kill" approach.

$$C_{(g,o)} = \begin{cases} C_{(g,o)} & \text{if } |C_{(g,o)}| \geq D \\ 0 & \text{if } |C_{(g,o)}| < D \end{cases} \tag{7}$$

Using Equation (7) (above), we see that the soft threshold method reduces wavelet coefficients both above and below the threshold. The hard threshold produces results with harsher edges, while the soft threshold produces smoother results. A new exponential threshold is developed to deal with the drawbacks of both discontinuous and constant deviation in decision making, taking into consideration the benefits of the soft, hard, semisoft, and Garrote threshold functions. The effectiveness of exponential threshold-based denoising is enhanced by this method. The exponential threshold function is defined mathematically as

$$C_{(g,o)} = \begin{cases} KNR(C_{(g,o)})(|C_{g,o}| - 1 & \text{if } |C_{(g,o)}| \geq D \\ 0 & \text{if } |C_{(g,o)}| < D \end{cases} \quad (8)$$

where $C_{(g,o)}$ may be easily manipulated using a shape parameter α. Since it is simply an ordinary integer, the scales may be set any way we want, and each signal will have its own value. It is important to carefully consider each element of Equation (9) since even little adjustments can significantly affect the amount of background noise. When the function's α value approaches 0, it becomes a soft threshold. With 'α' at infinity, the function exhibits a severe cutoff. We may adjust the following settings in this exponential thresholding technique: 'α' and D. These adjusting factors are chosen by the optimization procedure. In order to maximize both smoothing and detail retention, we use two separate goal functions.

4.4. NIMWVSO-Based Noise Removal

Optimizing using NIMWVSO helps in determining the best settings for the models ('α' and D) of the exponential threshold function.

$$\vartheta_{(g,o)} = \begin{cases} KNR(C_{(g,o)})\{(|C_{g,o}| - \frac{D}{exp^3[\alpha(|C_{g,o}|-D]/D}\} & \text{if } |C_{(g,o)}| \geq D \\ 0 & \text{if } |C_{(g,o)}| < D \end{cases} \quad (9)$$

That is, each particle a_j is constructed such that $a_j = (D_{11}, D_{12}, \ldots D_{ji})$, where D_{ji} is the jth particle's ith tweak factor. Two tuning variables t, β and d, are selected for this suggested task. One such method is NIMWVS optimization, which has found usage in many different scientific and practical contexts with positive results. Here, any change in inertia weight will result in a shift in the wave particle's position. The bigger the worth, the more accessible it is globally, yet the less feasible it is to mine locally. Results may be enhanced by using dynamic values rather than fixed ones. In this case, a more constrained radius for the search window, R_{search}, is convolved around a noisy $pixel_j$ dependent upon the found threshold. Utilizing the proposed based optimization statistics criterion, $pixel_i$ is similar to $pixel_j$. The radii of the local and global windows are similar, O_j and O_i, centered at $pixel_j$ and $pixel_I$, respectively. Similarity between $pixel_j$ and all non-local neighboring $pixel_I$ uses a fitness function that is optimized for a certain geographical area to determine its value. The starting location is determined by the density of the swarming pixels. At this stage, the degree of similarity between windows is evaluated. For each non-local window O_i, an optimization-based approach is employed to determine the value of O_j. Looking for nearby, comparable non-local pixels may give a fair approximation of a noise-free pixel. Edge pixels often have extremely distinct values from the surrounding pixels and serve to visually separate two parts of a picture at first. Non-local neighbors, those that are not themselves part of an edge, are used to estimate noise-free pixels since they cannot distort those edges. These distorted edges may lead to incorrect diagnosis of illness using ultrasonic data. Due to the inherent uncertainty in noisy ultrasound images, it is challenging to locate similar patches or locations beyond the immediate vicinity of the central patch, O_j. To address these unknowns, tuning functions are created using an optimization-based approach. These functions incorporate the mean ratio and the variance ratio denoted as G_θ and $G_{(\tau^2)}$ respectively for the patches O_j and O_i. These ratios are then utilized to determine the mutual resemblance grade. The similarity of the non-local window is then calculated as the sum of all of these similarities, O_i. With the information we have on the error threshold ratio, we may be able to pinpoint where the mistakes are being made. For regions with a greater membership degree, the local and non-local areas resemble one another more closely, but for regions with a lower membership degree, the O_i belong to a different location; therefore, despeckling throws away those pixels. The similarity mechanism is based on the trapezoidal-shaped function of Equation (11).

$$W(a: Z_1, Z_2, Z_3, Z_4) = \begin{cases} 0 & a \leq Z_1 \\ \frac{a-z_1}{z_1-Z_1} & Z_1 \leq a \leq Z_2 \\ 1 & Z_2 \leq a \leq Z_3 \\ \frac{Z_4-a}{Z_4-Z_3} & Z_3 \leq a \leq Z_4 \\ 0 & Z_4 \leq a \end{cases} \quad (10)$$

For the trapezoidal function, the input x-vector is denoted by an. The scalar factors are constants Z_1, Z_2, Z_3, and Z_4. Here, Z_1 and Z_4 denote the trapezoidal function's bottom and top, respectively, whereas Z_2 and Z_3 denote its upper and lower bounds, respectively. The rigorous steps are used to derive these components and evaluate how similar O_j and O_i are as input windows. All comparable regions outside of the immediate area have now been counted. They are first restored after being smoothed using noise estimates based on optimal local statistics. Using the definition of the local linear minimum mean square error, we may generate the noise-free region $w(a)$.

$$J_{LLMMSE}(a) = P(J(a)) + \frac{\tau_j^2(a)}{\tau_n^2(a)}[n(a) - P(n(a))] \quad (11)$$

where $J_{LLMMSE}(a)$ is the estimation of noise free image $J(a)$; $\tau_j^2(a)$ and $\tau_n^2(a)$ noise in the picture n, and the $J(a)$ variance (a). The expectations of the ideal picture $J(a)$ and the input noisy patch $n(a)$ are denoted by $P(J(a))$ and $P(n(a))$, correspondingly. These numbers are derived in the manner specified. Here, we use local statistics to compare non-locally similar patches and calculate the restored fitness value of a noisy pixel, j. Pixels that are visually identical also have the same statistical features. Euclidean distance are used to measure the proximity of two points on a map or at two different locations. The estimated noise level tends to cluster around low numbers rather than high ones. Zero-mean Gaussian distribution $(\theta = 0)$ and an estimated noise variance (τ^2) are used to identify extra-regional participation O_i:

$$\text{weight}(\tau_{ji}\tau, \theta) = p^{\frac{-(t_{ji}-\theta)^2}{2\tau^2}} \quad (12)$$

Euclidean distance t_{ji} among the local region 'j' and non-local region 'i' is given by

$$t_{ji} = \|O_j - O_i\| \quad (13)$$

The central pixel of patch O_j has the value calculated by adding the values of all neighboring pixels that are not included in the local region. The predicted noise-free value is pixel j as a consequence of the fuzzy centroid technique employed in the defuzzification step, and this is written as

$$pixel_l = \frac{1.0}{\sum_{g=1}^{N} weight_g} \sum_{g=1}^{N} (pixel_g X weight_g) \quad (14)$$

The value of $pixel_j$ estimates the restored pixel's value, where N is the number of non-locally comparable regions and local regions with similar values. $pixel_g$ is the value of the central pixel of window O_g, and $weight_g$ corresponds to the importance placed on the pixel with the highest degree of similarity as calculated by Equation (15).

"Case 1—Full Reference (FR) Measure"

Reference objective functions for the whole process include the peak-to-noise ratio (PSNR) and the mean structural similarity index metric (MSSSIM). Together, optimizing for these two aims produces a more distinct image overall while keeping the reaction smooth in otherwise similar regions. As the peak signal-to-noise ratio rises, so does the quality of the image following speckle reduction.

$$PSNR(J_D, J_G) = 10 \log_{10}[\frac{(J_G)^2_{peak}}{MSE}] \tag{15}$$

$$MSE(J_D, J_G) = \frac{1}{V_n} \sum_{j=1}^{V} \sum_{i=1}^{n} (J_g(j,i) - J_T(j,i))^2 \tag{16}$$

A further complete reference measure that places an emphasis on edge-preserving abilities is the mean structural similarity index. Two images' degree of resemblance is quantified using the structural similarity index metric (SSIM). The MSSIM index may be between 0 and 1, with 1 indicating excellent edge preservation. A demonstration of MSSIM's calculation is shown below.

$$MSSIM(J_T, J_G) = \frac{1}{V} \sum_{e=0}^{V-1} SSIM(J_T, J_G) \tag{17}$$

$$SSIM(J_T, J_G) = \frac{(2\theta_{jt}\theta_{IG} + Z_1)(2\pi_{j_T I_G} + Z_2)}{(\theta_{JT}^2 + \theta_{JG}^2 + Z_2)(\pi_{JT}^2 + \pi_{JG}^2 + Z_2)} \tag{18}$$

where V is the number of the image's local windows, JT and JG are the filtered and ground truth counterparts, and Z_1 and Z_2 are constants. The terms θ and π parallel the average and the deviation. The best solution is obtained by maximizing the objective functions $I(J)$ (such as PSNR and MSSIM), as shown in Equation (20)

$$J = arg(max(I(J))) \tag{19}$$

"Case 2—No Reference (NR) Measure"

The alpha–beta measure, which is derived from the ratio of the edge estimator and the despeckling evaluation index, is one example of a non-reference metric that may be used in MOPSO-tuned medical image despeckling (DEI). The estimator is then used to evaluate the filter's noise-reduction capability, and the DEI of the Edge Around Region is then used to assess the filter's edge-preserving abilities in this situation (EAR). Estimator examples include

$$\beta_{\gamma\gamma} = \beta|\tau_{ENL}| + (1-\beta)|\tau_\theta| + \gamma \tag{20}$$

$$\gamma = \frac{\sum_{j=1}^{S}((J_u)_{noisy} - (\vec{J}_u)_{noisy})((J_u)_{ratio} - (\vec{J}_u)_{ratio})}{\sum_{j=1}^{S}((J_u)_{noisy} - (\vec{J}_u)_{noisy})^2 \sum_{j=1}^{S}((J_u)_{ratio} - (\vec{J}_u)_{ratio})^2} \tag{21}$$

where J_u is the high-pass filtered image, $\bar{J}_u$ is the average of the filtered image, $\tau_E NL$. The mean of the ratio image is the Equivalent Number of Looks (ENL), which is calculated by subtracting the noisy picture from the ratio image. Typically, the estimator's values are between zero and one. A filter's ability to preserve edges is measured using the despeckling evaluation index (DEI), calculated by dividing the standard deviation of a narrower neighborhood window by that of a broader one. The DEI value must be negative. If the data in the window has a bigger standard deviation, there will be more edges. So, a lower DEI is associated with better edge preservation ability.

$$DEI = \frac{1}{V \bullet n} \sum_{a,b} \frac{min(std(C_{e,u}^v))}{std(C_a, b^N)} \tag{22}$$

To improve edge maintenance and eliminate noise, the goal function here should have small values. Therefore, it is necessary to minimize the objective function, as shown in Equation (24).

$$j = arg(min(I(J))) \tag{23}$$

Finally, the noises in the images are despeckled precisely.

5. Performance Analysis

The effectiveness of the approach that was recommended is analyzed in this section. Python was used as the operating system for the whole of the experiment. In order to show that the suggested network is superior to other conventional and well-known despeckling algorithms in terms of performance, the proposed network was compared with these other methods. Both actual ultrasounds and phantom images were used in the conducted experiments.

Figure 3 shows the denoised output of the Shepp–Logan phantom which was built as a reference standard for use in evaluating the accuracy of head CT image reconstruction simulations. The ISFWT-NIMWVSO technique was used to denoise this phantom, as seen in the picture. Subsequently, the real-time fetal image was processed to remove noise, as seen in Figure 3 and the comparison of the input sample and noise amplitude shown in Figure 4.

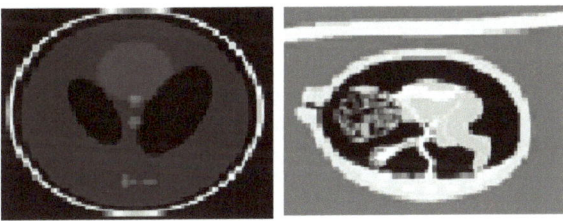

Figure 3. Denoised output.

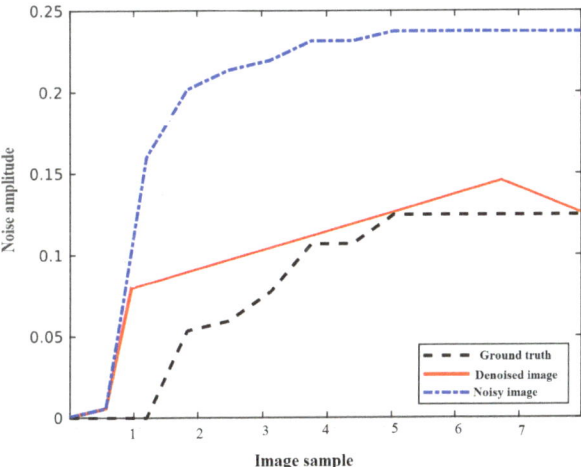

Figure 4. Image sample vs. noise amplitude.

In addition to this, we evaluated the estimate technique by applying it to phantom and fetal ultrasound images that had varying amounts of noise, and the results are shown in Table 1. We can observe that the suggested estimation technique has errors that are within acceptable ranges, since the estimated noise levels are somewhat higher than the actual low noise levels but slightly lower than the actual medium- and high-level estimates.

Table 1. Estimate Technique.

Read Noise Levels	Mean of Estimated Noise Level	Mean Estimated Error
0.1	0.09	0.01
0.2	0.18	0.02
0.3	0.3	0
0.4	0.4	0
0.5	0.5	0

Image Quality Evaluation Metrics

A novel algorithm for reducing speckle was recently shown. Several methods have been utilized to evaluate the efficiency of the proposed algorithm vs. the existing filters. Two common approaches to comparing results are quantitative assessments of image quality and qualitative evaluation, the latter of which is commonly carried out by the authors themselves. Significant effort has been made in recent years to establish objective metrics of image quality that correlate with assessments of how the quality is perceived. In order to evaluate filtering in relation to a speckle-free ideal reference, we use clinical and phantom images in addition to simulated ultrasonography as test data. However, it is difficult to tell how much enhancement was performed on an ultrasound image, and there is no universal way for doing so (Wang 2011). Quality evaluation metrics such as average difference (AD), Pratt's figure of merit (FOM), root mean square error (RMSE), signal-to-noise ratio (SNR), peak signal-to-noise ratio (PSNR), maximum difference (MD), normalized absolute error (NAE), normalized cross-correlation (NK), structural content (SC), coefficient of correlation (CoC), universal quality index (UQI), and quality index (QI) were applied to the final images in this study (MSSIM). In addition to serving as an index, the final metric incorporates a visibility error map, which allows for the examination of areas in the distorted image where deviations occur between the original and distorted versions. Furthermore, we introduce a novel evaluation measure called the Speckle Reduction Score, which assesses the degree of improvement achieved. This new measure (SRS) mixes the edge preservation evaluation with a local similarity map.

- Signal-to-noise ratio (SNR): A common method for determining how well coherent imaging suppresses noise when that noise is multiplicative. This is achieved by comparing the intensity of the desired signal to that of the surrounding noise.
- Root mean square error (RMSE): This is calculated by squaring the intensity value difference between the original and denoised images and then dividing that number by the image's size to obtain the root average.
- Peak signal-to-noise ratio (PSNR): This provides the image quality as a ratio of the original signal power to the signal power after denoising. A higher PSNR number indicates a better quality image.
- Pratt's figure of merit (FOM) (Pratt 2007): In particular, this assesses how effectively an image retains its borders. The method used to generate a binary edge map has a significant impact on the FOM; higher PSNR values suggest better image quality. The Canny edge detector, which optimizes the FOM, is used for all of the speckle-reduction methods so that the results may be fairly compared. The FOM may take on any value between 0 and 1, with 1 representing optimal edge preservation.
- Normalized cross-correlation (NK): Its value (as a correlation-based measure of picture quality) is 1 for pairs of identical images.
- Average difference (AD): The average noise reduction is determined by comparing the original and denoised versions of a single pixel.
- Maximum difference (MD): Image denoising to the greatest possible degree.
- Normalized absolute error (NAE): This is a measurement of how effectively an image can predict its own mistakes.
- Coefficient of correlation (CoC): illustrates the linear relationship between the original and denoised photos and the direction in which that relationship runs.

- Quality index based on local variance (QILV) (Aja-Fernandez 2006): This theory relies on the observation that the local variance distribution of a picture encodes a great deal of the image's structural information.
- Universal quality index (UQI) (Wang 2002): This is built on the idea that every distorted picture has three parts: a lack of correlation, distorted brightness, and distorted contrast.
- Laplacian mean square error (LMSE): Local contrast is an essential aspect of picture quality. Laplacian mean square error is the standard method for assessing picture local contrast.
- Mean structural similarity index map (MSSIM): We may use MSSIM to compare the lighting, contrast, and structure of two photos to see how closely they are alike (Wang, 2004). It may be used to discover comparable images for comparative purposes.
- Speckle Reduction Score (SRS): Several experiments have shown the usefulness of the MSSIM index, although there may be cases when the resulting quality measure does not agree with a subjective assessment based on visual data. A novel metric, the Speckle Reduction Score (SRS), is proposed and its computation is decomposed into two stages. The first stage is to determine the local similarity map, and the second is to combine the results from each map into a single value.

Table 2 synthesizes the results of applying the improved speckle filter algorithm to the simulated picture by calculating a number of performance measures. Each metric's optimal value is shown in bold. Figure 5 depicts performance analysis of the suggested mechanism.

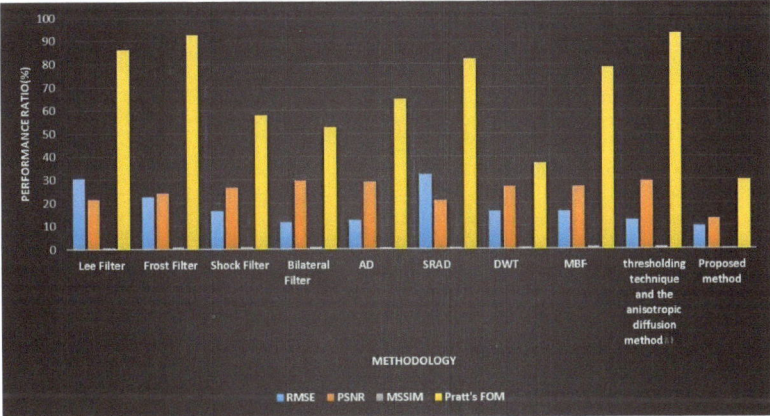

Figure 5. Performance analysis of the suggested mechanism.

Table 2. Comparative Performance Analysis.

Method	RMSE	PSNR	MSSIM	Pratt's FOM
Lee Filter [12]	30	21	0.783	86
Frost Filter [12]	23	24	0.88	93
Shock Filter [12]	17	27	0.877	58
Bilateral Filter [12]	12	30	0.882	53
AD [12]	13	29	0.78	65
SRAD [12]	32	21	0.757	82
DWT [12]	16	27	0.701	37
MBF [12]	16	27	0.861	78
Thresholding Technique and the Anisotropic Diffusion Method [12]	13	29	0.903	93
Proposed Method	10	13	0.2	30

Table 3 and Figure 6 compile the findings from several quality assessment techniques. Across the board, ISFWT-NIMWVSO filtering performs better than its competitors. As far as FOM is concerned, the suggested technique provides for more fulfilling results than do existing alternatives, enabling it to maintain its edge. Using the MSSIM, we can see that the suggested speckle filtering would maintain an appearance that is in line with how humans see things. The root mean squared error shows that the thresholding method employed in the multiresolution wavelet-based technique may keep the average error low all the way through the restoration procedure. By using optimization in place of a filter and a thresholding wavelet, our proposed method delivers the highest quantitative results. When the recommended method is implemented, the MSSIM index value dramatically rises. Thus, the proposed method yields an image that is very structurally similar to the standard. Since it is based on Pratt's FOM, this method is more advantageous. So, this demonstrates that the method may continue to evolve and improve. The suggested method outperforms the current one since it increases the values of Pratt's FOM, PSNR, and RMSE. The greatest noise reduction and edge retention is shown in Figure 6, thanks to the recommended method. The result of performance evaluation of the suggested mechanism is shown in Figure 7 and Table 4 compile the findings of performance metrics from existing and proposed method.

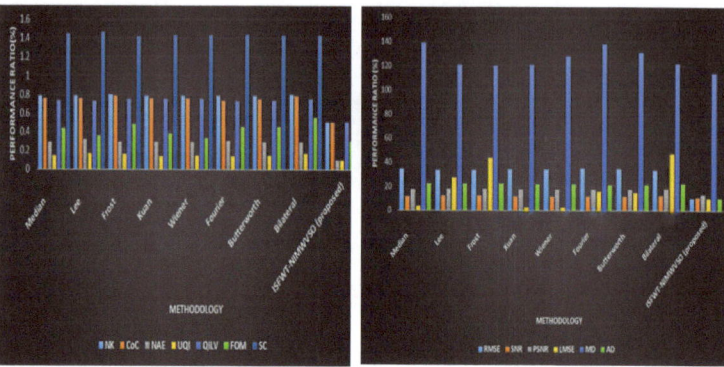

Figure 6. Performance evaluation.

As shown by the result obtained, the suggested methodology outperforms other existing speckle filter methodologies in use.

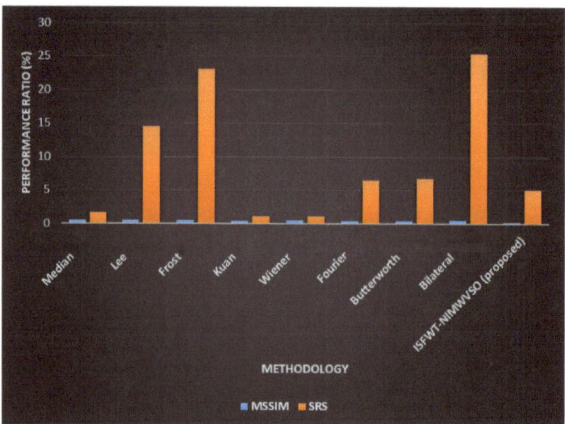

Figure 7. Performance evaluation.

Table 3. Proposed vs. existing comparative analysis.

Metrics	RMSE	SNR	PSNR	LMSE	MD	AD	NK
Median [21]	34.46	11.8	17.38	3.61	139	22.37	0.79
Lee [21]	33.28	12.03	17.74	27.43	121	22.31	0.79
Frost [21]	33.37	12.03	17.66	43.32	120	22.08	0.8
Kuan [21]	34.06	11.86	17.49	2.65	121	21.82	0.79
Wiener [21]	34.12	11.85	17.47	2.53	128	21.84	0.79
Fourier [21]	34.96	11.65	17.26	15.57	138	21.51	0.79
Butterworth [21]	34.29	11.8	17.43	14.76	131	21.43	0.79
Bilateral [21]	33.42	12.02	17.65	47.2	122	22.25	0.8
ISFWT-NIMWVSO (proposed)	10	11	13	10	114	10	0.5

Table 4. Proposed vs. existing comparative analysis.

Metrics	CoC	NAE	UQI	QILV	FOM	SC	MSSIM	SRS
Median [21]	0.76	0.29	0.15	0.74	0.44	1.45	0.47	1.68
Lee [21]	0.76	0.32	0.17	0.73	0.36	1.47	0.53	14.54
Frost [21]	0.79	0.29	0.16	0.75	0.48	1.42	0.53	23.09
Kuan [21]	0.76	0.29	0.14	0.75	0.38	1.43	0.44	1.17
Wiener [21]	0.76	0.29	0.15	0.75	0.33	1.43	0.47	1.18
Fourier [21]	0.74	0.3	0.14	0.73	0.45	1.44	0.42	6.47
Butterworth [21]	0.75	0.29	0.15	0.74	0.45	1.43	0.45	6.69
Bilateral [21]	0.79	0.29	0.17	0.75	0.55	1.43	0.54	25.38
ISFWT-NIMWVSO (proposed)	0.5	0.1	0.1	0.5	0.3	1.2	0.2	5

6. Conclusions

In this study, we compare and contrast several widely used algorithms and methods for speckle-noise reduction from medical ultrasound images. A revised set of metrics for evaluating despeckling performance is provided. Research evaluating various methods of noise suppression in ultrasound images employed both the fetal image and a noise-free synthetic image of a phantom. The image was manipulated using Field II to add the typical noise seen in ultrasound images. Finally, we showed the proposed speckle smoothing algorithms in action by comparing them to the noise-free image. This study compiles an inventory of strategies for diminishing speckle, all of which are evaluated using qualitative metrics. Experimental findings on both simulated and clinical ultrasound pictures show quantitatively that the proposed method is better in terms of PSNR, SSIM, SRS, and co-efficient of correlation. From what can be seen, the proposed approach outperforms the previous despeckling techniques in terms of reducing speckle noise and preserving clarity. In the future, we want to apply the proposed method to denoising other kinds of medical imaging, such as CT, MR, and PET scans, and to use deep learning to estimate the amount of speckle noise present in actual ultrasound images.

Author Contributions: Conceptualization, A.A. and R.A.; Methodology, P.M.; Software, M.A. and I.K.; Validation, A.A. and K.R.; Formal analysis, P.M., A.M.B. and I.K.; Investigation, R.A.; Resources, A.A.; Writing—original draft preparation, A.M.B.; Writing—review and editing, B.N.; Supervision, A.M.B. and K.R.; Project administration, K.R. All authors have read and agreed to the published version of the manuscript.

Funding: The Research Paper received funding from Deanship of Scientific Research, Taif University.

Institutional Review Board Statement: Not applicable.

Informed Consent Statement: Not applicable.

Data Availability Statement: The phantom picture used in our study, a modified Shepp-Logan image of size 200 × 200 was created using Matlab phantom function from the year 2013. The specific details and parameters of this modified Shepp-Logan phantom picture are available upon request.

Acknowledgments: The researchers would like to acknowledge Deanship of Scientific Research, Taif University for funding this work.

Conflicts of Interest: The Authors declare no conflict of interest regarding the publication of this research paper.

References

1. Shabana Sulthana, S.L.; Sucharitha, M. Kinetic Gas Molecule Optimization (KGMO)-Based Speckle Noise Reduction in Ultrasound Images. *Soft Comput. Signal Process.* **2022**, *10*, 447–455.
2. Karaoğlu, O.; Bilge, H.Ş.; Uluer, İ. Removal of speckle noises from ultrasound images using five different deep learning networks. *EST* **2022**, *29*, 101030. [CrossRef]
3. Shereena, V.B.; Raju, G. Modified non-local means model for speckle noise reduction in ultrasound images. *Congr. Intell. Syst.* **2022**, *10*, 691–707.
4. Jayasingh, R.; RJS, J.K.; Telagathoti, D.B.; Sagayam, K.M.; Pramanik, S.; Jena, O.P.; Bandyopadhyay, S.K. Speckle noise removal by SORAMA segmentation in Digital Image Processing to facilitate precise robotic surgery. *Int. J. Reliab. Qual. E-Healthc.* **2022**, *11*, 1–19.
5. Zeng, L.; Huang, M.; Li, Y.; Chen, Q.; Dai, H.N. Progressive Feature Fusion Attention Dense Network for Speckle Noise Removal in OCT Images. *IEEE/ACM Trans. Comput. Biol. Bioinform.* **2022**, *10*, 447–455. [CrossRef] [PubMed]
6. Bhonsle, D.; Rizvi, T.; Mishra, S.; Sinha, G.R.; Kumar, A.; Jain, V.K. Reduction of Ultrasound Images using Combined Bilateral Filter & Median Modified Wiener Filter. In Proceedings of the 2022 Second International Conference on Advances in Electrical, Computing, Communication and Sustainable Technologies, Bhilai, India, 21–22 April 2022 ; pp. 1–5.
7. Tătăranu, E.L.E.N.A.; Diaconescu, S.; Ivănescu, C.G.; Sarbu, I.; Stamatin, M. Clinical, immunological and pathological profile of infants suffering from cow's milk protein allergy. *Rom. J. Morphol. Embryol. Rev. Roum. Morphol. Embryol.* **2016**, *57*, 1031–1035.
8. Lather, M.; Singh, P. Contrast Enhancement and Noise Removal from Medical Images Using a Hybrid Technique. In *New Approaches for Multidimensional Signal Processing: Proceedings of International Workshop, NAMSP 2021*; Springer: Berlin/Heidelberg, Germany, 2022; Volume 10, pp. 223–232.
9. Pradeep, S.; Nirmaladevi, P. A review on speckle noise reduction techniques in ultrasound medical images based on spatial domain, transform domain and CNN methods. In *IOP Conference Series: Materials Science and Engineering*; IOP Publishing: Bristol, UK, 2021; Volume 10, p. 012116.
10. Joshi, K.; Memoria, M.; Singh, L.; Verma, P.; Barthwal, A. Multi-Modality Medical Image Fusion Using SWT & Speckle Noise Reduction with Bidirectional Exact Pattern Matching Algorithm. In *Disruptive Technologies for Society 5.0*; CRC Press: Boca Raton, FL, USA, 2021; Volume 10, pp. 339–359.
11. Nadeem, M.; Hussain, A.; Munir, A. Fuzzy logic based computational model for speckle noise removal in ultrasound images. *Multimed. Tools Appl.* **2019**, *78*, 18531–18548. [CrossRef]
12. Hermawati, F.A.; Tjandrasa, H.; Suciati, N. Hybrid Speckle Noise Reduction Method for Abdominal Circumference Segmentation of Fetal Ultrasound Images *Int. J. Electr. Comput. Eng.* **2018**, *8*, 2088–8708.
13. Ciongradi, C.I.; Sârbu, I.; Iliescu Halițchi, C.O.; Benchia, D.; Sârbu, K. Fertility of Cryptorchid Testis—An Unsolved Mistery. *Genes* **2021**, *12*, 1894. [CrossRef]
14. Ciongradi, C.I.; Filip, F.; Sârbu, I.; Iliescu Halițchi, C.O.; Munteanu, V.; Candussi, I.L. The Impact of Water and Other Fluids on Pediatric Nephrolithiasis. *Nutrients* **2022**, *14*, 4161. [CrossRef]
15. Duarte-Salazar, C.A.; Castro-Ospina, A.E.; Becerra, M.A.; Delgado-Trejos, E. Speckle noise reduction in ultrasound images for improving the metrological evaluation of biomedical applications: An overview *IEEE Access* **2020**, *8*, 15983–15999. [CrossRef]
16. Sui, X.; Ishikawa, H.; Selesnick, I.W.; Wollstein, G.; Schuman, J.S. Speckle noise reduction in OCT and projection images using hybrid wavelet thresholding. In Proceedings of the 2018 IEEE Signal Processing in Medicine and Biology Symposium, Philadelphia, PA, USA, 1 December 2018; pp. 1–6.
17. SL, S.S. Bayesian Framework-Based Adaptive Hybrid Filtering for Speckle Noise Reduction in Ultrasound Images Via Lion Plus FireFly Algorithm. *J. Digit. Imaging* **2021**, *34*, 1463–1477.
18. Ciongradi, C.I.; Benchia, D.; Stupu, C.A.; Iliescu Halițchi, C.O.; Sârbu, I. Quality of Life in Pediatric Patients with Continent Urinary Diversion-A Single Center Experience. *Int. J. Environ. Res. Public Health* **2022**, *19*, 9628. [CrossRef] [PubMed]
19. Castaneda, R.; Garcia-Sucerquia, J.; Doblas, A. Speckle noise reduction in coherent imaging systems via hybrid median–mean filter. *Opt. Eng.* **2021**, *60*, 123107. [CrossRef]
20. Choi, H.; Jeong, J. Speckle noise reduction in ultrasound images using SRAD and guided filter. In Proceedings of the 2018 International Workshop on Advanced Image Technology, Chiang Mai, Thailand, 7–9 January 2018; Volume 60, pp. 1–4.
21. Rosa, R. Performance analysis of speckle ultrasound image filtering. *Comput. Methods Biomech. Biomed. Eng. Imaging Vis.* **2016**, *4*, 193–201. [CrossRef]
22. Ramesh, T.R.; Lilhore, U.K.; Poongodi, M.; Simaiya, S.; Kaur, A.; Hamdi, M. Predictive Analysis of Heart Disease with Machine learning Approaches. *Malays. J. Comput. Sci.* **2022**, 132–148. [CrossRef]

23. Lilhore, U.K.; Poongodi, M.; Kaur, A.; Simaiya, S.; Algarni, A.D.; Elmannai, H.; Vijayakumar, V.; Tunze, G.B.; Hamdi, M. Hybrid Model for Detection of Cervical Cancer Using Causal Analysis and Machine Learning Techniques. *Comput. Math. Methods Med.* **2022**, *2022*, 4688327. [CrossRef]
24. Popa, Ș.; Apostol, D.; Bîcă, O.; Benchia, D.; Sârbu, I.; Ciongradi, C.I. Prenatally Diagnosed Infantile Myofibroma of Sartorius Muscle-A Differential for Soft Tissue Masses in Early Infancy. *Diagnostics* **2021**, *11*, 2389. [CrossRef] [PubMed]
25. Poongodi, M.; Hamdi, M.; Malviya, M.; Sharma, A.; Dhiman, G.; Vimal, S. Diagnosis and combating COVID-19 using wearable Oura smart ring with deep learning methods. *Pers. Ubiquitous Comput.* **2022**, *26*, 25–35. [CrossRef]
26. Ahila, A.; Poongodi, M.; Hamdi, M.; Bourouis, S.; Rastislav, K.; Mohmed, F. Evaluation of Neuro Images for the Diagnosis of Alzheimer's Disease Using Deep Learning Neural Network. *Front. Public Health* **2022**, *10*, 834032. [CrossRef]
27. Bourouis, S.; Band, S.S.; Mosavi, A.; Agrawal, S.; Hamdi, M. Meta-heuristic algorithm-tuned neural network for breast cancer diagnosis using ultrasound images. *Front. Oncol.* **2022**, *12*, 834028.

Disclaimer/Publisher's Note: The statements, opinions and data contained in all publications are solely those of the individual author(s) and contributor(s) and not of MDPI and/or the editor(s). MDPI and/or the editor(s) disclaim responsibility for any injury to people or property resulting from any ideas, methods, instructions or products referred to in the content.

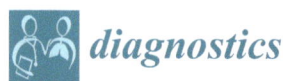

Article

A New Weighted Deep Learning Feature Using Particle Swarm and Ant Lion Optimization for Cervical Cancer Diagnosis on Pap Smear Images

Mohammed Alsalatie [1], Hiam Alquran [2,*], Wan Azani Mustafa [3,4,*], Ala'a Zyout [2], Ali Mohammad Alqudah [2], Reham Kaifi [5,6] and Suhair Qudsieh [7]

[1] King Hussein Medical Center, Royal Jordanian Medical Service, The Institute of Biomedical Technology, Amman 11855, Jordan; mhmdsliti312@gmail.com
[2] Department of Biomedical Systems and Informatics Engineering, Yarmouk University, Irbid 21163, Jordan; alzuet@yu.edu.jo (A.Z.); ali_qudah@hotmail.com (A.M.A.)
[3] Faculty of Electrical Engineering & Technology, Campus Pauh Putra, Universiti Malaysia Perlis, Arau 02600, Malaysia
[4] Advanced Computing (AdvCOMP), Centre of Excellence (CoE), Universiti Malaysia Perlis, Arau 02600, Malaysia
[5] College of Applied Medical Sciences, King Saud Bin Abdulaziz University for Health Sciences, Jeddah 21423, Saudi Arabia
[6] King Abdullah International Medical Research Center, Jeddah 22384, Saudi Arabia
[7] Department of Obstetrics and Gynecology, Faculty of Medicine, Yarmouk University, Irbid 21163, Jordan; suhair.qudsieh@yu.edu.jo
* Correspondence: heyam.q@yu.edu.jo (H.A.); wanazani@unimap.edu.my (W.A.M.)

Abstract: One of the most widespread health issues affecting women is cervical cancer. Early detection of cervical cancer through improved screening strategies will reduce cervical cancer-related morbidity and mortality rates worldwide. Using a Pap smear image is a novel method for detecting cervical cancer. Previous studies have focused on whole Pap smear images or extracted nuclei to detect cervical cancer. In this paper, we compared three scenarios of the entire cell, cytoplasm region, or nucleus region only into seven classes of cervical cancer. After applying image augmentation to solve imbalanced data problems, automated features are extracted using three pre-trained convolutional neural networks: AlexNet, DarkNet 19, and NasNet. There are twenty-one features as a result of these scenario combinations. The most important features are split into ten features by the principal component analysis, which reduces the dimensionality. This study employs feature weighting to create an efficient computer-aided cervical cancer diagnosis system. The optimization procedure uses the new evolutionary algorithms known as Ant lion optimization (ALO) and particle swarm optimization (PSO). Finally, two types of machine learning algorithms, support vector machine classifier, and random forest classifier, have been used in this paper to perform classification jobs. With a 99.5% accuracy rate for seven classes using the PSO algorithm, the SVM classifier outperformed the RF, which had a 98.9% accuracy rate in the same region. Our outcome is superior to other studies that used seven classes because of this focus on the tissues rather than just the nucleus. This method will aid physicians in diagnosing precancerous and early-stage cervical cancer by depending on the tissues, rather than on the nucleus. The result can be enhanced using a significant amount of data.

Keywords: Pap smear images; AlexNet; DarkNet-19; NasNet; support vector machine; random forest; cervical cancer; ant lion optimization; particle swarm optimization

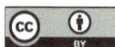

1. Introduction

Cervical cancer is a type of cancer that occurs in the cells of the cervix, the lower part of the uterus that connects to the vagina [1]. Worldwide, cervical cancer is the fourth most common cancer in women and the fourth leading cause of cancer-related deaths in women [1,2]. Most cervical cancers take years to progress to a severe stage; early symptoms are often limited to lower back and abdominal pain. Thus, the cancer may go undetected until it is so advanced that it is unresponsive to treatment [3]. The development of cervical carcinoma is preceded by a premalignant epithelial dysplasia called "cervical intraepithelial neoplasia" (CIN). Therefore, the term dysplasia is used to describe the precancerous changes, which are graded using a scale of one to three (mild, moderate, and severe dysplasia) based on how much of the cervical tissue looks abnormal. Precancerous changes can be detected using the Pap test and treated to prevent cancer from developing. Routine screening allows for the identification of precancerous lesions and early-stage cancers when interventions can be most effective. A Pap smear, also known as a Pap test or cervical cytology, is widely used as a screening procedure to detect cellular abnormalities in the cervix, including precancerous or cancerous changes at an early stage.

Currently, Pap smears are the most common method for identifying abnormal cervical cells [3,4]. Pap smears are prepared with an Ayre spatula or brush that is used to scrape cells from the cervix. Then, the collected cells are spread over a labeled glass slide before being submerged in 95% ethyl alcohol and delivered to pathology for histopathological analysis to look for abnormal cells that may develop into cancer or observe any inflammation or vaginal infections [5,6]. A cervical cell consists of two main components. One is the nucleus, which is in the cell's center and surrounded by cytoplasm. The nucleus is typically compact, nearly spherical, darker than the cytoplasm surrounding it, and intense. Dysplastic cells, also known as aberrant cells, are cells that do not develop and divide properly. Dysplastic cells exist at three levels: mild, moderate, and severe. A large percentage of mild dysplastic cells compared to severe dysplastic cells will resolve spontaneously without developing into malignant ones. The nuclei of squamous dysplastic cells are often bigger and darker and frequently stick together in clusters. The nuclei of severe dysplastic cells are often enlarged, covered in black granules, and malformed [7]. Figure 1 shows a sample of normal and abnormal cells.

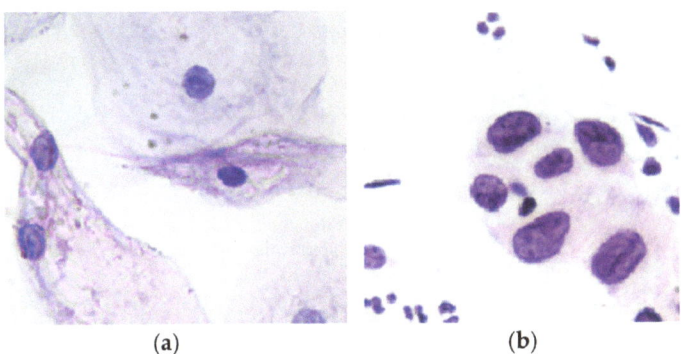

Figure 1. (**a**) Normal Pap smear. (**b**) Abnormal Pap smear 0.201 µm/pixel.

Pap smear image classification is an important method for diagnosing cervical cancer [8]. By analyzing cell images and categorizing the cells into one of seven classes, Pap smears for advanced cervical screening are a highly effective technique for precancerous cell detection. Computer-aided medical imaging systems have considerably benefited from remarkable advances in artificial intelligence (AI) technology [9]. Thus, this paper aims to take advantage of convolutional neural network (CNN) architectures and machine learning to analyze the classification of cervical Pap smear images to improve the reliability of the test results. Current classification systems use extracted nuclei or full Pap smear images to identify cervical cancer; the main limitation of this approach is that first the nuclei must be detected and excluded from images.

2. Literature Review

Many studies have applied computational methods to medical testing to reduce errors in evaluation. Some researchers have investigated the use of traditional machine-learning methods in classifying cervical cells [10]. The computer-assisted detection and classification (CAD) approach for cervical cancer utilizing Pap smear images was proposed by Sukumar et al. [11]. The nuclei cell area was segmented using morphological techniques. From the normal and abnormal cell nucleus, the Grey level, wavelet, and GLCM features were extracted. Using an adaptive neural fuzzy-based classifier (ANFIS) to train and classify these extracted features, they achieved an accuracy of 92.68%. Another study [12] presents the CAD technique for diagnosing cervical cancer utilizing Pap smear images. From Pap smear images, they extract LBP and gray features. The test pap smear cell image was classified into normal or abnormal cell images with a 99.1% accuracy using a hybrid classifier that included SVM and ANFIS. Using morphological techniques, the abnormal cell area was found and segmented.

A new technique for detecting cervical cancer in Pap smear images that show an overlap between the nucleus and inflamed cells was put forth by Muhimmah et al. [13], attaining up to a 95% sensitivity rate. Athinarayanan et al. [14] proposed a system with multiple stages proposed for cancer diagnosis and nuclei extraction. The Pap smear images were first treated to ensure noise removal during the preprocessing stage. These Pap smear images with little noise were used to extract texture features. The suggested system's classification phase came next, using RBF and kernel-based SVM classification with these extracted features. The classification step achieves an accuracy above 94%. On the other hand, Plissiti et al. [15] applied spectral clustering and fuzzy C-means methods for the classification of cervical cells, focusing only on the features extracted from the nucleus, ignoring the cytoplasm. The best classification, 90.58%, was obtained with K-PCA (Gaussian kernel). Mbaga et al. [16] used an SVM classifier in two kernel functions: the radial basis and polynomial kernel functions. The performance of the classifier when using the polynomial kernel was much better and higher when compared to the Gaussian kernel; the best accuracy attained with the polynomial kernel was 97.02% at a polynomial degree value of d = 5. Previous classification techniques have depended on manually extracted features. Zhang et al. [17] introduced a method to classify cervical cells based on deep features using ConvNets CNN. Their method was evaluated on both Pap smear and LBC datasets. When applied to the Herlev benchmark Pap smear dataset and evaluated using five-fold cross-validation, results showed that classification accuracy was 98.3%. An automated, comprehensive machine-learning technique has been proposed by Malli et al. [18]. The proposed technique gives the color and shape features of the nucleus and cytoplasm of the cervix cell. KNN and neural networks were trained with these features, and then unknown cervix cell samples were classified. Results showed an accuracy of 88.04% for KNN and 54% for ANN.

In 2020, Wang et al. [19] designed a PsiNet-TAP network to classify Pap smear images. It was optimized by modifying the convolution layer and pruning some convolution kernels that could interfere with the target classification task. The network was tested on 389 cervical Pap smear images, and the method achieved an accuracy of more than 98%. Ghoneim et al. [20] proposed a system based on a CNN-extreme-learning-machine (ELM) and investigated autoencoder (AE)-based classifiers and multi-layer perceptron (MLP), alternatives to the ELM. Experiments performed using the Herlev database achieved 99.5% accuracy for the detection problem (two classes) and 91.2% for the classification problem (seven classes). Alquran et al. [21] proposed an ensemble machine-learning model with deep learning features extracted using ResNet 10 beside to features selection method. The best accuracy achieved for seven classes was 92%. In another study, Chen et al. [22] suggested using lightweight hybrid loss-constrained CNNs for the classification of cervical cells at the finest level. The proposed combined supervision of hybrid loss function improved the CNNs' ability in categorizing cervical cells. ShufflenetV2 and GhostNet both achieved satisfactory classification using this approach (96.18% accuracy, 96.30% precision, 96.23% recall, and 99.08% specificity for ShufflenetV2 and 96.39% accuracy for GhostNet) [22]. Waly et al. proposed a system that uses intelligent deep CNN by using biomedical Pap smear images. First, they removed noise using a Gaussian filter. Then, they segmented the nuclei using the Tsallis entropy technique with dragonfly optimization and used SqueezeNet to extract features. Finally, classification was performed using weighted ELM. They achieved high accuracy, at 97.81% [23]. Fekri-Ershad and Ramakrishnan [24] suggested an effective multi-stage method for detecting cervical cancer in Pap smear images. First, the cytoplasm, including the nucleus, is removed from the intracellular fluid in the cervix cell using a straightforward thresholding method. The local textural elements are then described using a texture descriptor called modified uniform local ternary patterns (MULTP). Then, to classify the Pap smear images, a multi-layer feed-forward neural network is optimized. Recently, Deepa and Rao (2023) proposed a useful assistive tool for radiologists and clinicians to detect overlapped cervical cells using the CNN model with Rectified Linear Unit (ReLU) classifier. The model used 917 Pap smear cell images from the Herlev Dataset for training and testing, with 96% accuracy [25].

Reviews of the literature indicate that early cancer detection is essential for the treatment process in general; thus, early detection is also crucial for cervical cancer treatment. The Pap smear test is an important screening test for detecting cervical cancer, while the gold standard for diagnosing cervical cancer remains biopsy of cervical tissue. The Pap smear test has limitations. It may not detect all cases of cervical cancer or precancerous lesions. Therefore, regular screening is essential to maximize its effectiveness. The use of artificial intelligence techniques in medical imaging, such as ML, DL, and CNN, has gained popularity in recent years [26]. One constraint, though, is posed by morphological alterations and how they are intertwined with the cells' structural components. Algorithms using DL and ML have significantly improved the healthcare sector. Moreover, deep learning advancements have produced neural network algorithms that can now compete with humans in computer vision-like image classification. Previous studies have focused on whole Pap smear images or on extracted nuclei to detect cervical cancer. This study focused instead on the area surrounding the nucleus, which is affected by the presence or absence of cancerous cells. At times, the nucleus is not clear in Pap smear images. Therefore, the surrounding regions can significantly contribute to the classification task. This study excluded the nucleus from Pap smear images and then classified them based on automated extracted features using deep-learning algorithms, feeding the features into the ML algorithm to discriminate among seven classes of Pap smear images.

3. Materials and Methods

The first step was preparing the image dataset for the system implementation. The approach used for Pap smear image classification is shown in Figure 2: first, the deep-learning algorithms, feature extraction, and feature reduction; then, training the SVM kernel and RF kernel; and finally, the diagnosis of the Pap smear images for all scenarios whole image, without a nucleus, and only nucleus.

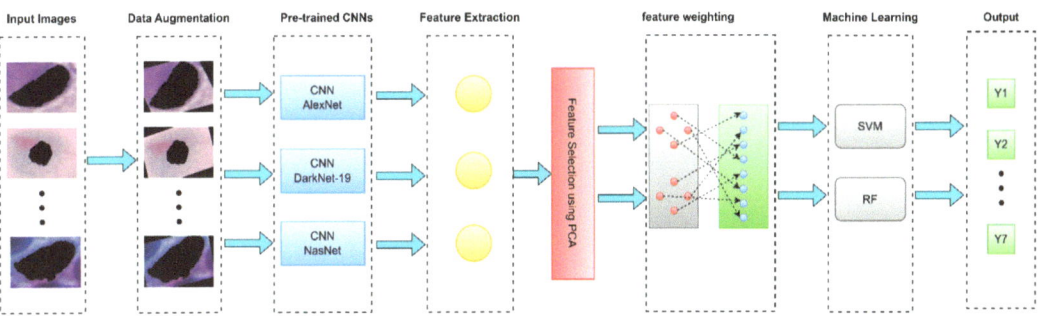

Figure 2. Block diagram of the proposed methodology.

3.1. Dataset

This study used the Herlev Pap smear dataset, consisting of 917 cell images, with each image containing one nucleus. To determine the effect of the surrounding region of the nucleus, the nucleus was excluded from each cell image. The dataset was collected by Herlev University Hospital (Denmark) and the Technical University of Denmark [27]. Table 1 shows the distribution of cervical images for each class; three are normal, and the rest are types of abnormal classes. Figures 3–5 show the normal classes for whole cell, with nucleus exclusion, and with exclusion surrounding region, respectively, while Figures 6–8 represent the abnormal classes for whole cell, with nucleus exclusion, and with exclusion surrounding region, respectively.

Table 1. Distribution of data.

Cell Type (Seven Classes)	Counts
Superficial squamous epithelial (Normal)	74
Intermediate squamous epithelial (Normal)	70
Columnar epithelial (Normal)	98
Mild squamous non-keratinizing dysplasia (Abnormal)	182
Moderate squamous non-keratinizing dysplasia (Abnormal)	146
Severe squamous non-keratinizing dysplasia (Abnormal)	197
Squamous cell carcinoma in situ intermediate (Abnormal)	150

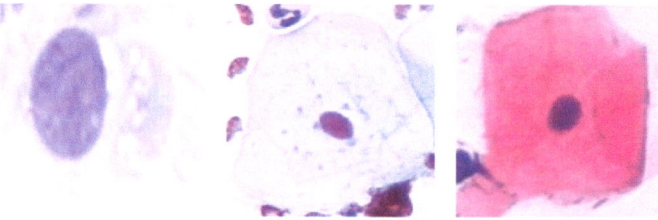

Figure 3. Normal classes for whole cell.

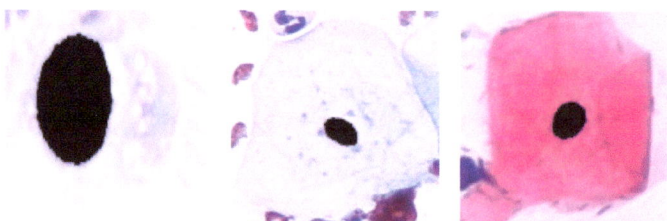

Figure 4. Normal classes with Nucleus exclusion.

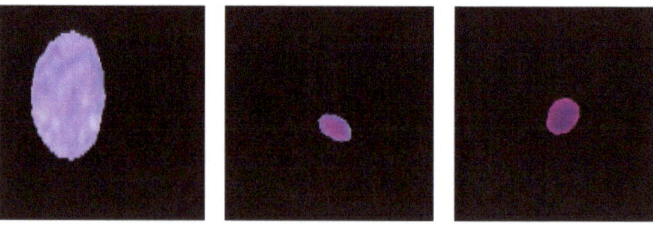

Figure 5. Normal classes with exclusion surrounding region.

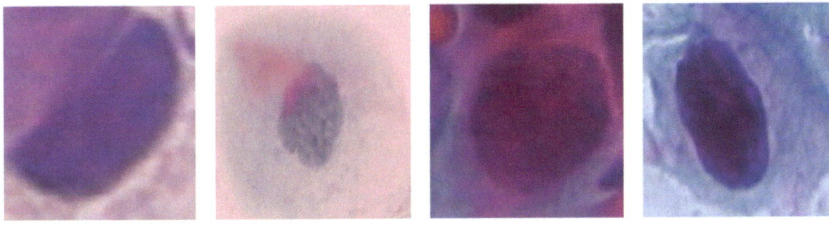

Figure 6. Abnormal classes for whole cell.

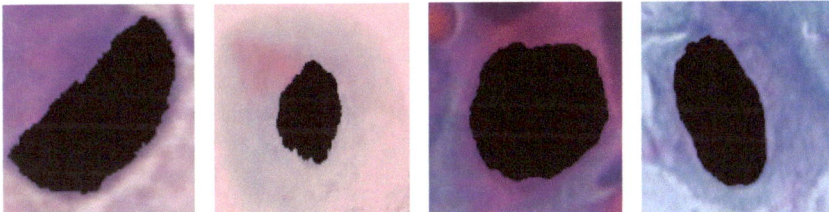

Figure 7. Abnormal Classes with Nucleus exclusion.

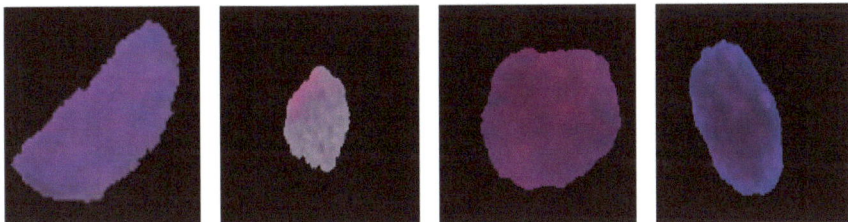

Figure 8. Abnormal Classes with exclusion surrounding region.

3.2. New Image Augmentation

A technique called data augmentation involves adding copies of already existing data that have been significantly altered or product synthetic data that have been generated from already existing data [28]. Data augmentation causes regularization and reduces overfitting. This study applied image augmentation to the dataset by rotating images at random angles between $[-20, 20]$, scaling images using various scale factors within $[0.1, 1]$, and translating images in both X and Y directions between $[-1, 1]$. The count of images before and after augmentation is shown in Table 2.

Table 2. Distribution of the dataset after augmentation.

Cell Type (Seven Classes)	Before Augmentation	After Augmentation
Superficial squamous epithelial (Normal)	74	200
Intermediate squamous epithelial (Normal)	70	200
Columnar epithelial (Normal)	98	200
Mild squamous non-keratinizing dysplasia (Abnormal)	182	200
Moderate squamous non-keratinizing dysplasia (Abnormal)	146	200
Severe squamous non-keratinizing dysplasia (Abnormal)	197	200
Squamous cell carcinoma in situ intermediate (Abnormal)	150	200

The augmentation procedure is performed in the same manner for all scenarios to ensure that the comparison is reasonable and under the same conditions. The number of images increases to 1400 (200 for each class for all cases).

3.3. Deep Learning Features

Deep learning techniques are widely employed across a variety of fields to address a wide range of complicated issues, including computer vision, speech recognition, and image processing. The most frequently used DL algorithms are CNN and Recurrent Neural Networks (RNN) [29]. The necessity for manual feature extraction is eliminated by the ability of CNN to extract the features of the input image. To extract the most representative features, three pre-trained CNN models are applied. The DL structures used were trained on the ImageNet dataset to differentiate among 1000 natural classes. Transfer learning methods were employed to render these structures compatible with the intended problem, which focused on identifying seven categories of cervical cells [26]. Transfer learning appeared by changing the image input size to be suitable with the input layer of each one and eliminating the last completely connected layer to leave seven neurons for seven classes. AlexNet, DarkNet-19, and Nasnet were used for feature extraction.

3.3.1. AlexNet

DL algorithms assist in automatically extracting features from a large dataset. The first CNN to use a GPU to improve performance was AlexNet. Five convolutional layers, three max-pooling layers, two normalization layers, two fully connected layers, and a single softmax layer make up the AlexNet architecture. The input size is typically stated as $224 \times 224 \times 3$, but, due to padding, it comes out to be $227 \times 227 \times 3$. To be appropriate through the first input layer, all images were modified [30]. Here, the top seven features are automatically extracted using the transfer learning strategy (Figure 9).

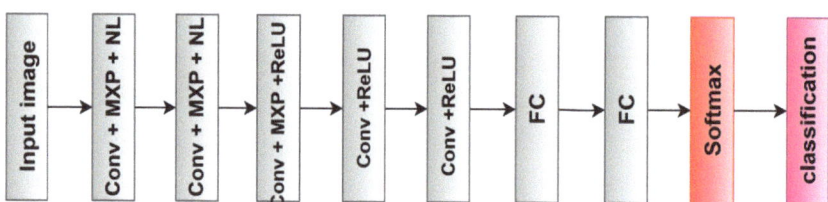

Figure 9. AlexNet architecture [30].

3.3.2. DarkNet-19

The CNN with 19 layers is known as DarkNet19. DarkNet19 consists of five max-pooling layers and 19 convolutional layers, ranging from many 1×1 CL to the smallest triangle parameters comprising 3×3. The deep feature was extracted at this stage using DarkNet19. Additionally, the input layer image size for DarkNet19 is 256×256. Figure 10 displays the structure of the neural network of DarkNet19 [31].

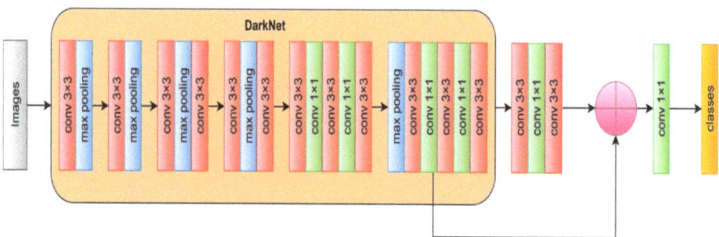

Figure 10. The structure of DarkNet-19 [32].

3.3.3. NasNet

NasNet is a new, optimizable deep neural network based on the reinforcement learning approach, which is the parent artificial intelligence (AI), making corrections and modifications of the weights, number of layers regularization methods of the child of AI. Its architecture is composed of two main blocks: controller recurrent neural network (CRNN) and CNN. There are three different versions: A, B, and C. Figure 11 demonstrates its basic idea [33]. In this stage, transfer learning is used, and the last layers are used to extract seven features.

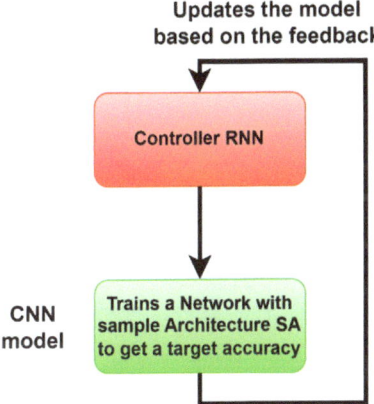

Figure 11. Controller RNN in NASNet architecture [33].

3.4. Principal Component Analysis (PCA)

The fundamental principle behind utilizing PCA as a feature selection method is to choose variables based on the magnitude (from biggest to lowest in absolute values) of the coefficients. Each variable contributes differently to each of the primary components, which are ranked in importance by their explained variance [34].

All previously pre-trained CNNs' 21 collected features are processed, and the 10 most promising features are chosen for additional processing and diagnosis. These independent features came from six NasNet features, two DarkNet-19 features, and the remaining features from AlexNet. The features reduction method is described in Table 3, and works by examining the number of features from each pretrained model, the total extracted features from all used CNN models by combination the extracted features, applying PCA, and then the most significant features by displaying the number of candidates features from each model.

Table 3. Number of features before and after PCA.

Pre-Trained Model	Number of Extracted Features	The Combination of Whole Features	Using PCA
AlexNet	7		2
DarkNet-19	7	21 features	2
NasNet	7		6
	21 features	21 features	10 features

3.5. Feature Weighting Method

The feature weighting aims to determine the relative value of each feature in relation to the classification job and provide it an appropriate weight. A vital feature would be given a higher weight than a less significant or irrelevant feature if the weighting were conducted appropriately. Feature weighting employs a continuous value and, as a result, has a higher degree of detail in assessing the relevance of feature rather than making a binary decision. It works better for tasks where certain features are more important than others [35].

Using the strategy of ant and lion hunting, Seyedali Mirjalili introduced ALO in 2015 [36]. The ALO algorithm is used to simultaneously obtain the best feature weights and parameter values for neural networks. The five main steps of this hunting strategy are the random walk of agents, trapping ants in a trap, building traps, tearing them down, and catching prey. Numerous ant lions and ants with randomly placed locations are present throughout the search area. Ants will travel randomly throughout the search area, potentially going through or around the traps, to mimic how ant lions and ants interact. The more skilled individual or "ant lion" will dig a deeper, sharper pit, and capture more ants. Ant lions, specifically the elite (best) ant lion, influence the random movements of ants. To ensure the variety and optimization ability of the algorithm, ants will change their positions according to ant lion and elite ant lion [37,38].

The Particle Swarm Optimization (PSO) starts by randomly initializing the particle positions. The fitness value of each particle was then determined based on the assessment function. Until the desired state is attained, this procedure will keep iterating. Each particle is impacted by two values during each iteration. The first is best value any particle has ever attained. The second value is the best overall value that all particles in the sample have. The particles updated their velocity and positions after achieving the two best results [39].

3.6. Classification

3.6.1. Support Vector Machine

SVM is a well-known ML approach that is used for both classification and regression. The SVM algorithm's objective is to establish the best line or decision boundary that can divide n-dimensional space into classes, allowing the quick classification of new data points. This optimal decision boundary is called a hyperplane. SVM selects the extreme vectors and points that aid in the creation of a hyperplane. Support vectors, which are used to represent these extreme instances, form the basis of the SVM method. Consider the diagram below, where a decision boundary or hyperplane is used to categorize two distinct categories. SVM uses the kernel trick, which maps the features to higher dimensional space to find the appropriate training model that can be generalized. The polynomial kernel is exploited in this study [40–42]. Figure 12 illustrates the principle of SVM.

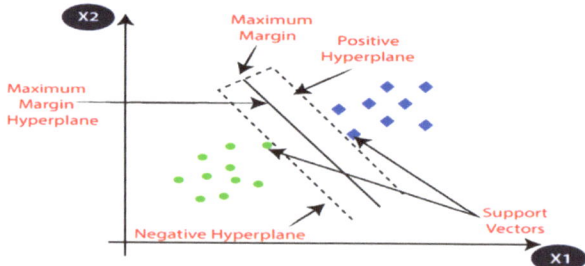

Figure 12. The principal operation of SVM classifier [40].

3.6.2. Random Forest (RF)

The decision tree (DT) is the random forest classifier's unit block. Each RF is made up of numerous independent DTs that work together to form an ensemble classifier. Several decision trees are grown and combined in the RF model to form a "forest." Another kind of algorithm used to categorize data is the decision tree. In the simplest terms, it works like a flowchart that shows a clear path to a choice or result; it begins at one point and branches out in two or more ways, with each direction giving a range of potential possibilities. While the trees are developing, the random forest adds more randomness to the model. When dividing a node, it looks for the best feature from a random subset of features rather than the most crucial one. A better model is often produced because of the great diversity caused by this process. Figure 13 describes the principal operation of RF classifier [43].

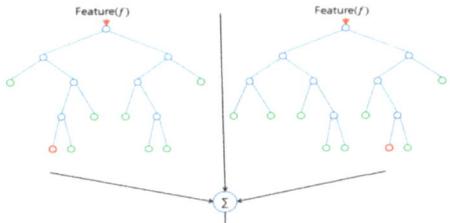

Figure 13. The principal operation of RF classifier [43].

4. Results

4.1. Ant Lion Optimization

Using ALO weighting algorithm after feature selection, we conducted three experiments, where once the image was whole, another time we segmented the nucleus, and the last one we excluded the nucleus. This method's main steps include data augmentation, automatic feature extraction utilizing transfer learning from several CNN structures, feature reduction via PCA, and a novel feature weighting technique. The 10 most significant features were extracted. These graphical features were ordered as follows: six features from NasNet, two from Darknet-19, and two from AlexNet. This distribution of the most significant features demonstrated that the NasNet extracted the most relevant features for classes and that is compatible with its deep structure. The K-fold cross validation techniques are used. Both SVM and RF were used to classify the images into seven classes based on the selected automated graphical features. A confusion matrix is a table that lists how many predictions a classifier made correctly and incorrectly. It is employed to evaluate a classification model's effectiveness. With the measurement of performance metrics like accuracy, precision, recall, and F1-score, it can be utilized to assess a classification model's effectiveness [38]. Figure 14 illustrates the results of the confusion matrix of RF with ALO weighting method.

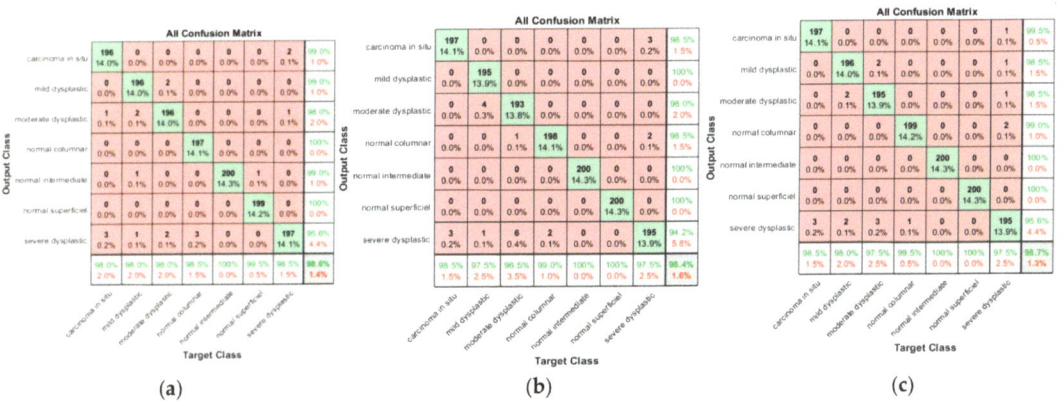

Figure 14. Confusion matrix for ALO-RF for various scenarios; (**a**) For nucleus only, (**b**) Whole cell exclusion, (**c**) for nucleus only.

By using the corresponding matrices [42], the evaluation of the classifiers are performed.

$$Accuracy = \frac{TP + TN}{TP + FN + FP + TN}$$

$$Precision = \frac{TP}{TP + FP}$$

$$Sensitivity = \frac{TP}{TP + FN}$$

$$F1 - Score = \frac{2 \times Precision \times Sensitivity}{Precision + Sensitivity}$$

Figure 14a shows that 196 carcinomas in situ cases were classified correctly, with three cases misclassified as severe and one as dysplastic. The sensitivity obtained was 98%, and the positive predictive value was 99%. From 200 mild dysplastic cases, 196 were classified correctly, with a true positive rate of 98%. There were four misclassified cases: two as moderate dysplastic and two as normal and severe dysplastic, respectively. The precision of the mild category was 99%. The results for moderate dysplastic were 98% as recall and PPV was 98%. For normal columnar, the sensitivity was 98.5%, with three cases misclassified cases one as severe dysplastic. On the other hand, the precision was 98%. However, promising results were achieved in normal intermediate normal columnar and normal superficial classes, with almost 100% recall and precision. The last class was severe superficial; here, the lowest sensitivity reached 95.6%, with three cases misclassified as carcinoma in situ, one misclassified as mild dysplastic, two misclassified as moderate dysplastic, and three as normal intermediate. The proposed approach provides promising results, with an accuracy of 98.6% and an overall misclassification rate of 1.4%.

Figure 14b shows that one hundred and ninety-seven carcinomas in situ cases were classified correctly, with three cases misclassified as severe dysplastic. The sensitivity and precision obtained were 98.6%. Four mild dysplastic cases were misclassified as moderate dysplastic and 195 out of 200 mild dysplastic cases were classified correctly, with a true positive rate of 97.5. The precision of the mild category was 100%. The results for moderate dysplastic were 96.5% as recall, with six misclassified cases as severe and one as columnar. In addition, the PPV was 98%, where four mild dysplastic cases were incorrectly classified as moderate. For normal columnar, the sensitivity was 99%, with two cases misclassified as severe. On the other hand, the precision was 98.5%, with two cases classified as severe and one as moderate dysplastic. However, promising results were achieved in both normal intermediate and normal superficial classes, with 100% recall and precision. The last class was severe superficial; here, the sensitivity reached to 97.5%, with three cases misclassified as carcinoma in situ and two misclassified as normal columnar. However, the moderate precision obtained in the severe dysplastic class reached 94.2%. The proposed approach provides promising results, with an accuracy of 98.4% and an overall misclassification rate of 1.6%.

Figure 14c shows that 190 of 200 carcinomas in situ cases were classified correctly, with three cases misclassified as sever dysplastic. The sensitivity obtained was 98.5%, and the positive predictive value was 99.5%. Of 200 mild dysplastic cases, 196 were classified correctly, with a true positive rate of 98%, with four misclassified cases: two as moderate dysplastic and the other two as severe dysplastic. The precision of the mild category was 98%. The results for moderate dysplastic were 97.5% as recall and PPV was 98.5%, where two mild dysplastic cases were incorrectly classified as moderate and another one as severe. For normal columnar, the sensitivity was 99.5%, with one case misclassified as severe. On the other hand, the precision was 99%, with two cases classified as severe. However, promising results were achieved in both normal intermediate and normal superficial classes, with 100% recall and precision. The last class was severe superficial, where sensitivity reached 97.5%, with five cases misclassified as carcinoma in situ, mild, moderate, and two misclassified as normal columnar. The proposed approach provides promising results, with an accuracy of 98.7% and an overall misclassification rate of 1.3%.

As is clear from Figure 15a, 198 cases were classified correctly among 200 cases, with two cases misclassified as severe dysplastic. The obtained sensitivity was 99%, and the positive predictive value was 98.5%. Two severe dysplastic cases were misclassified as carcinoma in situ. Of 200 mild dysplastic cases, 196 were classified correctly, with a true positive rate of 98%; there were only four misclassified cases (one as moderate and three as severe). The precision of the mild category was 99.5%. The maintained results for moderate dysplastic are 97.5% as recall and two misclassified case, as mild and three cases as severe dysplastic. In addition, the PPV was 99%; one severe dysplastic case and one mild case were classified as moderate. For normal columnar, normal intermediate, and normal superficial, the promising results were obtained with the highest sensitivity and a precision of 100%. The last class was severe superficial, with a sensitivity reaching 97.5%, with three cases being misclassified as carcinoma in situ, one as normal columnar, and one as moderate. However, the precision in the severe dysplastic class reached 96.1%. The proposed approach provided promising results, with an accuracy of 98.9% and an overall misclassification rate reaching 1.1%.

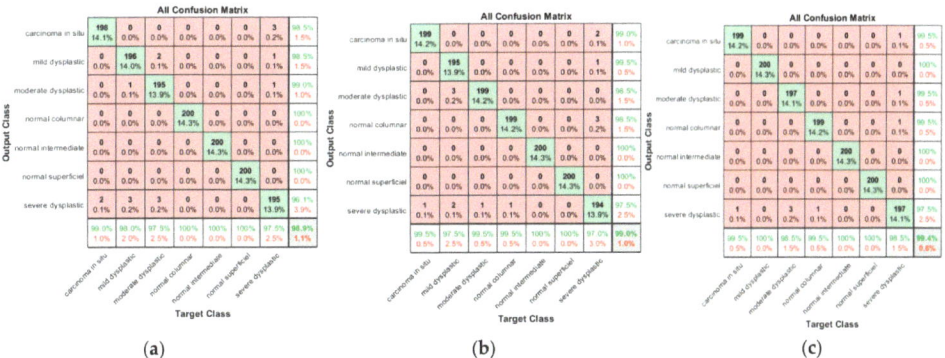

Figure 15. Confusion matrix for ALO-SVM for various scenarios; (a) for nucleus exclusion (b) For Whole cell, (c) for nucleus only.

As is clear from Figure 15b, 199 carcinomas in situ cases were classified correctly among 200 cases, with one case misclassified as severe dysplastic. The obtained sensitivity was 99.5%, and the positive predictive value was 99%. While two severe dysplastic was misclassified as carcinoma in situ, 195 mild dysplastic cases were classified correctly, with a true positive rate of 97.5%; there were only five misclassified cases: three as moderate dysplastic and the other as severe dysplastic. The precision of the mild category was 99.5%. Just one severe case was misclassified as mild dysplastic. The maintained results for moderate dysplastic are 99.5% as recall and one misclassified case as mild. In addition, the PPV was 98.3%, where three mild was incorrectly classified as moderate. For normal columnar, the sensitivity was 99.5%, with one case misclassified as severe. Nevertheless, the precision obtained in the columnar class was 98.5%, with three severe cases being misclassified as normal columnar. However, promising results were obtained in both normal intermediate and normal superficial classes, with 100% recall and precision. The last class was severe superficial, with a sensitivity reaching 97%, with one case being misclassified as carcinoma in situ, two as mild, with three misclassified cases as normal columnar. However, the precision obtained in the severe dysplastic class reached 97.5%. The proposed approach provided promising results, with an accuracy of 99% and an overall misclassification rate reaching 1%.

As is clear from Figure 15c, 199 carcinoma in situ cases were classified correctly from 200 cases, with one case misclassified as severe dysplastic. The obtained sensitivity was

99.5%, and the positive predictive value was 99%. One severe dysplastic was misclassified as carcinoma in situ. The promising results in mild dysplastic cases showed 200 cases classified correctly, with a true positive rate of 100%. The precision of the mild category was 100%. The maintained results for moderate dysplastic are 98.5% as recall, with three cases misclassified as severe. In addition, the PPV was 99.5%, where one severe dysplastic case was incorrectly classified as moderate. For normal columnar, the sensitivity was 99.5%, with one case misclassified as severe and one as carcinoma in situ. The precision obtained in the columnar class was 99.5%. Promising results were obtained in both normal, intermediate, and normal superficial classes, with 100% recall and precision. The last class was severe superficial, with a sensitivity reaching 98.5%. Three cases were misclassified as carcinoma in situ, one as moderate, and one as normal columnar. The lowest precision obtained in the severe dysplastic class reached 97.5%, where five cases were misclassified as severe dysplastic: three from moderate, one from carcinoma in situ, and one from normal columnar. The proposed approach provided promising results, with an accuracy of 99.4% and an overall misclassification rate reaching 0.6%.

4.2. Particle Swarm Optimization

The same selected features are weighted swarm optimization method for various scenarios. The following confusion matrices illustrated the outcomes of the RF and SVM.

Figure 16a shows that 199 carcinomas in situ cases were classified correctly, with one case misclassified as sever dysplastic. The sensitivity obtained was 99.5%, and the positive predictive value was 99%. Of 200 mild dysplastic cases, 189 were classified correctly, with a true positive rate of 94.5%; there were eleven cases misclassified as severe dysplastic. The precision of the mild category was 96.9%. The best achieved results in sensitivity term for moderate dysplastic, normal columnar, and normal superficial were 100%; the same value in precision was achieved, but the moderate achieved 98.5%, where three case were misclassified as moderate (one from carcinoma in situ, one from normal columnar, and the last one comes from severe dysplastic). The last class was severe dysplastic; here, the sensitivity reached 95.0%, with five cases misclassified as mild, two as carcinoma in situ, two misclassified as moderate dysplastic, and one as normal intermediate. The proposed approach provides promising results, with an accuracy of 98.1% and an overall misclassification rate of 1.9%.

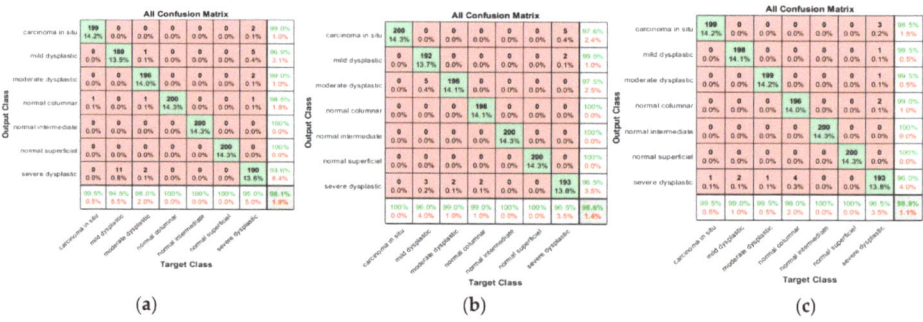

Figure 16. Confusion matrix for SVM for various scenarios; (**a**) for nucleus only (**b**) For Whole cell, (**c**) for nucleus exclusion.

As is clear from Figure 16b, 200 carcinomas in situ cases were classified correctly among 200 cases, with an obtained sensitivity of 100%; the positive predictive value was 97.6%. Five severe dysplastic was misclassified as carcinoma in situ, one hundred ninety-two mild dysplastic cases were classified correctly, with a true positive rate of 96%; three cases were misclassified as severe dysplastic. The precision of the mild category was 99.0%; two severe class were misclassified as mild dysplastic. The maintained results for moderate dysplastic are 99% as recall and two misclassified cases as severe. In addition, the PPV was

97.5%, with five mild cases incorrectly classified as moderate. For normal columnar, the sensitivity was 99.0%, with two cases misclassified as severe. Nevertheless, the precision obtained in the columnar class was 100%. Promising results were obtained in both normal intermediate and normal superficial classes, with 100% recall and precision. The last class was severe superficial, with a sensitivity reaching 96.5%, with five cases being misclassified as carcinoma in situ and two as mild. The precision obtained in the severe dysplastic class reached 96.5%. The proposed approach provided promising results, with an accuracy of 98.6% and an overall misclassification rate reaching 1.4%.

Figure 16c shows that 199 of 200 carcinomas in situ cases were classified correctly, with one case misclassified as severe dysplastic. The sensitivity obtained was 99.5%, and the positive predictive value was 98.5%. Of 200 mild dysplastic cases, 198 were classified correctly, with a true positive rate of 99%; two misclassified cases were classified as severe dysplastic. The precision of the mild category was 99.5%. The results for moderate dysplastic were 99.5% as recall and PPV was 99.5%, where one mild dysplastic case was incorrectly classified severe. For normal columnar, the sensitivity was 98%, with four cases misclassified as severe. The precision was 99%, with two cases classified as severe. Promising results were achieved in both normal intermediate and normal superficial classes, with 100% recall and precision. The last class was severe superficial. Sensitivity reached 96.5%, with three cases misclassified as carcinoma in situ, one as mild, one as moderate, and two misclassified as normal columnar. The proposed approach provides promising results, with an accuracy of 98.9% and an overall misclassification rate of 1.

As is clear from Figure 17a, 198 cases were classified correctly among 200 cases, with two cases misclassified as severe dysplastic. The obtained sensitivity was 99%, and the positive predictive value was 98.5%. Three severe dysplastic were misclassified as carcinoma in situ. Of 200 mild dysplastic cases, 196 were classified correctly, with a true positive rate of 98%. There were four misclassified cases (two as moderate, one as normal intermediate, and one as severe). The precision of the mild category was 99.5%. The maintained results for moderate dysplastic are 97.5% as recall and four cases were misclassified as severe dysplastic. The PPV was 99%, and two mild cases were classified as moderate. For normal columnar the sensitivity is 100% and precision is 99.5%. For normal intermediate and normal superficial, promising results were obtained with the highest sensitivity and precision of almost 100%. The last class was severe superficial, with a sensitivity reaching 98%, with three cases being misclassified as carcinoma in situ and one as normal columnar and one as moderate. The precision in the severe dysplastic class reached 96.6%. The proposed approach provided promising results, with an accuracy of 98.8% and an overall misclassification rate reaching 1.2%.

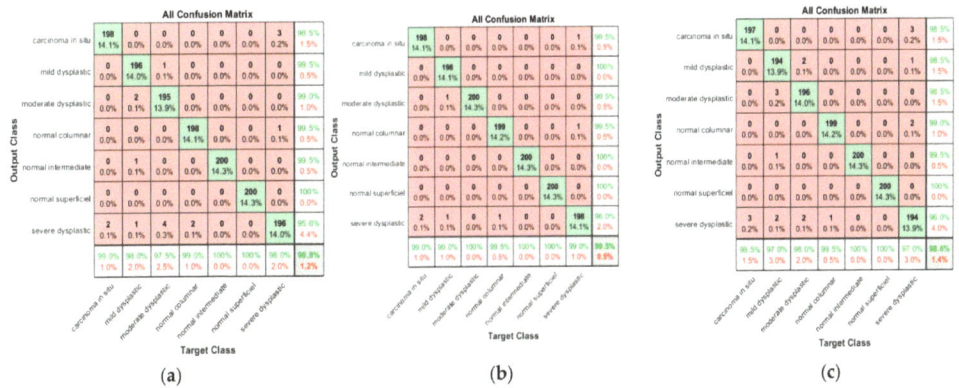

Figure 17. Confusion matrix for SVM for various scenarios; (**a**) for nucleus exclusion, (**b**) For Whole cell, (**c**) for nucleus only.

As is clear from Figure 17b, 198 carcinomas in situ cases were classified correctly among 200 cases, with obtained sensitivity was 99%; the positive predictive value was 99.5%. While one severe dysplastic was misclassified as carcinoma in situ, 198 mild dysplastic cases were classified correctly, with a true positive rate of 99%, with only one misclassified as severe dysplastic. The precision of the mild category was 100%. The maintained result for moderate dysplastic are 100% as recall. The PPV was 99.5%, where one mild case was incorrectly classified as moderate. For normal columnar, the sensitivity was 99.5%, with one case misclassified as severe. The precision obtained in the columnar class was 99.5%. Promising results were obtained in both normal intermediate and normal superficial classes, with 100% recall and precision. The last class was severe superficial, with a sensitivity reaching 99%, with one case being misclassified as carcinoma in situ and one case as normal columnar. The precision obtained in the severe dysplastic class reached 98%. The proposed approach provided promising results, with an accuracy of 99.5% and an overall misclassification rate reaching 0.5%.

Figure 17c shows that 197 of 200 carcinomas in situ cases were classified correctly, with three cases misclassified as severe dysplastic. The sensitivity obtained was 98.5%, and the positive predictive value was 98.5%. Of 200 mild dysplastic cases, 194 were classified correctly, with a true positive rate of 97%; two cases were misclassified as severe dysplastic and three misclassified cases as moderate. The precision of the mild category was 98.5%. The results for moderate dysplastic were 98.0% as recall and PPV was 98.5%, with three mild dysplastic case incorrectly classified as moderate. For normal columnar, the sensitivity was 99.5%, with one case misclassified as severe. The precision was 99%, with two cases misclassified as severe. Promising results were achieved in both normal intermediate and normal superficial classes, with almost 100% recall and precision. The last class was severe superficial. Sensitivity reached 97%, with three cases misclassified as carcinoma in situ, one as mild, and two misclassified as normal columnar. The proposed approach provides promising results, with an accuracy of 98.6% and an overall misclassification rate of 1.4%.

It is obvious from the previous discussion that the performance of Swarm optimization after feature selection is better than ALO, either in SVM or RF classifiers. The best scenario is obtained in nucleus exclusion case. This indicates the effectiveness of the surrounding region on the diagnosis of the cervical cells.

As is clear from previous results, the combination of automated features with the ML classifiers beside various weighting algorithms was capable of distinguishing among various classes of cervical cells, thus establishing the effectiveness of focusing the difference of using whole cell, nucleus exclusion, and nucleus only. The results of using the two types of classifiers with deep features with NasNet and the most common pre-trained CNNs AlexNet and DarkNet-19 beside two types of optimization techniques are compared with the literature. Table 4 represents the study, the proposed method, number of classes, the data set used, and their results.

As is clear from the table, the proposed method is capable of distinguishing among the seven classes. This study encourages the use of cytoplasm features instead of whole cell or nucleus region, which is easier than studying the nuclei in Pap smear cells. This study may lead to a good approach in cases where the shape of the nucleus cannot be handled or is unreachable by various image processing techniques and in which taking patches from the cytoplasm and passing the proposed model can expect or guide the class of the Pap smear image sample. The proposed approach achieved the highest accuracy among literature either using whole cell or without nucleus. The maintained results approved the ability of the proposed method to diagnose cervical cells into seven classes without further processing to segment the nucleus. The diagnosis can be performed using cytoplasm or whole cell. This approach yields to preserves time and effort.

Table 4. The comparison between the proposed study and the literature.

Ref.	Method	Number of Classes	Type of Dataset	Result
[11]	Shape and gray co-occurrence features; they employed the adaptive neuro fuzzy inference system	Normal and Abnormal	Herlev	Accuracy reached 92.68%
[12]	Utilized texture features for processed Pap smear images	Normal and Abnormal	Herlev	Accuracy reached 99.1%
[14]	Texture features of nucleus	Normal and Abnormal	Herlev	Accuracy reached 94%
[15]	Spectral features of the nucleus with K-PCA	Normal and Abnormal	Herlev	Accuracy reached 90.58%
[17]	Deep features, using ConvNets CNN	Normal and Abnormal	Herlev	Accuracy reached 98.3%
[18]	Color and shape features of nucleus and cytoplasm of the cervix cell beside machine learning	Normal and Abnormal	Herlev	Accuracy reached 88.04%
[20]	CNN-ELM-based system and an autoencoder (AE)-based classifiers and multi-layer perceptron (MLP),	Seven classes	Herlev	Accuracy reached 91.2%
[21]	Deep features with feature selection combined with ensemble machine learning model	Seven classes	Herlev	Accuracy reached 92%
[22]	Hybrid Loss-Constrained Lightweight Convolutional Neural Networks for Cervical Cell Classification	Seven classes	Herlev	Accuracy reached 96.39%
[23]	Optimal deep convolution neural network for cervical cancer diagnosis model	Seven classes	Herlev	Accuracy reached 97.81%
[24]	Uniform local ternary patterns and feed forward multilayer network optimized by genetic algorithm	Seven classes	Herlev	-
[25]	Classification of normal and abnormal overlapped squamous cells in Pap smear image	Seven classes	Herlev	Accuracy reached 96%
This Study	**Deep features with feature weighting method (ALO, PSO)**	Seven classes	Herlev	Accuracy reached **99.5%**

5. Conclusions

A new method that may lower the mortality rate from cervical cancer among women is the detection of the disease using Pap smear images. Determination of the type of cervical cancer depends on the cell nuclei visible in a Pap smear image. Sometimes, however, the nuclei may be difficult to visualize, in which case the area surrounding the nucleus may help in the diagnosis of Pap smear images. This study aims to compare the performance of using whole cell, nucleus region, or cytoplasm region only in order to distinguish the type of cervical cell, due to some limitations on segmentation of nucleus and the challenges of delineating the nucleus region. Therefore, the proposed approach focuses on comparing the effectiveness of three scenarios: whole cell, surrounding region, and nucleus only. The proposed approach does not require pre-processing of the images. This study directed the most significant automated features at the region surrounding the nucleus, nucleus, and whole cell. Based on our knowledge, this is the first study comparing the various types of regions for seven classes beside utilizing various optimization algorithms (AntLion and swarm optimization methods). The obtained results enhance the capability of the researcher to take a patchy image from the cytoplasm and diagnose the pap smear images without requiring additional processing around the nucleus features or whole cell properties. The proposed system achieved an accuracy for seven classes of 99.5% using the SVM classifier and swarm optimization, after selecting the ten most significant deep features, the weighting algorithm optimize the effectiveness of each feature to distinguishing of various classes. These features are intrinsic to each class because they are automated, deeply extracted, graphical features. The utilization of feature-reduction techniques and weighting algorithms enhance the accuracy beside to complexity and computation time. This automated system may help physicians when the nucleus is not clear to include the whole cell or the surrounding regions only. This CAD system can be beneficial to the doctors and physicians in rural countries.

Author Contributions: Conceptualization, M.A. and H.A.; methodology, M.A., H.A. and A.M.A.; software, M.A., A.Z., A.M.A. and H.A.; validation, H.A., A.Z. and W.A.M.; formal analysis, H.A., A.Z.; investigation, A.Z., H.A., M.A. and W.A.M.; resources, A.Z.; data curation, A.Z.; writing—original draft preparation, A.Z., H.A., W.A.M., M.A., A.M.A. and S.Q.; writing—review and editing, R.K., W.A.M. and S.Q.; visualization, R.K., A.Z. and H.A.; supervision, H.A.; project administration, H.A.; funding acquisition, H.A. and W.A.M. All authors have read and agreed to the published version of the manuscript.

Funding: This work was supported funding by the Ministry of Higher Education Malaysia under the Fundamental Research Grant Scheme (FRGS/1/2021/SKK0/UNIMAP/02/1).

Institutional Review Board Statement: Not applicable.

Informed Consent Statement: Not applicable.

Data Availability Statement: The dataset analyzed during the current study was derived from the Herlev Pap Smear dataset, which consists of 917 manually isolated Pap smear cell images. This dataset has been publicly available online since 2006. It is available on the corresponding website: (http://mde-lab.aegean.gr/index.php/downloads) (accessed on 10 March 2021).

Conflicts of Interest: The authors declare no conflict of interest.

References

1. Bora, K.; Chowdhury, M.; Mahanta, L.B.; Kundu, M.K.; Das, A.K. Automated classification of Pap smear images to detect cervical dysplasia. *Comput. Methods Programs Biomed.* **2017**, *138*, 31–47. [CrossRef] [PubMed]
2. Sung, H.; Ferlay, J.; Siegel, R.L.; Laversanne, M.; Soerjomataram, I.; Jemal, A.; Bray, F. Global cancer statistics 2020: GLOBOCAN estimates of incidence and mortality worldwide for 36 cancers in 185 countries. *CA Cancer J. Clin.* **2021**, *71*, 209–249. [CrossRef] [PubMed]
3. Tsai, M.-H.; Chan, Y.-K.; Lin, Z.-Z.; Yang-Mao, S.-F.; Huang, P.-C. Nucleus and cytoplast contour detector of cervical smear image. *Pattern Recognit. Lett.* **2008**, *29*, 1441–1453. [CrossRef]
4. William, W.; Ware, A.; Basaza-Ejiri, A.H.; Obungoloch, J. A pap-smear analysis tool (PAT) for detection of cervical cancer from pap-smear images. *Biomed. Eng. Online* **2019**, *18*, 16. [CrossRef] [PubMed]
5. Sachan, P.L.; Singh, M.; Patel, M.L.; Sachan, R. A Study on cervical cancer screening using pap smear test and clinical correlation. *Asia-Pacific J. Oncol. Nurs.* **2018**, *5*, 337–341. [CrossRef] [PubMed]
6. Thippeveeranna, C.; Mohan, S.S.; Singh, L.R.; Singh, N.N. Knowledge, Attitude and Practice of the Pap Smear as a Screening Procedure Among Nurses in a Tertiary Hospital in North Eastern India. *Asian Pac. J. Cancer Prev.* **2013**, *14*, 849–885. [CrossRef] [PubMed]

7. Taha, B.; Dias, J.; Werghi, N. Classification of cervical-cancer using pap-smear images: A convolutional neural network approach. In Proceedings of the Medical Image Understanding and Analysis: 21st Annual Conference, MIUA 2017, Edinburgh, UK, 11–13 July 2017; Springer International Publishing: Berlin/Heidelberg, Germany; pp. 261–272.
8. Liu, W.; Li, C.; Xu, N.; Jiang, T.; Rahaman, M.M.; Sun, H.; Wu, X.; Hu, W.; Chen, H.; Sun, C.; et al. CVM-Cervix: A hybrid cervical Pap-smear image classification framework using CNN, visual transformer and multilayer perceptron. *Pattern Recognit.* **2022**, *130*, 108829. [CrossRef]
9. Alias, N.A.; Mustafa, W.A.; Jamlos, M.A.; Alquran, H.; Hanafi, H.F.; Ismail, S.; Ab Rahman, K.S. Pap Smear Images Classification Using Machine Learning: A Literature Matrix. *Diagnostics* **2022**, *12*, 2900. [CrossRef]
10. Diniz, D.N.; Rezende, M.T.; Bianchi, A.G.C.; Carneiro, C.M.; Luz, E.J.S.; Moreira, G.J.P.; Ushizima, D.; Medeiros, F.; Souza, M.J.F. A deep learning ensemble method to assist cytopathologists in pap test image classification. *J. Imaging* **2021**, *7*, 111. [CrossRef]
11. Sukumar, P.; Gnanamurthy, R.K. Computer Aided Detection of Cervical Cancer Using Pap Smear Images Based on Adaptive Neuro Fuzzy Inference System Classifier. *J. Med. Imaging Health Inform.* **2016**, *6*, 312–319. [CrossRef]
12. Sukumar, P.; Gnanamurthy, R.K. Computer aided detection of cervical cancer using Pap smear images based on hybrid classifier. *Int. J. Appl. Eng. Res. Res. India Publ.* **2015**, *10*, 21021–21032.
13. Muhimmah, I.; Kurniawan, R. Analysis of features to distinguish epithelial cells and inflammatory cells in Pap smear images. In Proceedings of the 2013 6th International Conference on Biomedical Engineering and Informatics, Hangzhou, China, 16–18 December 2013; pp. 519–523.
14. Athinarayanan, S.; Srinath, M.V. Robust and efficient diagnosis of cervical cancer in Pap smear images using textures features with RBF and kernel SVM classification. *System* **2006**, *6*, 8.
15. Plissiti, M.E.; Nikou, C. Cervical cell classification based exclusively on nucleus features. In Proceedings of the Image Analysis and Recognition: 9th International Conference, ICIAR 2012, Aveiro, Portugal, 25–27 June 2012; Springer: Berlin/Heidelberg, Germany Part II. ; pp. 483–490.
16. Mbaga, A.H.; ZhiJun, P. Pap smear images classification for early detection of cervical cancer. *Int. J. Comput. Appl.* **2015**, *118*, 10–16.
17. Zhang, L.; Lu, L.; Nogues, I.; Summers, R.M.; Liu, S.; Yao, J. DeepPap: Deep Convolutional Networks for Cervical Cell Classification. *IEEE J. Biomed. Health Inform.* **2017**, *21*, 1633–1643. [CrossRef] [PubMed]
18. Malli, P.K.; Nandyal, S. Machine learning technique for detection of cervical cancer using k-NN and artificial neural network. *Int. J. Emerg. Trends Technol. Comput. Sci. IJETTCS* **2017**, *6*, 145–149.
19. Wang, P.; Wang, J.; Li, Y.; Li, L.; Zhang, H. Adaptive Pruning of Transfer Learned Deep Convolutional Neural Network for Classification of Cervical Pap Smear Images. *IEEE Access* **2020**, *8*, 50674–50683. [CrossRef]
20. Ghoneim, A.; Muhammad, G.; Hossain, M.S. Cervical cancer classification using convolutional neural networks and extreme learning machines. *Futur. Gener. Comput. Syst.* **2020**, *102*, 643–649. [CrossRef]
21. Alquran, H.; Mustafa, W.A.; Abu Qasmieh, I.; Yacob, Y.M.; Alsalatie, M.; Al-Issa, Y.; Alqudah, A.M. Cervical Cancer Classification Using Combined Machine Learning and Deep Learning Approach. *Comput. Mater. Contin.* **2022**, *72*, 5117–5134. [CrossRef]
22. Chen, W.; Shen, W.; Gao, L.; Li, X. Hybrid Loss-Constrained Lightweight Convolutional Neural Networks for Cervical Cell Classification. *Sensors* **2022**, *22*, 3272. [CrossRef]
23. Waly, M.I.; Sikkandar, M.Y.; Aboamer, M.A.; Kadry, S.; Thinnukool, O. Optimal Deep Convolution Neural Network for Cervical Cancer Diagnosis Model. *Comput. Mater. Contin.* **2022**, *70*, 3295–3309.
24. Fekri-Ershad, S.; Ramakrishnan, S. Cervical cancer diagnosis based on modified uniform local ternary patterns and feed forward multilayer network optimized by genetic algorithm. *Comput. Biol. Med.* **2022**, *144*, 105392. [CrossRef] [PubMed]
25. Deepa, T.P.; Rao, A.N. Classification of normal and abnormal overlapped squamous cells in pap smear image. *Int. J. Syst. Assur. Eng. Manag.* **2023**, 1–13. [CrossRef]
26. Alquran, H.; Alsalatie, M.; Mustafa, W.A.; Abdi, R.A.; Ismail, A.R. Cervical Net: A Novel Cervical Cancer Classification Using Feature Fusion. *Bioengineering* **2022**, *9*, 578. [CrossRef] [PubMed]
27. Albuquerque, T.; Cruz, R.; Cardoso, J.S. Ordinal losses for classification of cervical cancer risk. *PeerJ Comput. Sci.* **2021**, *7*, e457. [CrossRef] [PubMed]
28. Tawalbeh, S.; Alquran, H.; Alsalatie, M. Deep Feature Engineering in Colposcopy Image Recognition: A Comparative Study. *Bioengineering* **2023**, *10*, 105. [CrossRef] [PubMed]
29. Alsalatie, M.; Alquran, H.; Mustafa, W.A.; Yacob, Y.M.; Alayed, A.A. Analysis of Cytology Pap Smear Images Based on Ensemble Deep Learning Approach. *Diagnostics* **2022**, *12*, 2756. [CrossRef] [PubMed]
30. Alom, M.Z.; Taha, T.M.; Yakopcic, C.; Westberg, S.; Sidike, P.; Nasrin, M.S.; Van Esesn, B.C.; Awwal, A.A.S.; Asari, V.K. The history began from alexnet: A comprehensive survey on deep learning approaches. *arXiv* **2018**, arXiv:1803.01164.
31. Al-Haija, Q.A.; Smadi, M.; Al-Bataineh, O.M. Identifying phasic dopamine releases using darknet-19 convolutional neural network. In Proceedings of the 2021 IEEE International IOT, Electronics and Mechatronics Conference (IEMTRONICS), Toronto, ON, Canada, 21–24 April 2021; pp. 1–5.
32. Wu, W.; Guo, L.; Gao, H.; You, Z.; Liu, Y.; Chen, Z. YOLO-SLAM: A semantic SLAM system towards dynamic environment with geometric constraint. *Neural Comput. Appl.* **2022**, *34*, 6011–6602. [CrossRef]
33. Radhika, K.; Devika, K.; Aswathi, T.; Sreevidya, P.; Sowmya, V.; Soman, K.P. Performance analysis of NASNet on unconstrained ear recognition. In *Nature Inspired Computing for Data Science*; Springer: Cham, Switzerland, 2020; pp. 57–82.

34. Valpola, H. From neural PCA to deep unsupervised learning. In *Advances in Independent Component Analysis and Learning Machines*; Academic Press: Cambridge, MA, USA, 2015; pp. 143–171.
35. Zeng, X.; Martinez, T.R. Feature weighting using neural networks. In Proceedings of the 2004 IEEE International Joint Conference on Neural Networks (IEEE Cat. No. 04CH37541), Budapest, Hungary, 25–29 July 2004; IEEE: Piscataway, NJ, USA, 2004; Volume 2, pp. 1327–1330.
36. Mirjalili, S. The ant lion optimizer. *Adv. Eng. Softw.* **2015**, *83*, 80–98. [CrossRef]
37. Dalwinder, S.; Birmohan, S.; Manpreet, K. Simultaneous feature weighting and parameter determination of neural networks using ant lion optimization for the classification of breast cancer. *Biocybern. Biomed. Eng.* **2020**, *40*, 337–351. [CrossRef]
38. Khader, A.; Alquran, H. Automated Prediction of Osteoarthritis Level in Human Osteochondral Tissue Using Histopathological Images. *Bioengineering* **2023**, *10*, 764. [CrossRef] [PubMed]
39. Dongoran, A.; Rahmadani, S.; Zarlis, M. Feature weighting using particle swarm optimization for learning vector quantization classifier. *J. Phys. Conf. Ser.* **2018**, *978*, 012032. [CrossRef]
40. Sweilam, N.H.; Tharwat, A.A.; Moniem, N.A. Support vector machine for diagnosis cancer disease: A comparative study. *Egypt. Inform. J.* **2010**, *11*, 81–92. [CrossRef]
41. Vichianin, Y.; Khummongkol, A.; Chiewvit, P.; Raksthaput, A.; Chaichanettee, S.; Aoonkaew, N.; Senanarong, V. Accuracy of support-vector machines for diagnosis of Alzheimer's disease, using volume of brain obtained by structural MRI at Siriraj hospital. *Front. Neurol.* **2021**, *12*, 640696. [CrossRef] [PubMed]
42. Farhadian, M.; Shokouhi, P.; Torkzaban, P. A decision support system based on support vector machine for diagnosis of periodontal disease. *BMC Res. Notes* **2020**, *13*, 337. [CrossRef] [PubMed]
43. Louppe, G. Understanding random forests: From theory to practice. *arXiv* **2014**, arXiv:1407.7502.

Disclaimer/Publisher's Note: The statements, opinions and data contained in all publications are solely those of the individual author(s) and contributor(s) and not of MDPI and/or the editor(s). MDPI and/or the editor(s) disclaim responsibility for any injury to people or property resulting from any ideas, methods, instructions or products referred to in the content.

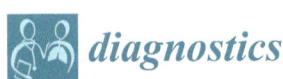

Article

NeuPD—A Neural Network-Based Approach to Predict Antineoplastic Drug Response

Muhammad Shahzad [1,†], Muhammad Atif Tahir [1,†], Musaed Alhussein [2], Ansharah Mobin [1,†], Rauf Ahmed Shams Malick [1] and Muhammad Shahid Anwar [3,*]

[1] FAST School of Computing, National University of Computer and Emerging Sciences (NUCES-FAST), Karachi 75030, Pakistan; mshahzad@nu.edu.pk (M.S.); atif.tahir@nu.edu.pk (M.A.T.); k190958@nu.edu.pk (A.M.); rauf.malick@nu.edu.pk (R.A.S.M.)

[2] Department of Computer Engineering, College of Computer and Information Sciences, King Saud University, P.O. Box 51178, Riyadh 11543, Saudi Arabia; musaed@ksu.edu.sa

[3] Department of AI and Software, Gachon University, Seongnam-si 13120, Republic of Korea

* Correspondence: shahidanwar786@gachon.ac.kr

† These authors contributed equally to this work.

Abstract: With the beginning of the high-throughput screening, in silico-based drug response analysis has opened lots of research avenues in the field of personalized medicine. For a decade, many different predicting techniques have been recommended for the antineoplastic (anti-cancer) drug response, but still, there is a need for improvements in drug sensitivity prediction. The intent of this research study is to propose a framework, namely **NeuPD**, to validate the potential anti-cancer drugs against a panel of cancer cell lines in publicly available datasets. The datasets used in this work are Genomics of Drug Sensitivity in Cancer (GDSC) and Cancer Cell Line Encyclopedia (CCLE). As not all drugs are effective on cancer cell lines, we have worked on 10 essential drugs from the GDSC dataset that have achieved the best modeling results in previous studies. We also extracted 1610 essential oncogene expressions from 983 cell lines from the same dataset. Whereas, from the CCLE dataset, 16,383 gene expressions from 1037 cell lines and 24 drugs have been used in our experiments. For dimensionality reduction, Pearson correlation is applied to best fit the model. We integrate the genomic features of cell lines and drugs' fingerprints to fit the neural network model. For evaluation of the proposed **NeuPD** framework, we have used repeated K-fold cross-validation with 5 times repeats where K = 10 to demonstrate the performance in terms of root mean square error (RMSE) and coefficient determination (R^2). The results obtained on the GDSC dataset that were measured using these cost functions show that our proposed **NeuPD** framework has outperformed existing approaches with an RMSE of 0.490 and R^2 of 0.929.

Keywords: NeuPD; cell lines; gene expression; machine learning; neural networks; drug response prediction; XGBoost

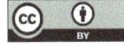

1. Introduction

The field of precision medicine in cancer has attracted serious attention from researchers at different stages. The identification of underlying genomic features that lead to mutations has become an effective research area. The identification of specific mutations, methylation, copy number variants (CNVs), and gene expression are considered important contributors in cancer studies. The specific changes in particular genes may result in specific resistance to generally available drugs. On the other hand, as complexities develop at the individual level, they demand specific interventions for the particular target in the area of precision medicine. The identification of specific genes and the association of biomarkers with particular diseases require evidence-based studies to report the drug response accordingly. In the presence of hundreds of drugs, particularly for cancer, it is important to evaluate the specific response against the specific biomarkers and expression level of particular tumors. Moreover, to identify the most appropriate drugs, the method is being applied at the individual level for better results. This paper presents drug response prediction, which is a crucial topic in the field of cancer precision medicine. Precision medicine refers to the treatment that is best suited to the individual based on their multi-omics characteristics [1]. A drug might have a positive or negative effect on a patient's body due to differences in individual biological characteristics. As conducting drug trials on each individual for large-scale research is expensive, time consuming, and challenging [2], we have worked on cell lines of tumor samples which are taken from the GDSC [3] and CCLE [4] datasets. These datasets contain multi-omics data such as gene expression, mutation, methylation, copy number variants, and so on for different cancer cell lines.

The deep learning-based techniques in the drug sensitivity prediction problem have been in use for a couple of years. Ref. [5] performed a systematic review of the literature covering 105 research papers that focused on using machine learning and deep learning techniques to predict the response of anti-cancer drugs. The review described multiple methods designed to enhance and categorize the response of cancer types to drug treatment. Due to the remarkable results of the deep learning models, we have also adopted the same technique. Our novelty in the proposed work is choosing the top 10 drugs' chemical features with gene expression features to train our proposed model. These drugs have top modeling performance according to previous studies. This makes our proposed model simple and more robust in the drug sensitivity prediction problem.

Recently, the DREAM challenge has been opened, which attracts researchers and data scientists to use these datasets to solve the drug response prediction problem [6]. Many predictive models have been proposed to contribute to this problem, such as [7–18]. Some of the work includes anti-cancer drug repositioning [19–21]. Most of these works focus on the prediction of drug sensitivity to a panel of cancer cell lines using gene expression data. The drug sensitivity is measured in terms of the half-maximal inhibitory concentrations IC_{50} value in (μM) units. In addition, the lower IC_{50} value means that the drug is more sensitive or more effective against the disease, whereas a higher IC_{50} value means drug resistance or that it is not effective.

Many predictive models have been used to solve the drug sensitivity prediction problem. All of these computation models use multiple omics datasets to predict drug sensitivity. Recently, ref. [22] proposed a set of guidelines for the proper use of machine learning models with gene expression data. Moreover, the emergence of these computational methods has had a significant influence on the identification of new applications for existing drugs [23]. Furthermore, these computational approaches have greatly facilitated a more systematic and rational approach to drug development processes, resulting in reduced timeframes for bringing drugs to market [24]. In summary, through the utilization of computational models and the integration of various data sources, these methodologies facilitate expedited and more effective drug screening, personalized treatment decision making, drug repurposing, prediction of drug toxicity, and identification of drug resistance. This advancement holds immense potential for advancing the efficiency and efficacy of healthcare interventions.

The authors in [25] proposed a DNN-PNN fresh parallel DL method to predict drug sensitivity by combining the strengths of two deep learning models. The first uses a DNN with a continuous gene expression profile as input, while the second uses a deep neural network based on a product and its discrete drug fingerprint traits. With higher prediction accuracy, faster convergence, and greater stability, the DNN-PNN outperforms both conventional and cutting-edge machine learning models, according to extensive experiments.

In [26], the authors used random forest to predict drug activity for cell lines based on chemical and genomic information. In contrast, Chiu et al. [27] recommended a DeepDR model that predicted drug response based on the cancer cell lines. This model comprises deep neural networks and a dataset taken from "TCGA: The Cancer Genome Atlas". The model predicted values for 265 given drugs and was tested on 622 cell lines. The mean square error was 1.96 on the testing sample set. Another computational approach named ProGENI [28] detects genes that exhibit the strongest correlation with variations in drug response among diverse individuals. This method relies on gene expression data and distinguishes itself from existing approaches by additionally leveraging prior knowledge of protein–protein and genetic interactions. Random walk techniques are employed within ProGENI to incorporate this prior knowledge effectively. Another study was conducted using 678 drugs on only three cell lines. On both pathway and genetic levels, DNN performs better than the other model of SVM [29]. The limitation was that they used only three cell lines.

Deep learning is widely used to interpret the concepts based on deep layers to extract the representations of the data: see Refs. [30–33]. A deep learning model named DeepPredictor is proposed in [34] that predicts drug sensitivity using CCLE data. The results claim that the DeepPredictor performed better, and the coefficient of determination gave a value ranging from 0.68 to 0.75.

Another model named DeepDSC for drug sensitivity in cancer was proposed based on deep learning [35]. Their study obtained a dataset from GDSC and CCLE. The recommended model consisted of two stages. In the first stage, an autoencoder is used to extract the cell line features from gene expression data. In the second and final stage, the features will be presented as input to the deep neural network for sensitivity prediction. The validation was performed like [34] on the given datasets. The performance was measured by the coefficient of determination and the root mean square error (RMSE). The value of the coefficient of determination shows that it performed better than previous ones with R^2 0.78 for the GDSC and CCLE datasets; as we discussed in [34], the maximum value achieved was 0.75, indicating that DeepDSC might help cancer therapy and predict drug responses in the future.

An approach was taken for the purpose of classifying drug responses using regression. The proposed model AutoBorutaRF [36] was built to predict drug response. For the feature selection, the Boruta algorithm was used to improve the prediction. Dr.VAE [37] was a generative model that concurrently trains drug-induced changes on transcriptomic data and on drug response. As the term implies, the technique employs a VAE to generate latent representations of pre-treatment gene expression and match them with post-treatment gene expression in terms of prediction. In order to forecast drug reactions, both latent models are then put into a logistic regression classifier. Dr. VAE outperformed many traditional classification methods in terms of cross-validated AUROC ratings. As compared to our proposed work, Dr. VAE used drug sensitivity data as a classification problem, i.e., responders or non-responders, whereas we treated drug response as a regression problem because the discretizing sensitivity score loses some information.

MOLI [38] is another deep learning model that encodes mutation, copy number variants (CNVs), and gene expression data separately and concatenates them to represent cancer cell lines for drug classification. MOLI was trained on the GDSC dataset and tested on patient-derived xenografts. They have achieved up to a 0.75 AUC score on TCGA Cisplatin data with gene expression data. Whereas in our proposed method, we have reached a 0.490 IC50 value on the GDSC dataset for the top ten selected drugs, which is quite higher than many recent models.

A bit of a different approach was described in [39], which follows the deep learning concept along with a drug synergy named DeepSynergy. DeepSynergy is the mapping of input vectors to a single output that is known as the synergy score and predicts the scores of drugs for cancer cell lines. This proposed new model was compared with support vector machines, random forests, and boosting machines, and it proved to show better results with an increase of 7.2%.

For predicting drug response, a hybrid graph convolutional network model called DeepCDR was created [40]. This proposed method outperformed different techniques of classification and regression, such as ridge regression and random forest. The DeepDCDR achieved a 1.058 RMSE. A study of cultured cell line sensitivity and drug profiles was conducted to predict the inhibition patterns of the drugs along with the cell line profiles [10].

Although these methods can work reasonably well on CCLE and GDSC datasets with full genomic features set along with a maximum number of drugs, the downside of these methods is that they were limited to a casual integration of genomic and drug features. This drawback can lead to increased computational complexity and potentially make it difficult for readers to discern the key contributing factors in drug sensitivity prediction. Hence, there is a pressing need for a solution that enables a more comprehensive understanding of the integration between targeted drugs and genomic features while also facilitating the evaluation of biological significance.

To address this issue and take inspiration from the swift advancement of deep learning technology, this paper introduces a novel deep learning framework, **NeuPD**, designed for the prediction of drug sensitivity on cancer cell line data taken from GDSC and CCLE. Our approach involves the fusion of genomic profiles of cell lines and chemical profiles of compounds, forming a comprehensive architecture for predicting drug sensitivity.

In this research work, the data are extracted from GDSC, which is then preprocessed by applying a Mix–Max Scaler for normalization and then Pearson's correlation for dimensionality reduction. Standard machine learning approaches, which are elastic net, XGBoost, and neural networks, are applied to the preprocessed data and then compared, giving rise to the proposed model, which is a deep neural network named **NeuPD** to assist medical practitioners and researchers in cancer therapeutics by working on essential cancer genes and the top 10 anti-cancer drugs. Different evaluation measures are used to verify the results.

To be precise, the novelty of our proposed model can be summarized in the following directions:

- Our contribution to modeling the drug sensitivity prediction problem is the selection of the top 10 drugs of interest. These drugs have been deduced from previous studies based on achieving top modeling performance. We took these drugs' chemical features to integrate them with genomic features and trained our proposed deep neural network. The remarkable performance of our model shows that deep learning can enhance the work on drug response prediction. Our proposed approach has achieved outstanding results when compared with previous models.
- Our model has been applied to GDSC and CCLE datasets and was tested using RMSE, MAE, and R^2 scores. By comparing the results, the lowest RMSE score shows the achievable part of our proposed model.

The structure of the rest of the paper is as follows: Section 2 presents the Material and Methods, Section 3 discusses the experimental environment, and Section 4 presents the results and discussion. Finally, the conclusion and future work are presented in Section 5.

2. Materials and Methods

2.1. Materials

To predict the drug sensitivity on unseen cancer cell lines, a deep learning neural network named NeuPD is proposed. As an input, gene expression data for cell lines, drug response data, and drug compound fingerprints were integrated into the model.

The drug response data were collected from the public repository of Genomics of Drug Sensitivity in Cancer (GDSC) (https://www.cancerrxgene.org/, accessed on 5 March 2023) and Cancer Cell Line Encyclopedia (CCLE), while data related to genes are collected from COSMIC Cancer Gene Census (https://cancer.sanger.ac.uk/cosmic/, accessed on 5 March 2023, [41]).

2.1.1. GDSC

This is the largest publicly available repository for drug response in cell lines. The baseline dataset contains 17,737 genes from 1018 human cell lines, and the drug response data contain IC$_{50}$ measurements of 198 anti-cancer drugs across more than 500 human cell lines for each of them, respectively. The IC$_{50}$ was converted to Log$_e$-IC$_{50}$, and smaller values of Log$_e$-IC$_{50}$ mean a better response: that is, more cancer cells are dying. The compound structures for 10 drugs in 2D structures were collected from PubChem (https://pubchem.ncbi.nlm.nih.gov/, accessed on 5 March 2023, [42]) in Structure-Data File (SDF) which contains a compound structure-data file format that can link data with one or more chemical structures. It is commonly referred to as SDF, .sdf, or SD file. The structures are illustrated in Figure 1.

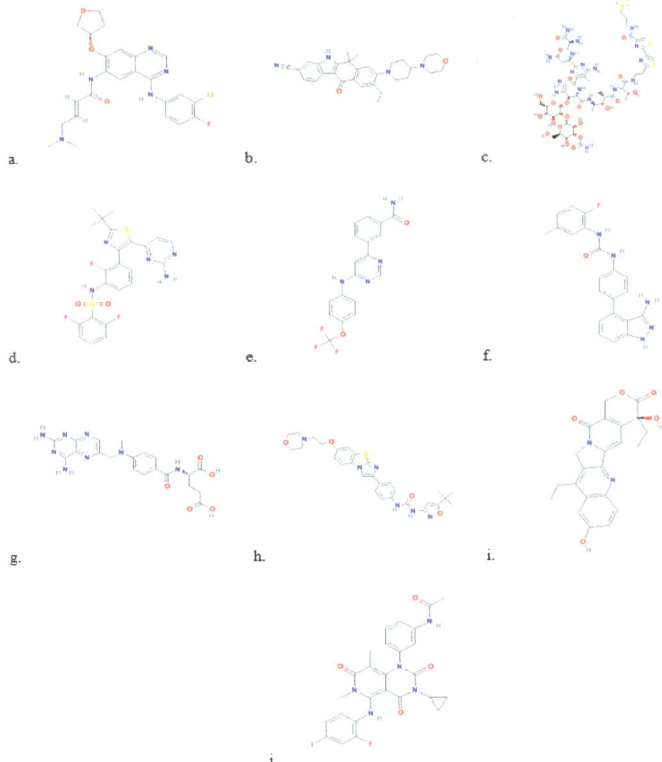

Figure 1. GDSC drugs 2D structures (**a**) Afatinib, (**b**) Alectinib, (**c**) Bleomycin, (**d**) Dabrafenib, (**e**) GNF-2, (**f**) Linifanib, (**g**) Methotrexate, (**h**) Quizartinib, (**i**) SN-38, and (**j**) Trametinib.

The collected structures were processed for hashed count Morgan fingerprints of 256 bits, making the obtained drug feature vectors length of 256. The final matrix consists of drug responses, gene expressions, and drug features which are then further processed for the training of the model. The list of all selected drugs along with their PubChem Compound ID number is given in Table 1.

Table 1. GDSC drug names and PubChem ID.

Drug Name	PubChem CID
Afatinib	10184653
Alectinib	49806720
Bleomycin (50 uM)	5460769
Dabrafenib	44462760
GNF-2	5311510
Linifanib	11485656
Methotrexate	126941
Quizartinib	24889392
SN-38	104842
Trametinib	11707110

2.1.2. CCLE

This contains 16,383 gene identifiers of 1037 cell lines that were downloaded from the CCLE website. The drug responses were given in values of IC_{50}. The 2D compound structures for 24 drugs were collected in the same way as GDSC, making the feature vector of size 256. The structures are illustrated in Figure 2.

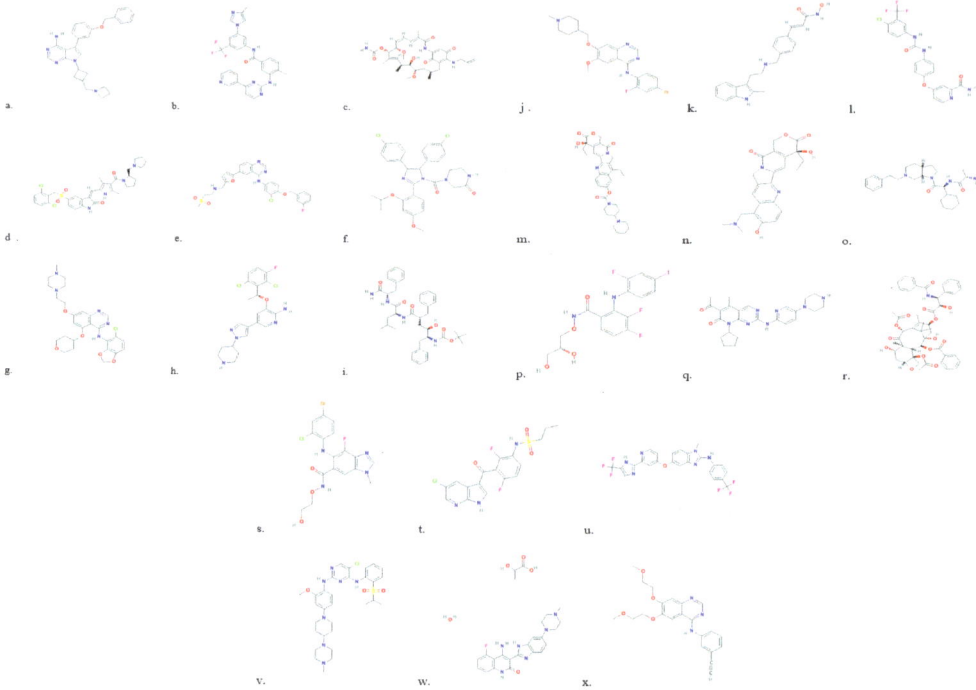

Figure 2. CCLE drugs 2D structures: (**a**) AEW541, (**b**) Nilotinib, (**c**) 17-AAG, (**d**) PHA-665752, (**e**) Lapatinib, (**f**) Nutlin-3, (**g**) AZD0530, (**h**) PF2341066, (**i**) L-685458, (**j**) ZD-6474, (**k**) Panobinostat, (**l**) Sorafenib, (**m**) Irinotecan, (**n**) Topotecan, (**o**) LBW242, (**p**) PD-0325901, (**q**) PD-0332991, (**r**) Paclitaxel, (**s**) AZD6244, (**t**) PLX4720, (**u**) RAF265, (**v**) TAE684, (**w**) TKI258, (**x**) Erlotinib.

The list of all selected drugs along with their PubChem Compound ID number is given in Table 2.

Table 2. CCLE drug names and PubChem ID.

Drug Name	PubChem ID	Drug Name	PubChem ID
AEW541	11476171	Irinotecan	60838
Nilotinib	644241	Topotecan	60700
17-AAG	6505803	LBW242	11503417
PHA-665752	10461815	PD-0325901	9826528
Lapatinib	208908	PD-0332991	5330286
Nutlin-3	216345	Paclitaxel	36314
AZD0530	10302451	AZD6244	10127622
PF2341066	11626560	PLX4720	24180719
L-685458	5479543	RAF265	11656518
ZD-6474	3081361	TAE684	16038120
Panobinostat	6918837	TKI258	135611162
Sorafenib	216239	Erlotinib	176870

2.2. Datasets Preprocessing

Before the model training, we performed normalization to scale the numerical data without distorting its actual shape. For this step, we have used the Min–Max Scaling method using Equation (1) in which the data are scaled to a range of 0–1. Each value at the features is processed in a way that the minimum value will be transformed into the value of 0, and thus, the maximum value will scale to the value of 1.

$$x_{scaledvalue} = \frac{x - min(x)}{max(x) - min(x)} \quad (1)$$

Equation (1) is the mathematical formula for the Min–Max Scaler where x is a single feature of the data.

After normalization, we have reduced the size, i.e., 10 drugs instead of 198 drugs from the GDSC dataset. We selected these drugs based on the top-ranked cancer drugs with the process defined in [43]. The selection of these drugs followed two criteria: Firstly, they were identified as the most suitable candidates for modeling based on all the feature selection methods employed. Secondly, they exhibited a noteworthy superiority in modeling when compared to the other type of feature selection methods, either genome-wide or biologically driven. Among the selected drugs, five demonstrated superior modeling performance when utilizing genome-wide features, whereas the remaining five exhibited better modeling outcomes with biologically driven features. This gives us the best top 10 modeled drugs. From the GDSC dataset, 851 cell lines against 10 selected drugs as response data have been extracted. From the CCLE dataset, we took 24 drug responses against 491 cell lines.

The total samples with all available *drugs* X *cell − lines* in the final data matrices are given in Table 3.

Table 3. Preprocessed Data.

Dataset	Drugs	Cell Lines	Data Points
GDSC	10	851	8510
CCLE	24	491	11,784

2.3. Cell Line Features Selection

For both CCLE and GDSC datasets, cell line features are expressed as a vector of gene expression values which are quite larger than the drug Morgan feature vector of 256 bits. So, to avoid the dominance of gene expression features over the drug features during model training, we have reduced the gene expression features by using dimensionality reduction. To achieve this objective, we used the Pearson correlation coefficient (PCC) method to obtain the optimized gene expression features up to 500 feature vectors. To find the correlation between all pairs of variables, a Pearson correlation matrix was calculated.

This will give us a table of correlation coefficients, one for each pair of variables. Its range lies between −1 and 1, where −1 means a negative correlation, 0 means no correlation, and +1 means a positive correlation. PCC measures the linear relationship between two variables. The focus will be on variables having a high correlation coefficient. Equation (2) is the mathematical formula for calculating the Pearson correlation coefficient.

$$P = \frac{\sum_{n=1}^{N}(x_i - x')(y_i - y')}{\sqrt{\sum_{n=1}^{N}(x_i - x')^2}\sqrt{\sum_{n=1}^{N}(y_i - y')^2}} \quad (2)$$

Let us assume that there are N samples, i.e., cancer cell lines in dataset S, where P is the correlation coefficient, x_i here represents the gene expression values as x-variables in the sample, x' is the mean of the gene expression values of the x-variables, y_i represents the drug sensitivity (IC_{50}) values of the y-variables to the panel of cancer cell lines samples, and y' is the mean of the IC_{50} values of the y-variables. If $P > 0$, then it implies a positive relation, $P < 0$ implies that it is a negative correlation, while $P = 0$ represents that there is no correlation between the two variables.

2.4. NeuPD

With the increase of more neural units and layers, a feedforward deep neural network (DNN) would be able to produce a more universal approximator [44]. In many scientific areas, the powerful modeling technique has been extensively used [20,21,45,46]. These neural network-based modeling capabilities have been applied in drug sensitivity prediction problems for a couple of years. In spite of high-dimensional pharmacogenomics profile data, DNN has achieved remarkable results both in regression and classification tasks. In the regression task, DNN is used to predict drug sensitivity value in terms of IC_{50} value. While in the classification task, drug sensitivity values are discretized. However, ref. [14] has pointed out that the drug sensitivity prediction as a classification task loses more information than that of the regression task. Moreover, representing drug sensitivity data as a regression problem has also outperformed the classification problem. Based on these facts, we have used IC_{50} values as regression values to train our proposed deep learning model.

Figure 3 gives the overall workflow diagram of our proposed model, which is a NeuPD. The work is undertaken on two different datasets, i.e., GDSC and CCLE. These datasets contain different numbers of cell lines with gene expression values as cell line feature vectors. There were around 20,000 genes in both datasets, from which we further extracted 1610 essential oncogenes expressions based on CRISPR experiment [47]. The gene expressions were first normalized using the method defined in Equation (1), and then, the Pearson correlation method was applied to further reduce the cell lines features up to 500 features vector. The reason for this reduction is to make gene expression features close to the drug's Morgan fingerprint features in terms of vector length. Moreover, to build final input matrices, drug features with known drug responses to a panel of cancer cell lines were integrated.

2.5. Experimental Environment

All methods are implemented using Python3 Scikit-learn, Keras, and TensorFlow libraries. For the process of forming hash values of Morgan fingerprints, an environment of RDKit is built for importing the required modules. The code is created in Python 3.9 on a 4.9 GHz Intel Core i7 CPU with 16 GB RAM equipped with high-performance NVIDIA GeForce MX130 GPU, using Google Colab and a Jupyter Notebook.

The architecture is then implemented using Keras embedded with four layers excluding the input and output layer, each having a weight less than the previous layer. The input dimension assigned in an input layer is 756, which comprises 500 dimensions for the reduced gene expressions data and 256 for the Morgan fingerprints. The first layer contains 1000 neural units, the second layer contains 800 neural units, the third layer contains

500 neural units, and the fourth contains 100 neural units. The activation function used for all hidden layers is ReLU (Rectified Linear Activation Function).

In the output layer, a weight of 1 neural unit is applied with no activation function, so the output range will not be restricted to a specific range. The loss function applied is of root mean square error to measure the magnitude of error in the applied model.

To overcome the issue of overfitting, early stopping is used with patience of 30, and a dropout rate of 0.1 is set after each layer. By the term dropout, it means to randomly select some neurons to omit during training.

Evaluation Measures

There are many different metrics used for measuring the performance of the model and measuring the magnitude of the error. The functions which are used to measure the error are known as loss functions. Some of the metrics used in this thesis work are RMSE, MAE, coefficient of determination (R^2), and MSE.

- RMSE Among all these metrics, RMSE is the loss function that is used to measure the error of the model as it is more suitable and accurate to measure the drug response model. RMSE is calculated by taking the difference between the predicted and target variable and then taking the root of the value, giving only positive values. The formula of RMSE is given in (3) where y_i is the target variable that is drug response and y_i' is the predicted variable that is the features and N is the total size of the test data. $(y_i - y_i')$ is the target and predicted drug sensitivity data.

$$\sqrt{\frac{\sum(y_i - y_i')^2}{N}} \tag{3}$$

- MSE: It is the measure of the average squared difference between the predicted values and the actual value.
- MAE: It is the mean absolute error that measures the magnitude of errors between the predicted and actual value of the dataset.
- R^2: It is the coefficient of determination and is used to measure the predictive performance in our model which is NeuPD. It explains how much divergence of one variable can occur by its relationship to the other variable.

To be specific with the training details, the Keras framework is used based on the backend of TensorFlow and validated with 10-fold cross-validation by taking one fold for validation and remaining folds for training that were repeated ten times, as illustrated in Figure 4.

We applied 10-fold cross-validation. The ReLU activation function is used in the full connection layer for the network structure in the feature extraction stage. The optimizer used is Adamax.

2.6. Summarized Model

A flowchart of the **NeuPD** is illustrated in Figure 3.

The process starts by gathering the data from different public repositories of GDSC and CCLE. The data are then normalized using Min–Max Scaler. For reducing the dimension, Pearson correlation is applied to reduce it to a dimension of 500. The datasets are preprocessed by extracting essential genes, the top 10 best-modeled drugs, and extracting the 2D structure of drugs from the PubChem repository. The 2D structures are converted into Morgan fingerprints to identify the drug features. The final matrix consists of chemical features that are the Morgan fingerprints and genomic features that are the gene expression. The drug features are of 256 bits, and the gene expression dimension as mentioned above is 500, making the final matrix of size 756. The final matrix consists of gene expressions and drug features versus the target variable, which is the drug response. The model is fitted by tuning different parameters, which are already defined. The fitted model is trained in the proposed NeuPD, and predictions are made by adding new data and evaluating the results using different metrics or loss functions of RMSE, MSE, MAE, and R^2.

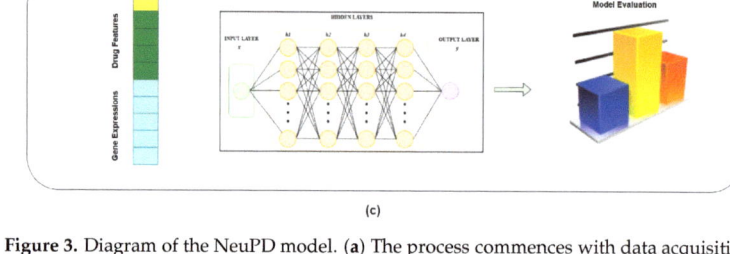

Figure 3. Diagram of the NeuPD model. (**a**) The process commences with data acquisition from the CCLE and GDSC datasets, which is followed by a selection of oncogenes' expression data and then data normalization followed by PCC-based gene feature selection. (**b**) Extracting 2D drug structures from PubChem datasets, converting them into Morgan fingerprints as drug features and finally merging them with gene expression data to produce the final response data. (**c**) Both genomic and drug features are concatenated together as the input to train the neural network model. The model performance is evaluated in terms of RMSE and R^2.

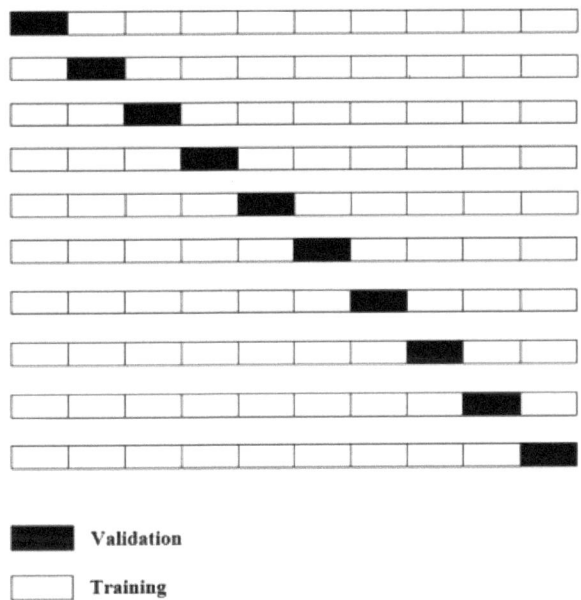

Figure 4. 10-fold cross-validation.

3. Results

To achieve less biased results in performance analysis, we used 10-fold cross-validation in performance analysis of the NeuPD trained on the datasets of GDSC and CCLE. An average is taken for all loss functions to achieve the final results accordingly. The mean of the values is taken across the genes, novel cell lines, and drug responses. Different ML-based techniques are used to validate and compare the results obtained on GDSC and CCLE datasets.

3.1. Baseline Methods

Apart from the proposed method, two competing machine learning techniques are also used to compare the results, which are outlined below.

1. **Elastic Net**

   It is a regularized linear regression model having L1 and L2 penalty functions. It is a further extension to the regular linear regression by adding regularization penalties during the training phase to the loss function. It has two hyperparameters: *alpha* and *lambda*. *Alpha* can be set by declaring *l1_ratio* and *lambda* by *alpha*. A default value of 0.5 is assigned for *"l1_ratio"* and for *"alpha"*, a full weighting is used of 1.0, as there were no major changes in the results when different values were tried. Previous studies used the elastic net as a technique to predict drug response [48,49]. This elastic net model was implemented using the sklearn library applied to the processed dataset by using a repeated 10-fold cross-validation five times. To evaluate the results, loss functions were used of RMSE, MSE, MAE, and R^2.

2. **XGBoost**

   It is a gradient boosting library that is implemented under the framework of gradient boosting. It is beneficial as it provides a parallel way to solve data-related issues in a fast and precise way. This model supports Scikit-learn advanced features along with regularization. In a SciPy environment, it can be easily installed using pip. The command to install xgboost is: *sudo pip install xgboost*.

XGBoost gives a wrapper class, which means that the models can be treated as classifiers or regressors in the Scikit framework. The models for the classifier and regressor are "XGBClassifier" and "XGBRegressor". To make predictions, a **model.predict()** function is used, which is a Scikit-Learn built-in function. After fitting the model, evaluation is performed using different metrics.

3.2. Comparison on CCLE Dataset

As already discussed, the CCLE dataset consists of 16,383 gene expressions for 1037 cell lines and 24 drugs. The results achieved from cross-validation were compared with the state-of-the-art study [50] in which the CCLE dataset was used, giving an RMSE of 5.378 for the elastic net, while the RMSE achieved in our research is 3.202 for elastic net and 2.074 for XGBoost. NeuPD showed a much lower value of RMSE than the elastic net and XGBoost, which is 1.784. The methods comparison based on root mean square error (RMSE), mean absolute error (MAE), mean square error (MSE), and coefficient of determination (R^2) is given in Table 4 below.

Table 4. Results on CCLE Dataset.

Method	RMSE	MSE	MAE	R^2
Elastic Net	±3.202	±10.25	±2.972	0.281
XGBoost	±2.074	±4.308	±1.491	0.317
NeuPD	**±1.784**	**±3.192**	**±1.568**	**0.543**

3.3. Comparison on GDSC Dataset

As already described above, these data contain 983 cell lines related to 1610 genes for 10 drugs. The final matrix thus is made up of drug responses, gene expressions, and Morgan fingerprint for 10 drugs that are 256 bits.

The results achieved outperformed the results by having an RMSE of 0.490, while the coefficient of determination R^2 is 0.929. The closer the R^2 is to 1, the better it fits the value. The RMSE achieved is 1.784 for CCLE. The lesser the value of RMSE, the better the model is because it means that the error value is less, and in precision medicine, we need an approach that gives less error as compared to other approaches.

The methods comparison based on RMSE, MAE, coefficient of determination (R^2), and MSE is given in Table 5.

Table 5. Results on GDSC Dataset.

Method	RMSE	MSE	MAE	R^2
Elastic Net	±2.419	±5.851	±2.020	0.532
XGBoost	±1.337	±1.794	±0.953	0.609
NeuPD	**±0.490**	**±0.246**	**±0.392**	**0.929**

By comparing the results with two other approaches performed—elastic net and XGBoost—it can be seen that the elastic net again performs worse than XGBoost and NeuPD by having the RMSE value of 2.419 and R^2 of 0.532, which means it did not fit the model well. Meanwhile, XGBoost performed much better than the elastic net, having an RMSE of 1.337 but for the R^2, not much improvement was seen, as the value differs by only 0.1. The proposed model, again, outperformed the other baseline methods used in this research.

The results of both datasets are given in Figure 5.

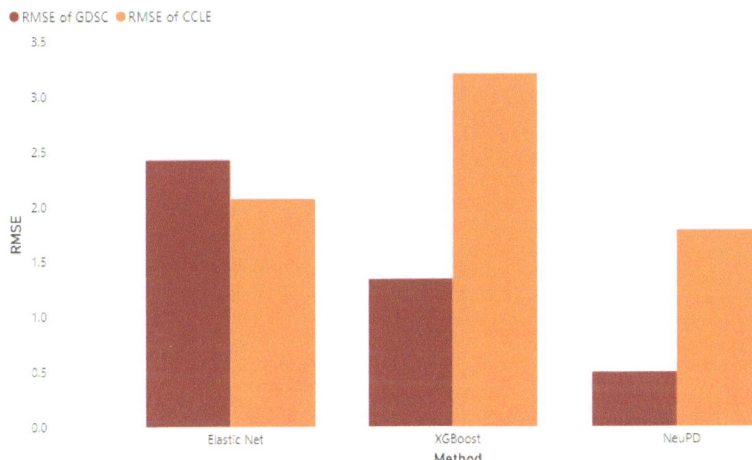

Figure 5. RMSE comparison for GDSC and CCLE dataset.

3.4. Comparisons to Previous Studies

The RMSE achieved by applying NeuPD is 0.490 and the R^2 achieved is 0.929. By looking at previous studies, the comparison can be made for the results achieved with other existing relevant models. All these existing studies used 10-fold cross-validation to calculate their RMSE scores. The RMSE achieved was 0.52 ± 0.01 and R^2 was 0.78 ± 0.01 by using neural networks with 10-fold cross-validation [35]. A model named DeepCDR [40] achieved an RMSE of 1.058 ± 0.006. In a matrix factorization approach [51], an RMSE of 1.73 was achieved for the GDSC dataset. A study using the GDSC dataset along with Morgan fingerprints achieved a lower RMSE of 0.75 ± 0.01 and R^2 of 0.74 ± 0.01 [10]. The results are given in Table 6 below.

Table 6. Results on GDSC Dataset.

Dataset	Method	RMSE
GDSC	SRMF [51]	±1.73
	DeepCDR [40]	±1.058
	PGM [10]	±0.75
	DeepDSC [35]	±0.52
	NeuPD	**±0.490**
CCLE	Ridge Regression [50]	±6.576
	Random Forest [50]	±5.738
	Elastic Net [50]	±5.378
	Lasso [50]	±5.333
	NeuPD	**±1.784**

The performance of the proposed NN-based NeuPD model was compared to the elastic net (EN) regression and XGBoost. By looking at the results, NeuPD achieved the best results compared with other baseline models and different studies. To lessen the chance of overfitting, early stopping is also used in which the training phase was stopped if the validation loss did not decrease after 500 epochs. The performance of each algorithm was evaluated by using the root mean square error (RMSE). The best value of RMSE is 0.490, which was achieved for the GDSC dataset over 10 drugs. For the CCLE dataset, the least value achieved for RMSE is 1.784. So, in these datasets, the proposed model performed better for GDSC than CCLE.

4. Discussion

The abundance of cancerous control and disease datasets at the genomic and proteomics levels allow us to better understand the drug and disease appropriateness. The genomic data including the gene expression level have been found to be an important biomarker toward the state and nature of cancer disease. The medicine prescription has entered the era of precision medicine that aimed to prescribe the most appropriate drug for the target disease sample based on the association with respective genomic biomarkers.

The availability of cancer cell lines, in particular, allowed AI experts to predict associations among hundreds of available drugs and associated genes through ML and DL tools. Several DL models have been proposed to identify the right drug for the GDSC and CCLE datasets. Drugs' chemical compositions are being used to represent drug features.

There are numerous recent computational methods such as [7–9,35] that potentially contributed to the drug sensitivity prediction problem. Despite the effectiveness of these methods on CCLE and GDSC datasets using complete genomic features and a wide range of drugs, they have a limitation when it comes to integrating genomic and drug features causally. This limitation results in increased computational complexity and can make it challenging for the scientific community to identify the key factors influencing drug sensitivity prediction.

In this research work, we proposed a deep learning model named **NeuPD** that predicts the antineoplastic drug sensitivity of cancer cell lines. Our proposed model was trained on GDSC and CCLE datasets downloaded from the public repository. The data were normalized by applying Mix–Max Scaler, and then Pearson's correlation was applied for dimensionality reduction. For the drug features, the 2D structures were downloaded for each drug from PubChem for both the GDSC and CCLE drugs. The structures were then converted into hash values using Morgan fingerprints. For the training of the model, gene expressions are selected as cell line genomic features, and Morgan fingerprints are selected as chemical features of compounds. Both cell line features and drug features were combined as the inputs for the NeuPD.

The results have shown that **NeuPD** outperformed previous state-of-the-art models and techniques by having the lowest value of RMSE which is 0.490 and the highest value of the coefficient of determination R^2, which is 0.929. Moreover, the performance of the proposed model was evaluated using 10-fold cross-validation.

The present research work has also a few limitations, i.e., the size of the data and the applied DL tools employed during the course of the study. The applicability of our research findings is based on the available current state-of-the-art published results and the associated data. The biological scientific community is publishing tremendous results on an (almost) weekly basis, which demands the inclusion of the newly published results in a continuously updated mode. This inclusive nature demands extensive evaluation matrices of our results in consideration of the current state of the art. Secondly, high dimensionality is a challenge to the applicability of our research at a clinical level. In future, this work can be extended by integrating additional molecular features such as mutations, copy number variations, and methylation along with the gene expression data. Furthermore, incorporating explainability and interpretability into the framework would enable explicit extraction of biological significance from the obtained results.

5. Conclusions

In the recent past, the identification of appropriate drugs for particular genomic markers was found to be important in diagnostics and the prescription of drugs accordingly. Several machine learning and deep learning methods are being used to predict a significantly reduced subset of hundreds of available drugs. This study performed experiments on cancerous datasets extracted from different tissues and identified the most appropriate drugs for particular gene expression levels. The implemented and tested **NeuPD** method outperformed the existing state of the art and was helpful in predicting associations among the drugs for respective biomarkers across the different types of cancer disease. The study is aimed to develop results that have the potential to be employed by clinical practitioners in the future.

Author Contributions: Conceptualization, R.A.S.M. and M.A.T.; methodology, M.S.; software, A.M.; validation, M.A.T. and M.S.; formal analysis, M.A.; investigation, M.S. and M.S.A.; resources, M.A.T.; data curation, M.S.; writing—original draft preparation, M.S. and A.M.; writing—review and editing, M.S., A.M., M.S., M.A.T. and M.S.A.; visualization, M.S.; supervision, M.A.T.; project administration, M.A.; funding acquisition, M.A. All authors have read and agreed to the published version of the manuscript.

Funding: This research is funded by Research Supporting Project Number (RSPD2023R553, King Saud University, Riyadh, Saudi Arabia

Institutional Review Board Statement: Not applicable.

Informed Consent Statement: Not applicable.

Data Availability Statement: The datasets used in this research are available at https://www.cancerrxgene.org, https://cancer.sanger.ac.uk/cosmic, https://pubchem.ncbi.nlm.nih.gov, https://drive.google.com/drive/folders/1RqPDQ5eKAEAG1i5hQpHFv2qBQ_qnSKJw?usp=sharing (accessed on 5 March 2023).

Acknowledgments: This research is funded by Research Supporting Project Number (RSPD2023R553, King Saud University, Riyadh, Saudi Arabia.

Conflicts of Interest: The authors declare no conflict of interest.

Abbreviations

The following abbreviations are used in this manuscript:

CCLE	Cancer Cell Line Encyclopedia
GDSC	Genomics of Drug Sensitivity in Cancer
MAE	Mean Absolute Error
MSE	Mean Squared Error
R^2	Coefficient of Determination
RMSE	Root Mean Square Error

References

1. Chan, I.S.; Ginsburg, G.S. Personalized medicine: Progress and promise. *Annu. Rev. Genom. Hum. Genet.* **2011**, *12*, 217–244. [CrossRef]
2. Weinstein, J.N.; Collisson, E.A.; Mills, G.B.; Shaw, K.R.; Ozenberger, B.A.; Ellrott, K.; Shmulevich, I.; Sander, C.; Stuart, J.M. The cancer genome atlas pan-cancer analysis project. *Nat. Genet.* **2013**, *45*, 1113–1120. [CrossRef]
3. Yang, W.; Soares, J.; Greninger, P.; Edelman, E.J.; Lightfoot, H.; Forbes, S.; Bindal, N.; Beare, D.; Smith, J.A.; Thompson, I.R.; et al. Genomics of Drug Sensitivity in Cancer (GDSC): A resource for therapeutic biomarker discovery in cancer cells. *Nucleic Acids Res.* **2012**, *41*, D955–D961. [CrossRef]
4. Barretina, J.; Caponigro, G.; Stransky, N.; Venkatesan, K.; Margolin, A.A.; Kim, S.; Wilson, C.J.; Lehár, J.; Kryukov, G.V.; Sonkin, D.; et al. The Cancer Cell Line Encyclopedia enables predictive modelling of anticancer drug sensitivity. *Nature* **2012**, *483*, 603–607. [CrossRef]
5. Singh, D.P.; Kaushik, B. A systematic literature review for the prediction of anticancer drug response using various machine-learning and deep-learning techniques. *Chem. Biol. Drug Des.* **2023**, *101*, 175–194. [CrossRef]
6. Costello, J.C.; Heiser, L.M.; Georgii, E.; Gönen, M.; Menden, M.P.; Wang, N.J.; Bansal, M.; Ammad-Ud-Din, M.; Hintsanen, P.; Khan, S.A.; et al. A community effort to assess and improve drug sensitivity prediction algorithms. *Nat. Biotechnol.* **2014**, *32*, 1202–1212. [CrossRef]
7. Yingtaweesittikul, H.; Wu, J.; Mongia, A.; Peres, R.; Ko, K.; Nagarajan, N.; Suphavilai, C. CREAMMIST: An integrative probabilistic database for cancer drug response prediction. *Nucleic Acids Res.* **2023**, *51*, D1242–D1248. [CrossRef]
8. Zhu, E.Y.; Dupuy, A.J. Machine learning approach informs biology of cancer drug response. *BMC Bioinform.* **2022**, *23*, 184. [CrossRef]
9. Ren, S.; Tao, Y.; Yu, K.; Xue, Y.; Schwartz, R.; Lu, X. De novo Prediction of Cell-Drug Sensitivities Using Deep Learning-based Graph Regularized Matrix Factorization. In Proceedings of the Pacific Symposium on Biocomputing 2022, Big Island of Hawaii, HI, USA, 3–7 January 2022; World Scientific: Singapore, 2022; pp. 278–289.

10. Cortés-Ciriano, I.; van Westen, G.J.; Bouvier, G.; Nilges, M.; Overington, J.P.; Bender, A.; Malliavin, T.E. Improved large-scale prediction of growth inhibition patterns using the NCI60 cancer cell line panel. *Bioinformatics* **2016**, *32*, 85–95. [CrossRef]
11. Turki, T.; Wei, Z. A link prediction approach to cancer drug sensitivity prediction. *BMC Syst. Biol.* **2017**, *11*, 94. [CrossRef]
12. Huang, C.; Mezencev, R.; McDonald, J.F.; Vannberg, F. Open source machine-learning algorithms for the prediction of optimal cancer drug therapies. *PLoS ONE* **2017**, *12*, e0186906. [CrossRef]
13. Azuaje, F. Computational models for predicting drug responses in cancer research. *Briefings Bioinform.* **2017**, *18*, 820–829. [CrossRef]
14. Jang, I.S.; Neto, E.C.; Guinney, J.; Friend, S.H.; Margolin, A.A. Systematic assessment of analytical methods for drug sensitivity prediction from cancer cell line data. In *Biocomputing 2014*; World Scientific: Singapore, 2014; pp. 63–74.
15. Garnett, M.J.; Edelman, E.J.; Heidorn, S.J.; Greenman, C.D.; Dastur, A.; Lau, K.W.; Greninger, P.; Thompson, I.R.; Luo, X.; Soares, J.; et al. Systematic identification of genomic markers of drug sensitivity in cancer cells. *Nature* **2012**, *483*, 570–575. [CrossRef]
16. Chen, J.; Zhang, L. A survey and systematic assessment of computational methods for drug response prediction. *Briefings Bioinform.* **2021**, *22*, 232–246. [CrossRef] [PubMed]
17. Tan, M.; Özgül, O.F.; Bardak, B.; Ekşioğlu, I.; Sabuncuoğlu, S. Drug response prediction by ensemble learning and drug-induced gene expression signatures. *Genomics* **2019**, *111*, 1078–1088. [CrossRef]
18. Zhang, N.; Wang, H.; Fang, Y.; Wang, J.; Zheng, X.; Liu, X.S. Predicting anticancer drug responses using a dual-layer integrated cell line-drug network model. *PLoS Comput. Biol.* **2015**, *11*, e1004498. [CrossRef]
19. Cheng, F.; Hong, H.; Yang, S.; Wei, Y. Individualized network-based drug repositioning infrastructure for precision oncology in the panomics era. *Briefings Bioinform.* **2017**, *18*, 682–697. [CrossRef]
20. Luo, H.; Wang, J.; Li, M.; Luo, J.; Ni, P.; Zhao, K.; Wu, F.X.; Pan, Y. Computational drug repositioning with random walk on a heterogeneous network. *IEEE/ACM Trans. Comput. Biol. Bioinform.* **2018**, *16*, 1890–1900. [CrossRef] [PubMed]
21. Luo, H.; Li, M.; Wang, S.; Liu, Q.; Li, Y.; Wang, J. Computational drug repositioning using low-rank matrix approximation and randomized algorithms. *Bioinformatics* **2018**, *34*, 1904–1912. [CrossRef]
22. Sharifi-Noghabi, H.; Jahangiri-Tazehkand, S.; Smirnov, P.; Hon, C.; Mammoliti, A.; Nair, S.K.; Mer, A.S.; Ester, M.; Haibe-Kains, B. Drug sensitivity prediction from cell line-based pharmacogenomics data: Guidelines for developing machine learning models. *Briefings Bioinform.* **2021**, *22*, bbab294. [CrossRef]
23. Keiser, M.J.; Setola, V.; Irwin, J.J.; Laggner, C.; Abbas, A.I.; Hufeisen, S.J.; Jensen, N.H.; Kuijer, M.B.; Matos, R.C.; Tran, T.B.; et al. Predicting new molecular targets for known drugs. *Nature* **2009**, *462*, 175–181. [CrossRef] [PubMed]
24. Mogire, R.M.; Akala, H.M.; Macharia, R.W.; Juma, D.W.; Cheruiyot, A.C.; Andagalu, B.; Brown, M.L.; El-Shemy, H.A.; Nyanjom, S.G. Target-similarity search using Plasmodium falciparum proteome identifies approved drugs with anti-malarial activity and their possible targets. *PLoS ONE* **2017**, *12*, e0186364. [CrossRef] [PubMed]
25. Chen, S.; Yang, Y.; Zhou, H.; Sun, Q.; Su, R. DNN-PNN: A parallel deep neural network model to improve anticancer drug sensitivity. *Methods* **2023**, *209*, 1–9. [CrossRef]
26. Lind, A.P.; Anderson, P.C. Predicting drug activity against cancer cells by random forest models based on minimal genomic information and chemical properties. *PLoS ONE* **2019**, *14*, e0219774. [CrossRef] [PubMed]
27. Chiu, Y.C.; Chen, H.I.H.; Zhang, T.; Zhang, S.; Gorthi, A.; Wang, L.J.; Huang, Y.; Chen, Y. Predicting drug response of tumors from integrated genomic profiles by deep neural networks. *BMC Med. Genom.* **2019**, *12*, 143–155.
28. Emad, A.; Cairns, J.; Kalari, K.R.; Wang, L.; Sinha, S. Knowledge-guided gene prioritization reveals new insights into the mechanisms of chemoresistance. *Genome Biol.* **2017**, *18*, 1–21. [CrossRef]
29. Aliper, A.; Plis, S.; Artemov, A.; Ulloa, A.; Mamoshina, P.; Zhavoronkov, A. Deep learning applications for predicting pharmacological properties of drugs and drug repurposing using transcriptomic data. *Mol. Pharm.* **2016**, *13*, 2524–2530. [CrossRef]
30. Chen, Y.; Zhang, L. How much can deep learning improve prediction of the responses to drugs in cancer cell lines? *Briefings Bioinform.* **2022**, *23*, bbab378. [CrossRef]
31. Baptista, D.; Ferreira, P.G.; Rocha, M. Deep learning for drug response prediction in cancer. *Briefings Bioinform.* **2021**, *22*, 360–379. [CrossRef]
32. Goodfellow, I.; Bengio, Y.; Courville, A. *Deep Learning*; MIT Press: Cambridge, MA, USA, 2016.
33. LeCun, Y.; Bengio, Y.; Hinton, G. Deep learning. *Nature* **2015**, *521*, 436–444. [CrossRef]
34. Wang, Y.; Li, M.; Zheng, R.; Shi, X.; Li, Y.; Wu, F.; Wang, J. Using deep neural network to predict drug sensitivity of cancer cell lines. In Proceedings of the International Conference on Intelligent Computing, Wuhan,China, 15–18 August 2018; Springer: Berlin/Heidelberg, Germany, 2018; pp. 223–226.
35. Li, M.; Wang, Y.; Zheng, R.; Shi, X.; Wu, F.; Wang, J. DeepDSC: A deep learning method to predict drug sensitivity of cancer cell lines. *IEEE/ACM Trans. Comput. Biol. Bioinform.* **2019**, *18*, 575–582. [CrossRef]
36. Xu, X.; Gu, H.; Wang, Y.; Wang, J.; Qin, P. Autoencoder based feature selection method for classification of anticancer drug response. *Front. Genet.* **2019**, *10*, 233. [CrossRef] [PubMed]
37. Rampášek, L.; Hidru, D.; Smirnov, P.; Haibe-Kains, B.; Dr, Goldenberg, A. VAE: Improving drug response prediction via modeling of drug perturbation effects. *Bioinformatics* **2019**, *35*, 3743–3751. [CrossRef] [PubMed]
38. Sharifi-Noghabi, H.; Zolotareva, O.; Collins, C.C.; Ester, M. MOLI: Multi-omics late integration with deep neural networks for drug response prediction. *Bioinformatics* **2019**, *35*, i501–i509. [CrossRef]

39. Preuer, K.; Lewis, R.P.; Hochreiter, S.; Bender, A.; Bulusu, K.C.; Klambauer, G. DeepSynergy: Predicting anti-cancer drug synergy with Deep Learning. *Bioinformatics* **2018**, *34*, 1538–1546. [CrossRef]
40. Liu, Q.; Hu, Z.; Jiang, R.; Zhou, M. DeepCDR: A hybrid graph convolutional network for predicting cancer drug response. *Bioinformatics* **2020**, *36*, i911–i918. [CrossRef]
41. Tate, J.G.; Bamford, S.; Jubb, H.C.; fSondka, Z.; Beare, D.M.; Bindal, N.; Boutselakis, H.; Cole, C.G.; Creatore, C.; Dawson, E.; et al. COSMIC: The catalogue of somatic mutations in cancer. *Nucleic Acids Res.* **2019**, *47*, D941–D947. [CrossRef]
42. Kim, S.; Thiessen, P.A.; Bolton, E.E.; Chen, J.; Fu, G.; Gindulyte, A.; Han, L.; He, J.; He, S.; Shoemaker, B.A.; et al. PubChem substance and compound databases. *Nucleic Acids Res.* **2016**, *44*, D1202–D1213. [CrossRef]
43. Koras, K.; Juraeva, D.; Kreis, J.; Mazur, J.; Staub, E.; Szczurek, E. Feature selection strategies for drug sensitivity prediction. *Sci. Rep.* **2020**, *10*, 1–12.
44. Hornik, K.; Stinchcombe, M.; White, H. Multilayer feedforward networks are universal approximators. *Neural Netw.* **1989**, *2*, 359–366. [CrossRef]
45. Bhaskar, K.; Singh, S.N. AWNN-assisted wind power forecasting using feed-forward neural network. *IEEE Trans. Sustain. Energy* **2012**, *3*, 306–315. [CrossRef]
46. An, N.; Zhao, W.; Wang, J.; Shang, D.; Zhao, E. Using multi-output feedforward neural network with empirical mode decomposition based signal filtering for electricity demand forecasting. *Energy* **2013**, *49*, 279–288. [CrossRef]
47. Wang, T.; Birsoy, K.; Hughes, N.W.; Krupczak, K.M.; Post, Y.; Wei, J.J.; Lander, E.S.; Sabatini, D.M. Identification and characterization of essential genes in the human genome. *Science* **2015**, *350*, 1096–1101. [CrossRef] [PubMed]
48. Ding, M.Q.; Chen, L.; Cooper, G.F.; Young, J.D.; Lu, X. Precision oncology beyond targeted therapy: Combining omics data with machine learning matches the majority of cancer cells to effective therapeutics. *Mol. Cancer Res.* **2018**, *16*, 269–278. [CrossRef] [PubMed]
49. Basu, A.; Mitra, R.; Liu, H.; Schreiber, S.L.; Clemons, P.A. RWEN: Response-weighted elastic net for prediction of chemosensitivity of cancer cell lines. *Bioinformatics* **2018**, *34*, 3332–3339. [CrossRef] [PubMed]
50. Li, Q.; Shi, R.; Liang, F. Drug sensitivity prediction with high-dimensional mixture regression. *PLoS ONE* **2019**, *14*, e0212108. [CrossRef] [PubMed]
51. Wang, L.; Li, X.; Zhang, L.; Gao, Q. Improved anticancer drug response prediction in cell lines using matrix factorization with similarity regularization. *BMC Cancer* **2017**, *17*, 513. [CrossRef]

Disclaimer/Publisher's Note: The statements, opinions and data contained in all publications are solely those of the individual author(s) and contributor(s) and not of MDPI and/or the editor(s). MDPI and/or the editor(s) disclaim responsibility for any injury to people or property resulting from any ideas, methods, instructions or products referred to in the content.

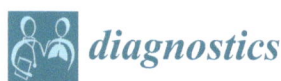

Article

Analysis of the Effectiveness of Metaheuristic Methods on Bayesian Optimization in the Classification of Visual Field Defects

Masyitah Abu [1], Nik Adilah Hanin Zahri [1,*], Amiza Amir [1], Muhammad Izham Ismail [2], Azhany Yaakub [3], Fumiyo Fukumoto [4] and Yoshimi Suzuki [4]

1. Center of Excellence for Advance Computing, Faculty of Electronic Engineering & Technology, Universiti Malaysia Perlis, Kangar 01000, Malaysia
2. Institute of Engineering Mathematics, Faculty of Applied and Human Sciences, Universiti Malaysia Perlis, Arau 02600, Malaysia
3. Department of Ophthalmology & Visual Science, Universiti Sains Malaysia, Kubang Kerian 16150, Malaysia
4. Graduate Faculty of Interdisciplinary Research, University of Yamanashi, Kofu 400-0016, Japan
* Correspondence: adilahhanin@unimap.edu.my

Abstract: Bayesian optimization (BO) is commonly used to optimize the hyperparameters of transfer learning models to improve the model's performance significantly. In BO, the acquisition functions direct the hyperparameter space exploration during the optimization. However, the computational cost of evaluating the acquisition function and updating the surrogate model can become prohibitively expensive due to increasing dimensionality, making it more challenging to achieve the global optimum, particularly in image classification tasks. Therefore, this study investigates and analyses the effect of incorporating metaheuristic methods into BO to improve the performance of acquisition functions in transfer learning. By incorporating four different metaheuristic methods, namely Particle Swarm Optimization (PSO), Artificial Bee Colony (ABC) Optimization, Harris Hawks Optimization, and Sailfish Optimization (SFO), the performance of acquisition function, Expected Improvement (EI), was observed in the VGGNet models for visual field defect multi-class classification. Other than EI, comparative observations were also conducted using different acquisition functions, such as Probability Improvement (PI), Upper Confidence Bound (UCB), and Lower Confidence Bound (LCB). The analysis demonstrates that SFO significantly enhanced BO optimization by increasing mean accuracy by 9.6% for VGG-16 and 27.54% for VGG-19. As a result, the best validation accuracy obtained for VGG-16 and VGG-19 is 98.6% and 98.34%, respectively.

Keywords: metaheuristic method; Bayesian optimization; acquisition function; VGGNet; visual field defect

Citation: Abu, M.; Zahri, N.A.H.; Amir, A.; Ismail, M.I.; Yaakub, A.; Fukumoto, F.; Suzuki, Y. Analysis of the Effectiveness of Metaheuristic Methods on Bayesian Optimization in the Classification of Visual Field Defects. *Diagnostics* 2023, 13, 1946. https://doi.org/10.3390/diagnostics13111946

Academic Editors: Wan Azani Mustafa, Ahsan Khandoker and Hiam Alquran

Received: 6 March 2023
Revised: 24 May 2023
Accepted: 30 May 2023
Published: 2 June 2023

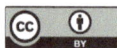

Copyright: © 2023 by the authors. Licensee MDPI, Basel, Switzerland. This article is an open access article distributed under the terms and conditions of the Creative Commons Attribution (CC BY) license (https://creativecommons.org/licenses/by/4.0/).

1. Introduction

Deep learning (DL) is a subfield of machine learning (ML) involving the training of artificial neural networks to automatically learn complex features and representations of the input data, allowing them to perform various tasks such as image and speech processing from large amounts of data [1]. Transfer learning utilizes a previously trained neural network model to improve the training of a new deep learning model on a related task [2,3]. The pre-trained model is adapted or fine-tuned using less training data for the new task or problem. Transfer learning can be beneficial when there is insufficient training data or when training a new model is time-consuming or computationally costly.

The error of a deep learning model can be minimized by selecting the optimal set of hyperparameters to maximize the model's performance on the validation set. This optimal set of hyperparameters can be retrieved efficiently and effectively through optimization to achieve high performance in a particular task [4]. In DL, optimization significantly enhances the model's performance by minimizing the errors or maximizing accuracy as an objective function during training. In the case of transfer learning, optimization is applied to fine-tune a previously trained model to improve a new related task.

Many previous works have proposed Bayesian Optimization (BO) [5–8] as an optimization method that uses a probabilistic model of the objective function. This probabilistic model, also called a surrogate model, searches the optimal set of hyperparameters and predicts the model's performance at untested points in the hyperparameter space. The performance of the surrogate model will be evaluated at different parameter settings by maximizing the Expected Improvement (EI) of the surrogate model. First, the EI is measured to identify how much the objective function is expected to improve the model's performance, or in other words, it measures the potential gain that can be obtained by evaluating the model at a new set of hyperparameters. Then, the acquisition function in BO is used to determine which set of hyperparameters should be evaluated next by balancing the trade-off between exploring regions of the search space where little is known and exploiting regions where the objective function is believed to be optimal [9]. However, the repeated process of evaluating the acquisition function in BO and updating the surrogate model can cause the computational cost to become prohibitively expensive due to increasing dimensionality, making it more challenging to achieve the global optimum.

In recent years, DL and transfer learning have become popular image classification techniques due to their high performance and ability to learn complex features from large amounts of data, and BO has grown in popularity as an optimization method. Previously, Shankar et al. [10] proposed a hyperparameter tuning of the BO framework to deal with the hyperparameter estimation problem in ML for diabetic retinopathy classification. They evaluate the performance of the CNN model with different hyperparameter settings, including batch size, learning rate, number of epochs, and weight decay. On the other hand, Hung et al. [9] have discussed contextual bandit problems, specifically in EI Contextual bandit problems involve making a decision based on contextual information with the goal of maximizing a reward for BO. From the experiment results, their proposed method outperformed other existing contextual bandits in Upper Confidence Bound (UCB) and Thompson Sampling (TS) by achieving a cumulative reward. Another related work was conducted by Abu et al. [11]. The authors discussed a thorough analysis of the transfer learning method when the hyperparameter tuning was performed using BO in a visual field defect classification problem.

Inspired by previous works [12–14], this study aims to expand their investigation by incorporating the metaheuristics methods on EI function BO for multi-class classification of VF defects. The metaheuristics can be broadly classified into four categories of swarm-based algorithms [5,15], evolutionary algorithms [16,17], physics-based algorithms [16,18], and human-based algorithms [16]. These algorithms are based on the behavior of a population of social organisms. These algorithms simulate the behavior of a swarm of agents collaborating to find the best solution to an optimization problem. Previously, a metaheuristics method, the PSO method, was employed by Li et al. [5] to optimize the hyperparameter of BO in the Random Forest (RF) classifier, Adaptive Boosting (AdaBoost), and Extreme Gradient Boosting (XGBoost). A few works in medical imaging examine the classification of a specific eye disease. For instance, Omer et al. [19] combined DL and metaheuristic methods to diagnose diabetic retinopathy. In another work, Nagaraja et al. [20] proposed a metaheuristic method to optimize the Principal Component Analysis (PCA) and HHO to optimize the CNN method for detecting diabetic retinopathy. Most previous research has focused on optimizing the binary classification problem using fundus images.

Therefore, this work aims to enhance the efficiency and accuracy of multi-class image classification by integrating the BO acquisition function with the metaheuristic approach. This work incorporates the Swarm-based algorithms [5], namely Particle Swarm Optimization (PSO) [5,21], Artificial Bee Colony (ABC) Optimization [13,22], Harris Hawks Optimization (HHO) [23], and SFO [24], with the acquisition function EI in BO. The metaheuristic functions are expected to enhance the acquisition function by optimizing the Exploration (mean) and Exploitation (variance) of the posterior distribution of the objective function. These four methods were chosen because swarm-based metaheuristic methods have produced remarkable results in solving complex optimization problems [25]. Furthermore, it is due to their capability of decentralized control of search agents to explore the search environment more effectively [25]. The novelty of this work can be summarized as follows:

1. To optimize the exploration and exploitation process by incorporating with the swarm-based metaheuristic methods (PSO, ABC, HHO, and SFO) with BO default acquisition function, EI.
2. To conduct a comprehensive investigation and analysis of the performance of the acquisition function in BO when incorporated with four different metaheuristic methods against the VGGNet pre-trained models.
3. To evaluate the performance of VGGNet pre-trained models after the BO enhancement in a multi-class image classification problem for VF defects images.

This paper is organized as follows: Section 1 presents the introduction of this work and some review of previous works. Section 2 explains the collection of datasets used in this work and the process of BO enhancement using the metaheuristic method. Section 3 discusses the experimental framework for conducting the effectiveness of the metaheuristic method in BO in classifying the visual field defect pattern using transfer learning. Lastly, Section 4 presents the conclusion and potential for future research.

2. Methodology

2.1. Data Collection

The work obtained 1200 visual field (VF) images from a public dataset. The first dataset is the Humphrey 10-2 Swedish Interactive Threshold Algorithm (SITA) [26,27]. The second dataset is Humphrey 24-2 from Rotterdam Eye Hospital [28,29] and the RT_dataset from Kucur et al. [30,31]. In addition, it included 68 VF images from the Department of Ophthalmology at Universiti Sains Malaysia (USM). All datasets will go through preprocessing to improve the quality and standardization of images, which can result in more accurate and efficient analysis. The dataset will then be divided 80:10:10 between the training, validation, and testing datasets. Table 1 presents the distribution of VF Defects from collected datasets.

Table 1. Distribution of visual field defects from collected datasets.

Type of Visual Field Defect	No. of Record
Central scotoma	204
Right/Left hemianopia	223
Right/left/upper/lower quadrantanopia	160
Tunnel vision	226
Superior/inferior defect field	181
Normal	274

2.2. Multi-Class Classification of VF Defect Using Transfer Learning

In this work, the multi-class classification task of VF defect is performed by using transfer learning (TL) techniques involving four pre-trained models: VGGNet [32], ResNet [33], MobileNet [34,35], and DenseNet [36]. The ImageNet database is the source dataset utilized in these pre-trained models, which includes various eye datasets in the ImageNet collection, including black and white and face images. The knowledge acquired by the pre-trained models was then transferred to the VF classification task, enabling the model to learn more quickly and perform better with less data. Only the VGGNet model is used because of its simple architecture. The framework of transfer learning in this study is shown in Figure 1.

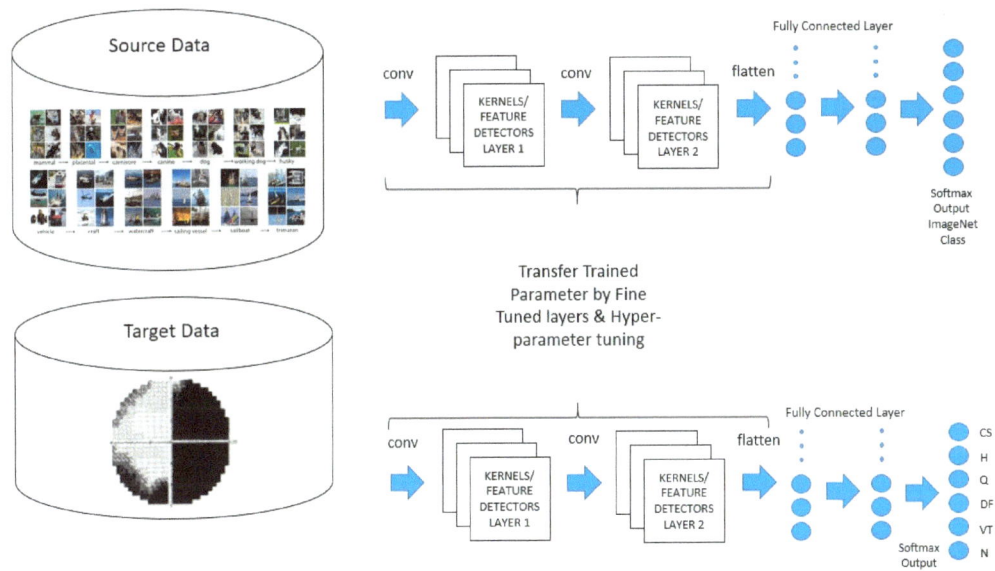

Figure 1. Transfer learning process on visual field defect.

2.3. Combination of Bayesian Optimization with Metaheuristics Methods

After the transfer learning model has been built, the layers and hyperparameters of the pre-trained model will be optimized using the BO technique to identify the optimal hyperparameter for the VF defect classification task. This study investigates and analyses the effect of a different set of hyperparameters and fine-tuned layers with two different pre-trained models using a total of 11 hyperparameters to be optimized, including fine-tuning layers. Fine-tuning will be performed by training the final few layers on the VF dataset while freezing or fixing the remaining layers. The goal of fine-tuning is to leverage the learned features from the pre-trained models to improve the model's performance on the VF classification task.

In BO, the utility functions are referred to as acquisition functions. The acquisition function helps achieve the optimum underlying function by exploring and exploiting regions where the uncertainty of the function is significant. The acquisition function is optimized to retrieve the next point for assessment [7,37,38]. Several acquisition functions have been developed to improve parameters in Bayesian to achieve the best estimation. The following are detailed descriptions of the acquisition functions used in this study:

- Expected Improvement (EI).

The EI [7,39] acquisition function is widely employed in BO because EI encourages the exploration of the search space by providing high values to points with high uncertainty. It also exploits promising regions by focusing on issues that have the potential to improve the current best solution. In addition, EI can capture the objective function's local structure, which can be important when the function is non-convex or has multiple local optima. An example of a non-convex hyperparameter is the number of hidden layers in a neural network. Equation (1) [7] represents the EI process:

$$EI(x) \equiv \mathbb{E}\left[f(x) - f\left(x_t^+\right)\right] \quad (1)$$

where
x_t^+ = the best point to observe before the next point.
x = default point to observe.

- Probability Improvement (PI).

The Probability Improvement (PI) acquisition function can identify the minimum value of the objective function [7]. The point where the objective function is most likely to outperform the default value is where it will be evaluated. It is equivalent to the utility function below that is connected to evaluating the objective function at a specific point with the default hyperparameters set as shown in Equation (2) [7]:

$$PI(x) = P(f(x) \geq f(x+)) = \varnothing(\mu(x) - f(x+)/\sigma(x)) \quad (2)$$

where
$f(x^+)$ = the max value already found.
$\mu(x)$ = the mean value of accuracy.
$\sigma(x)$ = the standard deviation of accuracy.
$\varnothing()$ = the accumulative density function of normal distribution.

- Upper Confidence Bound (UCB).

UCB [7] is an acquisition function that maximizes or minimizes the trade-off parameter and the marginal standard deviation of the objective function rather than the objective function itself [7]. Therefore, Equation (3) [7] is employed to express the UCB process:

$$UCB(x; \beta) = {}^{+}_{-}\mu(x) - \beta\sigma(x) \quad (3)$$

where
$\beta = \beta > 0$ is a trade-off parameter.
$\mu(x)$ = mean of the model.
$\sigma(x)$ = standard deviation of the model.

- Lower Confidence Bound (LCB).

LCB [40,41] aims to address the random bandit dilemma by balancing exploitation and exploration. It controls the trade-off between exploitation and exploration in a manner similar to the UCB process. The LCB process is described in Equation (4) [40,41]:

$$LCB(x) = -\{f(x) - \beta S(x)\} \quad (4)$$

where
β = the parameter managing the trade-off between exploitation and exploration.
$f(x)$ = objective function.
$s(x)$ = covariance of the objective function.

The enhancement of the acquisition function will only be tested using BO's default acquisition function, EI. The remaining acquisition functions will be used as a comparative assessment. In order to maximize the objective function, EI will be combined with four metaheuristic methods in a separate experiment setting, and the performance will be measured by the mean accuracy of BO iterations. The details of the metaheuristic method are explained below:

- Particle Swarm Optimization (PSO) [5,21] is an algorithm inspired by the behavior of a flock of birds or a school of fish. It is developed in the form of population-based stochastic optimization. In PSO, the optimal solution is obtained if the algorithm has reached convergence. If the algorithm has reached convergence, it is influenced by the particle's position and velocity.
- Artificial Bee Colony (ABC) Optimization [13,22] contains four phases: initialization phase, employed bee phase, onlooker bee phase, and scout bee phase. Different kinds of bees can change their roles iteratively until the termination condition is met. Note that there is an associated counter for each food source. If one food source is not improved, the increment of its corresponding counter is 1; otherwise, the counter resets to 0. If the quality of a solution has not been enhanced more than the limit (present parameter), the employed bee would be transformed into a scout bee.

- Harris Hawks Optimization (HHO) [23] is the cooperative behavior in which the chasing style of Harris' hawks in nature is called surprise pounce. HHO can reveal various chasing patterns based on the dynamic nature of scenarios and escaping patterns of the prey. The effectiveness of the HHO optimizer underwent 29 benchmark problems and several real-world engineering problems through a comparison with other nature-inspired techniques to check the optimizer's performance.
- Sailfish Optimization (SFO) [24] is inspired by a group of hunting sailfish. This method consists of two tips of populations, the sailfish population for intensification of the search around the best so far and the sardine population for diversification of the search space. This technique indicates competitive results for improving exploration and exploitation phases, avoiding local optima, and high-speed convergence, especially on large-scale global optimization.

In Bayesian Optimization, exploration $\mu(x)$ and exploitation $\sigma(x)$ are two opposing strategies used by the acquisition function to determine which set of hyperparameters to evaluate next. Exploration refers to the process of selecting hyperparameters that have a high potential for discovering new regions of the search space [42]. On the other hand, exploitation refers to the process of selecting hyperparameters that have the highest probability of improving the model's performance based on the information gathered [42]. The main issue is that computing a natural anticipated utility function with this acquisition function is impossible. The stopping criterion is met in BO when the maximum number of evaluations or a convergence threshold is met. By incorporating a metaheuristic approach to influence the point that BO chooses, the number of points with lesser accuracy can be decreased, and the performance of BO can be increased. In addition, the number of iterations is set during BO to obtain accuracy from different sets of hyperparameters. Hence, VF defect classification will serve as the basis for measuring the BO's performance to find the best hyperparameter.

This work observed the optimization of the EI acquisition function in BO using four swarm-based metaheuristic methods: PSO, ABC, HHO, and SFO. The metaheuristic methods optimize the mean and variance in the acquisition function to obtain many higher peak accuracies while evaluating the objective function. Here, the mean value determines the most promising point in the search space. In the meantime, the variance value is used to balance exploration and exploitation, which is extracted by the acquisition function based on the objective function, grouped as a population subject by the metaheuristic method, and used to maximize output. The mean and variance values estimated based on the observed values of the objective function at previous evaluation points are maximized using the swarm-based metaheuristic method. Finally, the mean and variance will be set as the candidate solutions that evolve to search for the optimal solution.

The pseudocode of the enhanced BO is shown in Algorithm 1. The section highlighted in bold outlines the proposed algorithm that incorporates the metaheuristics method into BO.

2.4. Evaluation

The performance of the four acquisition functions above was validated with VGGNet pre-trained models. Because the iteration number is set to 11, the mean accuracy (μ) value will be used to compare the 11 accuracies obtained from the experiments. The mean of the transfer learning accuracy over multiple runs of the algorithm is calculated to evaluate the accuracy of the optimization algorithm based on the following Equation (5).

$$\mu = \frac{\sum_{i=1}^{N} X_i}{N}, \tag{5}$$

where

N = the size of the iteration.
x_i = each accuracy value from the BO iteration.

μ = the iteration mean.

Algorithm 1: Psuedocode of the BO Enhancement: Enhance Bayesian Optimization with Metaheuristic Method
Required: An acquisition function
1: Inputs:
Bayesian Optimization process
2: While the stop criteria are not fulfilled, do the following:
3:     Select the next point to evaluate based on an acquisition function (Expected Improvement), which balances the exploration of new points and the the exploitation of promising areas of the search space until maximize accuracy is obtained: $$x^* = \underset{x \in X}{\mathrm{argmax}} f(x).$$
4:     Calculation of EI for each set of hyperparameters and fine-tuning layers using the probabilistic model provides: $$EI(x) = E[\max(0, f(x) - f(x^*))].$$
5:     Evaluate the mean $\mu(x)$ and variance $\sigma(x)$ of the probabilistic model at x. These values are estimated based on the observed values of the objective function at previous evaluation points.
6:     Initialize the population of mean $\mu(x)$ and variance $\sigma(x)$ of the probabilistic model at x.
7:     From the set of a population of mean $\mu(x)$ and variance $\sigma(x)$, maximize by me taheuristic method (PSO, ABC, HHO and SFO). The goal is to explore the search space and generate a diverse set of hyperparameters and fine-tuned layers solution.
8:     Evaluate the objective function for each new set of hyperparameters and fine-tuned layers solution in the population.
9:     Select the best hyperparameter and fine-tuned layers from the entire population based on the objective function values.
10: End while

3. Experimental Results and Discussion

Four different acquisition functions (EI, PI, LCB, and UCB) were initially used to optimize the pre-trained VGGNet models in BO. Then, the mean and variance of the EI acquisition function are enhanced using four metaheuristic techniques: PSO, ABC, HHO, and SFO. EI is selected for further enhancement as it is a default acquisition function for BO. The experiment was performed using KERAS and Scikit Optimize, a Python library for performing BO. The experiment was conducted on an Intel Core i7-10 processor with 8 GB of RAM and an RTX2080 graphics processing unit (GPU).

3.1. Validation Analyses of Pre-Trained Models Enhanced by Bayesian Optimization Based on Different Acquisition Functions

The validation accuracy of the VGG-16 and VGG-19 models using different acquisition functions in BO based on selected hyperparameters and fine-tuned layers is presented in Tables 2 and 3. Both tables compare the validation accuracy performance of the enhanced EI acquisition function based on the metaheuristic method compared to other acquisition functions. During the experiment, 11 hyperparameters selected by BO with fine-tuned layers were considered. The initial hyperparameters and fine-tune layer were set for the first iteration. Table 2 and 3 also include the comparison results of another metaheuristic optimization algorithm, the Covariance Matrix Adaptation Evolution Strategy (CMA-ES) [12]. Loshchilov and Hutter [12] mentioned that CMA-ES has the capacity to efficiently explore a high-dimensional search space and identify an optimal objective function solution. Additionally, therefore, the validation accuracy of CMA-ES is also included as a comparison.

Table 2. Validation accuracy of VGG-16 using different acquisition functions in Bayesian Optimization.

Acquisition Function	Iteration	Hyperparameter									Fine-Tuned Layer		Validation Accuracy (%)
		Feature Map	Filter Size	Activation Function	Pool Size	Optimizer	Learning Rate	Batch Size	Epoch	Dropout Rate	Upper Layer	Lower Layer	
CMA-ES [12]	1	45	1	ReLU	1	SGD	0.0001	25	49	0.3	FALSE	TRUE	20.55
	2	56	1	ReLU	2	ADAM	0.0053	20	189	0.8	FALSE	FALSE	20.55
	3	34	1	Sigmoid	1	SGD	0.0023	4	89	0.2	FALSE	TRUE	20.55
	4	53	3	Sigmoid	2	ADAM	0.0225	6	122	0.4	FALSE	FALSE	20.55
	5	51	1	ReLU	2	ADAM	0.0049	4	131	0.3	TRUE	TRUE	20.55
	6	42	3	Sigmoid	1	Adadelta	0.0711	4	127	0.3	TRUE	FALSE	20.55
	7	45	3	Sigmoid	2	Adadelta	0.0033	1	142	0.8	TRUE	TRUE	20.55
	8	61	2	ReLU	2	ADAM	0.0289	11	29	0.2	TRUE	TRUE	20.55
	9	48	2	ReLU	1	RMSprop	0.0028	16	105	0.6	FALSE	TRUE	20.55
	10	48	2	Sigmoid	2	ADAM	0.0031	17	105	0.6	FALSE	FALSE	15.67
	11	48	2	ReLU	2	RMSprop	0.0030	16	105	0.5	TRUE	TRUE	20.55
EI [39]	1	64	3	ReLU	2	ADAM	0.001	32	200	0.2	FALSE	FALSE	20.55
	2	58	2	ReLU	1	RMSprop	0.0009	24	29	0.5	TRUE	FALSE	95.97
	3	38	2	Sigmoid	1	ADAM	0.0022	10	51	0.2	TRUE	TRUE	20.55
	4	33	1	Sigmoid	1	Adadelta	0.0031	26	40	0.8	FALSE	FALSE	20.55
	5	38	2	Sigmoid	1	SGD	0.0117	13	23	0.7	TRUEs	FALSE	19.96
	6	46	2	Sigmoid	2	RMSprop	0.0019	18	34	0.6	TRUE	FALSE	20.55
	7	41	2	Sigmoid	2	ADAM	0.0003	11	76	0.9	FALSE	FALSE	20.55
	8	35	2	ReLU	1	ADAM	0.0007	29	94	0.1	FALSE	FALSE	96.74
	9	47	1	ReLU	2	RMSprop	0.0068	2	167	0.9	TRUE	TRUE	20.55
	10	56	2	ReLU	1	RMSprop	0.0264	6	97	0.4	TRUE	FALSE	18.81
	11	64	2	ReLU	2	SGD	0.0226	27	200	0.9	TRUE	TRUE	97.92
EI-PSO	1	64	3	ReLU	2	ADAM	0.001	32	200	0.2	FALSE	FALSE	20.55
	2	32	1	ReLU	2	ADAM	0.0006	9	42	0.1	FALSE	TRUE	94.75
	3	29	2	ReLU	2	Adadelta	0.0008	12	118	0.8	FALSE	FALSE	71.57
	4	17	2	Sigmoid	2	RMSprop	0.0774	10	156	0.4	TRUE	FALSE	17.16
	5	21	2	Sigmoid	1	RMSprop	0.0032	10	122	0.4	TRUE	FALSE	20.55
	6	24	2	ReLU	2	RMSprop	0.0002	7	180	0.7	FALSE	TRUE	97.80
	7	30	2	ReLU	1	RMSprop	0.0849	10	53	0.6	FALSE	FALSE	19.03
	8	32	3	Sigmoid	2	RMSprop	0.001	11	69	0.2	TRUE	FALSE	20.55
	9	25	1	Sigmoid	1	ADAM	0.0354	14	76	0.5	FALSE	TRUE	19.41
	10	18	1	Sigmoid	2	RMSprop	0.0297	9	164	0.8	TRUE	FALSE	19.96
	11	18	2	Sigmoid	2	ADAM	0.0001	14	128	0.9	FALSE	FALSE	20.55
EI-ABC	1	64	2	ReLU	2	ADAM	0.001	32	200	0.2	FALSE	FALSE	20.55
	2	19	2	ReLU	2	ADAM	0.0193	5	168	0.5	TRUE	TRUE	19.45
	3	29	1	Sigmoid	1	Adadelta	0.0231	5	141	0.8	FALSE	TRUE	20.55
	4	28	2	Sigmoid	2	ADAM	0.0213	15	30	0.6	FALSE	TRUE	15.93
	5	17	2	ReLU	2	Adadelta	0.0006	1	126	0.6	FALSE	TRUE	83.31
	6	26	2	Sigmoid	2	SGD	0.0014	6	75	0.7	FALSE	FALSE	20.00
	7	32	2	ReLU	2	SGD	0.0118	6	89	0.5	TRUE	FALSE	97.84
	8	18	1	ReLU	1	ADAM	0.0524	14	103	0.2	FALSE	TRUE	20.55
	9	26	1	ReLU	1	Adadelta	0.0009	11	184	0.5	TRUE	TRUE	71.19
	10	29	2	Sigmoid	2	RMSprop	0.0152	2	190	0.5	TRUE	TRUE	14.41
	11	22	2	ReLU	2	ADAM	0.0229	14	64	0.4	FALSE	TRUE	20.55
EI-HHO	1	64	3	ReLU	2	ADAM	0.001	32	200	0.2	FALSE	FALSE	20.55
	2	20	1	Sigmoid	1	SGD	0.0004	5	184	0.3	FALSE	FALSE	19.41
	3	30	3	Sigmoid	1	SGD	0.0005	1	193	0.4	FALSE	FALSE	20.55
	4	27	2	ReLU	2	RMSprop	0.0139	8	141	0.3	FALSE	FALSE	20.55
	5	22	2	ReLU	1	ADAM	0.0077	9	42	0.3	TRUE	FALSE	20.55
	6	23	2	ReLU	1	ADAM	0.0165	11	56	0.2	TRUE	FALSE	19.36
	7	18	2	ReLU	1	ADAM	0.0001	8	148	0.8	FALSE	TRUE	97.03

Table 2. Cont.

Acquisition Function	Iteration	Hyperparameter									Fine-Tuned Layer		Validation Accuracy (%)
		Feature Map	Filter Size	Activation Function	Pool Size	Optimizer	Learning Rate	Batch Size	Epoch	Dropout Rate	Upper Layer	Lower Layer	
	8	26	2	Sigmoid	2	ADAM	0.0002	10	159	0.7	FALSE	FALSE	20.55
	9	18	1	Sigmoid	2	ADAM	0.0103	13	89	0.3	TRUE	TRUE	20.55
	10	24	2	ReLU	2	SGD	0.0035	2	172	0.8	FALSE	TRUE	98.26
	11	18	3	ReLU	2	RMSprop	0.0006	15	53	0.5	FALSE	TRUE	96.53
	1	64	3	ReLU	2	ADAM	0.001	32	200	0.2	FALSE	FALSE	20.55
	2	30	2	ReLU	1	RMSprop	0.0018	11	93	0.6	TRUE	FALSE	94.87
	3	21	2	ReLU	1	Adadelta	0.0013	8	48	0.8	FALSE	FALSE	52.92
	4	25	2	Sigmoid	1	Adadelta	0.0791	3	164	0.4	FALSE	TRUE	20.55
EI-SFO	5	19	1	ReLU	2	SGD	0.034	9	58	0.8	TRUE	FALSE	92.84
	6	27	3	ReLU	2	RMSprop	0.0002	15	86	0.5	TRUE	TRUE	98.60
	7	25	1	ReLU	1	ADAM	0.0466	4	150	0.5	TRUE	FALSE	19.45
	8	19	3	Sigmoid	2	ADAM	0.0055	14	169	0.1	TRUE	FALSE	16.65
	9	29	1	Sigmoid	2	RMSprop	0.0279	14	23	0.3	TRUE	FALSE	20.55
	10	18	2	Sigmoid	2	RMSprop	0.0001	3	118	0.6	TRUE	TRUE	20.55
	11	30	1	Sigmoid	1	RMSprop	0.0001	9	77	0.1	TRUE	FALSE	20.55
	1	64	3	ReLU	2	ADAM	0.001	32	200	0.2	FALSE	FALSE	20.55
	2	50	3	Sigmoid	1	SGD	0.0906	1	46	0.8	FALSE	FALSE	15.68
	3	63	2	ReLU	2	RMSprop	0.0158	8	127	0.8	FALSE	FALSE	20.55
	4	62	2	ReLU	1	RMSprop	0.0278	8	74	0.8	TRUE	TRUE	20.55
	5	36	3	ReLU	1	RMSprop	0.0013	14	57	0.4	TRUE	FALSE	95.85
PI	6	33	2	Sigmoid	1	RMSprop	0.0007	2	44	0.8	TRUE	FALSE	20.55
	7	46	2	ReLU	1	Adadelta	0.0444	19	71	0.7	FALSE	FALSE	96.23
	8	46	3	Sigmoid	2	Adadelta	0.0071	17	95	0.5	TRUE	TRUE	20.55
	9	49	2	ReLU	1	RMSprop	0.0954	3	40	0.7	TRUE	FALSE	18.52
	10	47	3	Sigmoid	1	ADAM	0.0017	19	47	0.8	FALSE	FALSE	19.36
	11	44	3	Sigmoid	1	Adadelta	0.00717	27	116	0.4	TRUE	TRUE	20.55
	1	64	3	ReLU	2	ADAM	0.001	32	200	0.2	FALSE	FALSE	97.88
	2	61	2	ReLU	1	RMSprop	0.0029	22	143	0.6	FALSE	FALSE	20.55
	3	58	3	ReLU	2	SGD	0.0077	7	53	0.1	TRUE	FALSE	96.31
	4	44	3	ReLU	1	SGD	0.0075	14	162	0.2	FALSE	FALSE	96.86
	5	52	2	ReLU	1	ADAM	0.0023	1	115	0.9	FALSE	TRUE	20.55
UCB	6	53	2	Sigmoid	2	ADAM	0.0033	5	188	0.4	TRUE	TRUE	19.07
	7	51	2	Sigmoid	2	RMSprop	0.0164	7	99	0.5	FALSE	FALSE	16.19
	8	37	1	Sigmoid	1	ADAM	0.0001	21	172	0.6	TRUE	TRUE	20.55
	9	41	3	ReLU	2	RMSprop	0.0046	8	142	0.2	TRUE	FALSE	20.55
	10	60	2	Sigmoid	2	RMSprop	0.0017	25	173	0.5	TRUE	FALSE	20.55
	11	35	3	Sigmoid	2	ADAM	0.0383	29	52	0.9	FALSE	TRUE	17.46
	1	64	3	ReLU	2	ADAM	0.001	32	200	0.2	FALSE	FALSE	98.26
	2	40	3	ReLU	1	SGD	0.0313	9	14	0.3	FALSE	TRUE	94.28
	3	50	2	Sigmoid	2	ADAM	0.0498	21	167	0.1	FALSE	FALSE	18.31
	4	44	1	Sigmoid	1	ADAM	0.0010	10	34	0.9	FALSE	TRUE	20.55
	5	54	1	Sigmoid	2	RMSprop	0.0016	21	120	0.4	FALSE	TRUE	20.55
LCB	6	52	2	Sigmoid	1	RMSprop	0.0003	17	113	0.8	TRUE	TRUE	20.55
	7	54	1	Sigmoid	2	ADAM	0.0925	5	76	0.2	TRUE	FALSE	17.33
	8	39	2	ReLU	2	ADAM	0.0002	21	100	0.9	TRUE	FALSE	98.22
	9	64	2	Sigmoid	2	RMSprop	0.0087	29	59	0.4	FALSE	FALSE	16.91
	10	59	1	Sigmoid	2	RMSprop	0.0003	26	183	0.5	FALSE	TRUE	20.55
	11	55	1	ReLU	2	Adadelta	0.0791	32	105	0.8	FALSE	TRUE	93.43

Table 3. Optimization of VGG-19 using different acquisition functions in Bayesian Optimization.

Acquisition Function	Iteration	Hyperparameter									Fine-Tuned		Validation Accuracy (%)
		Feature Map	Filter Size	Activation Function	Pool Size	Optimizer	Learning Rate	Batch Size	Epoch	Dropout Rate	Upper Layer	Lower Layer	
CMA-ES [12]	1	37	2	ReLU	2	Adadelta	0.0001	3	192	0.4	TRUE	FALSE	20.55
	2	48	1	ReLU	2	RMSprop	0.0528	7	92	0.3	FALSE	TRUE	17.80
	3	42	3	ReLU	2	RMSprop	0.0193	3	79	0.8	FALSE	FALSE	20.55
	4	63	3	ReLU	2	RMSprop	0.0002	2	77	0.4	FALSE	TRUE	97.03
	5	58	2	Sigmoid	2	RMSprop	0.0436	14	173	0.3	TRUE	TRUE	17.58
	6	44	3	Sigmoid	1	RMSprop	0.0026	1	25	0.3	FALSE	TRUE	17.58
	7	32	1	Sigmoid	2	Adadelta	0.0016	7	13	0.5	TRUE	TRUE	20.55
	8	63	2	ReLu	2	RMSprop	0.0006	13	37	0.4	TRUE	TRUE	93.64
	9	48	2	Sigmoid	2	RMSprop	0.0041	16	105	0.7	FALSE	TRUE	20.55
	10	48	2	ReLU	1	ADAM	0.0023	16	105	0.4	FALSE	TRUE	20.55
	11	48	2	ReLU	1	Adadelta	0.0037	16	105	0.6	TRUE	FALSE	92.16
EI [39]	1	64	3	ReLU	2	ADAM	0.001	32	200	0.2	FALSE	FALSE	20.55
	2	39	2	Sigmoid	1	SGD	0.0041	32	60	0.4	TRUE	TRUE	19.11
	3	62	2	ReLU	1	ADAM	0.0019	3	110	0.8	TRUE	FALSE	20.55
	4	39	2	Sigmoid	1	RMSprop	0.0015	31	99	0.6	TRUE	TRUE	20.55
	5	44	3	ReLU	1	RMSprop	0.0724	27	90	0.3	FALSE	FALSE	19.96
	6	32	2	Sigmoid	1	ADAM	0.0003	1	154	0.4	TRUE	TRUE	20.55
	7	36	1	ReLU	2	RMSprop	0.0874	18	58	0.7	FALSE	TRUE	18.22
	8	52	3	Sigmoid	2	RMSprop	0.0846	3	97	0.8	TRUE	FALSE	17.37
	9	55	2	ReLU	1	RMSprop	0.0029	10	172	0.8	TRUE	TRUE	20.55
	10	53	2	Sigmoid	1	ADAM	0.0001	27	142	0.6	FALSE	TRUE	20.55
	11	51	1	Sigmoid	1	ADAM	0.0019	4	135	0.7	TRUE	TRUE	18.52
EI-PSO	1	64	3	ReLU	2	ADAM	0.001	32	200	0.2	FALSE	FALSE	20.55
	2	24	2	Sigmoid	2	ADAM	0.0068	4	53	0.2	FALSE	TRUE	18.26
	3	31	3	Sigmoid	2	Adadelta	0.0532	5	72	0.6	FALSE	TRUE	20.55
	4	21	1	Sigmoid	1	ADAM	0.0453	11	53	0.3	FALSE	TRUE	19.96
	5	24	1	ReLU	2	ADAM	0.0001	7	65	0.9	FALSE	FALSE	92.67
	6	26	3	ReLU	1	Adadelta	0.0019	9	192	0.2	FALSE	TRUE	95.64
	7	31	1	ReLU	2	Adadelta	0.0003	14	67	0.6	FALSE	TRUE	20.55
	8	21	1	Sigmoid	1	SGD	0.0004	4	147	0.3	TRUE	FALSE	20.55
	9	30	1	Sigmoid	1	RMSprop	0.0002	5	45	0.8	FALSE	FALSE	20.55
	10	18	3	ReLU	1	ADAM	0.0006	4	82	0.7	FALSE	FALSE	20.55
	11	28	3	ReLU	2	RMSprop	0.06234	12	174	0.2	FALSE	TRUE	19.96
EI-ABC	1	64	3	ReLU	2	ADAM	0.001	32	200	0.2	FALSE	FALSE	97.63
	2	21	2	Sigmoid	2	ADAM	0.0005	1	114	0.8	TRUE	TRUE	20.55
	3	25	2	ReLU	2	RMSprop	0.0001	7	14	0.7	TRUE	TRUE	94.19
	4	19	2	Sigmoid	2	RMSprop	0.0016	14	112	0.4	FALSE	TRUE	20.55
	5	17	3	Sigmoid	1	ADAM	0.0005	13	116	0.4	TRUE	FALSE	20.55
	6	26	1	Sigmoid	2	ADAM	0.0017	10	114	0.6	TRUE	FALSE	20.55
	7	32	2	Sigmoid	2	RMSprop	0.0003	8	144	0.9	FALSE	TRUE	20.55
	8	21	2	Sigmoid	2	Adadelta	0.0001	2	78	0.8	FALSE	FALSE	20.55
	9	23	1	ReLU	2	ADAM	0.0015	15	131	0.8	TRUE	FALSE	94.53
	10	16	3	Sigmoid	2	RMSprop	0.0018	14	169	0.2	FALSE	TRUE	20.55
	11	17	2	ReLU	1	RMSprop	0.0001	11	16	0.9	FALSE	TRUE	92.12
EI-HHO	1	64	3	ReLU	2	ADAM	0.001	32	200	0.2	FALSE	FALSE	20.55
	2	28	1	ReLU	1	ADAM	0.0056	4	174	0.6	FALSE	TRUE	20.55
	3	25	3	ReLU	1	SGD	0.0047	2	27	0.8	FALSE	TRUE	92.88
	4	19	2	ReLU	2	RMSprop	0.0053	4	76	0.23	TRUE	TRUE	20.55
	5	18	2	ReLU	1	ADAM	0.0312	12	94	0.7	TRUE	TRUE	20.00
	6	20	1	ReLU	2	ADAM	0.0042	6	115	0.5	FALSE	FALSE	20.55
	7	23	2	Sigmoid	2	Adadelta	0.0167	8	191	0.5	FALSE	FALSE	20.55

Table 3. Cont.

Acquisition Function	Iteration	Hyperparameter									Fine-Tuned		Validation Accuracy (%)
		Feature Map	Filter Size	Activation Function	Pool Size	Optimizer	Learning Rate	Batch Size	Epoch	Dropout Rate	Upper Layer	Lower Layer	
	8	18	2	Sigmoid	2	Adadelta	0.0007	14	52	0.7	TRUE	TRUE	20.55
	9	29	3	Sigmoid	2	RMSprop	0.0015	8	132	0.1	TRUE	TRUE	20.55
	10	22	1	Sigmoid	1	ADAM	0.0361	12	186	0.4	TRUE	FALSE	19.41
	11	26	2	Sigmoid	2	Adadelta	0.0333	10	140	0.1	TRUE	TRUE	20.55
	1	64	3	ReLU	2	ADAM	0.001	32	200	0.2	FALSE	FALSE	20.55
	2	20	1	ReLU	1	RMSprop	0.0343	10	124	0.7	TRUE	FALSE	20.00
	3	22	1	ReLU	1	RMSprop	0.0009	16	137	0.8	FALSE	FALSE	94.87
	4	20	2	Sigmoid	2	RMSprop	0.0768	13	134	0.8	TRUE	FALSE	18.77
	5	21	2	Sigmoid	2	SGD	0.0196	14	35	0.7	FALSE	FALSE	20.55
EI-SFO	6	27	3	Sigmoid	2	RMSprop	0.0080	7	191	0.7	FALSE	FALSE	17.58
	7	29	1	ReLU	2	RMSprop	0.0169	11	107	0.4	FALSE	TRUE	20.00
	8	19	2	ReLU	2	RMSprop	0.0677	12	173	0.2	FALSE	FALSE	19.37
	9	31	1	ReLU	2	ADAM	0.0005	5	111	0.5	FALSE	TRUE	95.55
	10	29	1	ReLU	1	ADAM	0.0004	5	55	0.5	TRUE	TRUE	95.89
	11	20	2	ReLU	2	ADAM	0.0003	7	107	0.6	TRUE	TRUE	98.35
	1	64	3	ReLU	2	ADAM	0.001	32	200	0.2	FALSE	FALSE	20.55
	2	51	3	Sigmoid	1	RMSprop	0.0007	14	83	0.7	TRUE	TRUE	20.55
	3	48	3	Sigmoid	1	RMSprop	0.0678	16	108	0.3	TRUE	TRUE	18.98
	4	35	1	ReLU	2	Adadelta	0.0001	8	147	0.5	TRUE	TRUE	20.55
	5	44	2	ReLU	1	RMSprop	0.0002	21	199	0.8	FALSE	FALSE	97.67
PI	6	50	2	ReLU	2	SGD	0.001	13	70	0.1	TRUE	TRUE	76.99
	7	54	3	ReLU	1	ADAM	0.001	4	41	0.2	TRUE	TRUE	97.12
	8	47	1	ReLU	2	SGD	0.0013	13	65	0.7	FALSE	TRUE	71.31
	9	58	1	ReLU	2	ADAM	0.0027	5	145	0.3	FALSE	FALSE	20.55
	10	40	2	Sigmoid	1	ADAM	0.0017	20	25	0.8	TRUE	TRUE	19.96
	11	40	1	ReLU	1	RMSprop	0.0372	29	23	0.9	FALSE	TRUE	19.41
	1	64	3	ReLU	2	ADAM	0.001	32	200	0.2	FALSE	FALSE	20.55
	2	46	1	Sigmoid	1	RMSprop	0.0255	14	195	0.7	TRUE	TRUE	16.95
	3	54	2	ReLU	1	ADAM	0.0028	5	112	0.5	TRUE	FALSE	20.55
	4	40	1	ReLU	2	RMSprop	0.0004	5	37	0.3	FALSE	TRUE	93.64
	5	57	1	Sigmoid	1	ADAM	0.0036	26	171	0.7	TRUE	TRUE	20.55
UCB	6	55	1	Sigmoid	2	ADAM	0.0006	16	160	0.1	TRUE	TRUE	20.55
	7	63	3	ReLU	2	ADAM	0.0022	5	129	0.8	TRUE	TRUE	20.55
	8	55	1	Sigmoid	2	ADAM	0.0002	18	180	0.4	FALSE	TRUE	20.55
	9	42	3	Sigmoid	2	ADAM	0.0249	3	92	0.4	TRUE	FALSE	15.47
	10	50	3	ReLU	1	ADAM	0.0022	14	112	0.8	TRUE	FALSE	20.55
	11	40	1	ReLU	2	RMSprop	0.0004	5	37	0.3	FALSE	TRUE	93.60
	1	64	3	ReLU	2	ADAM	0.001	32	200	0.2	FALSE	FALSE	20.55
	2	48	2	ReLU	2	SGD	0.0116	4	63	0.6	FALSE	TRUE	98.00
	3	39	2	Sigmoid	2	ADAM	0.0016	19	151	0.6	TRUE	TRUE	19.36
	4	53	2	Sigmoid	1	ADAM	0.0312	19	172	0.9	FALSE	TRUE	18.18
	5	64	2	ReLU	2	SGD	0.0002	10	16	0.2	TRUE	TRUE	20.55
LCB	6	59	1	Sigmoid	2	RMSprop	0.0002	11	130	0.8	TRUE	TRUE	20.55
	7	34	2	Sigmoid	2	Adadelta	0.0247	13	120	0.7	TRUE	FALSE	20.55
	8	33	2	Sigmoid	2	RMSprop	0.0003	6	56	0.6	TRUE	FALSE	20.55
	9	38	2	Sigmoid	2	ADAM	0.0042	16	95	0.2	FALSE	FALSE	19.96
	10	34	3	ReLU	2	RMSprop	0.0056	16	161	0.8	TRUE	FALSE	20.55
	11	52	1	ReLU	1	SGD	0.0004	27	110	0.6	TRUE	TRUE	32.46

The majority of the hyperparameters and fine-tuned layers in Table 2 indicate a validation accuracy of 20.55%, suggesting overfitting. This issue may occur because the pre-trained model is too complex for the VF defect image as a result of their small size or lack of diversity. Another possibility is that the set of hyperparameters is too extensive and involves all network layers, resulting in a complex network architecture. In some cases, tuning all layers of a pre-trained neural network achieved high accuracy in this classification task. It was observed that BO would adjust to a slower learning rate as more layers are tuned to prevent overwriting existing knowledge in earlier layers in order to preserve features that are likely to be useful for the new task.

The proposed method, EI-SFO, from both Tables 2 and 3 indicates the performance of EI when enhanced using SFO metaheuristic methods. SFO is used to maximize the mean and variance processes within the EI acquisition function, but its performance cannot surpass the performance of the LCB acquisition function in BO. This is because the LCB can efficiently search the hyperparameter in the search space by selecting the hyperparameter that is likely to perform well and have low uncertainty [43]. LCB selects the lowest expected value of the transfer learning and then calculates the sum of the mean and a scaled variance value. The scaling factor will control the exploration and exploration of BO, and the larger the scaling factor values will encourage more exploration. In contrast, smaller values of the scaling factor will encourage more exploitation.

On the other hand, it was observed that the SFO method maximized the mean and variance inside the EI acquisition function. The maximization of the mean and variance of EI induced the mean to select candidate solutions that are both promising and diverse. This helps the BO to explore a broader range of the search space, potentially leading to better solutions. When the mean is maximized, the surrogate model predicts that the current hyperparameter set will likely perform well. This is a sign that the optimization process exploits the most promising areas of the search space, and it can lead to faster convergence toward the optimal set of hyperparameters [43].

In contrast, when the variance is maximized, the surrogate model is uncertain about the performance of the current set of hyperparameters. This indicates that the optimization process is exploring new areas of the search space. However, it can also result in slower convergence since the optimizer may need to evaluate more hyperparameter configurations to gain enough information about the objective function. However, the maximized mean and variance can lead to exploring suboptimal regions of the search space. Consequently, the objective function must have a well-balanced mean and variance. When comparing the standard EI to EI-PSO, EI-ABC, EI-HHO, and EI-SFO on VGG-16, the incorporation of the metaheuristic method results in a significant improvement in mean accuracy evaluations.

3.2. Performance Analyses of Pre-Trained Models Enhanced by Bayesian Optimization Based on Different Acquisition Functions

In BO, four acquisition functions (EI, PI, UCB, and LCB) are commonly used to optimize the objective function. Therefore, these acquisition functions were tested to analyze the difference in terms of performance in the VF defect classification task. Since the VGGNet model presents the lowest performance in the default acquisition function, i.e., EI, this work focuses on optimizing this acquisition function with four metaheuristic methods (PSO, ABC, HHO, and SFO) to enhance the performance of BO.

Figure 2a demonstrates the performance accuracy distribution across 11 iterations of the VGG-16 pre-trained model based on different acquisition functions. In this work, the number of iterations is set to 11, which is the maximum number of iterations supported by the hardware computational capability in order to achieve optimal EI performance. In the box plot green triangle represent the mean of accuracy obtain from the 11 iteration and the circle is the accuracy outlier where's the 90% accuracy is not the majority in the 11 iteration. When optimizing hyperparameters in BO using the LCB acquisition function, LCB has shown the highest mean accuracy when compared to other acquisition functions. Without an outlier, the mean accuracy is 47.17%, with a maximum and minimum accuracy of 98.26% and 16.91%, respectively. The lower quartile value is 18.31, indicating that 25% of the obtained accuracy falls below 18.31% and 75% of the data for the upper quartile fall below 98.22. In contrast, UCB performed the worst in terms of accuracy distribution, regardless of the fact that the maximum accuracy achieved was 97.88%. The average accuracy achieved is 30.59%, with a median of 20.55% and a minimum of 16.81%.

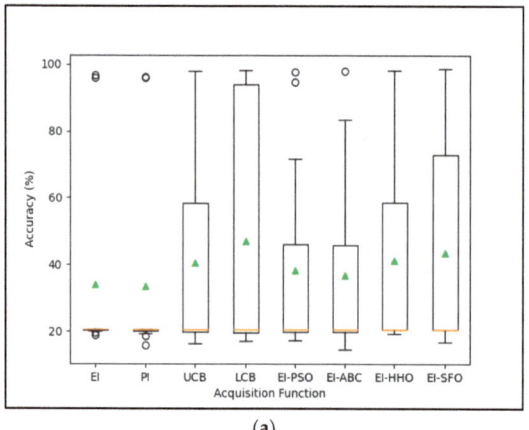
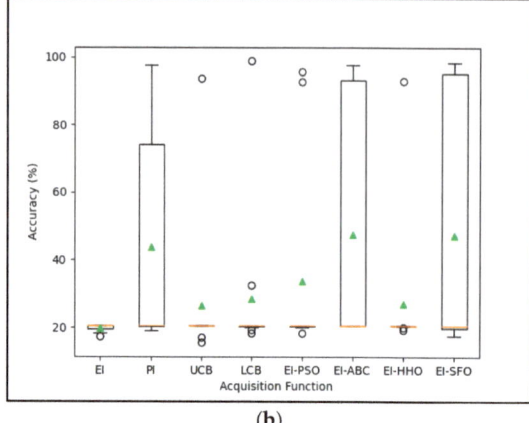

Figure 2. Comparison of performance accuracy distribution of VGGNet using difference acquisition function in Bayesian Optimization; (**a**) VGG-16; (**b**) VGG-19.

On the other hand, Figure 2b shows the range of performance accuracy across 11 iterations of the VGG-19 pre-trained model based on different acquisition functions. Based on the box plot, the EI-SFO method outperformed other metaheuristic methods with a mean accuracy of 47.40%, a maximum accuracy of 98.34%, and a minimum accuracy of 15.50%. The lower quartile value for the EI-SFO is 19.37%. The median is 20.55%, and the upper quartile value is 95.55%. In contrast, EI has the worst performance, with a mean accuracy of 19.86%, median accuracy of 20.55%, first quartile value of 18.96%, and third quartile value of 20.55%. The maximum accuracy is 20.55%, while the minimum achievable accuracy is 17.37%.

The following Table 4 compares the performance accuracy of enhanced BO and conventional methods. For the classification of VF defects, the performance of a pre-trained model enhanced by BO using the EI-SFO method is comparable to the performance of the LCB acquisition function for VGG-16. As for VGG-19, the mean accuracy is better compared to others, while the highest accuracy is almost identical to the LCB method. The mean evaluation of VGGNet is determined by the number of iterations set during BO in order to detect VF defects with optimal accuracy. The average precision rises as the metaheuristic method optimizes the EI acquisition function. Among the enhancements to EI, the EI-SFO method achieves the highest accuracy of 98.60% for VGG-16 and 98.34% for VGG-19. The experiment also included CMA-ES, one of the acquisition functions proposed by Loshchilov and Hutter [12], that exhibits superior performance in more complex optimization problems. However, the performance of both VGGNet models for the VF classification task suggests that overfitting occurred. This could be the result of an incompatible combination of hyperparameters and fine-tuning explored by the acquisition function.

In addition to a comparative analysis of performance accuracy, a confusion matrix analysis was also conducted. The confusion matrix consists of a square matrix with dimensions equal to the number of classes in the problem. Each cell in the matrix represents the precision that belongs to a particular actual class and is predicted to belong to a particular predicted class. The diagonal elements of the matrix represent the precision of correctly classified instances for each class. The off-diagonal component represents the precision of instances that are misclassified. The darker the blue color in confusion matrix the higher the accuracy. The confusion matrix was constructed using the classification result of six types of VF defects observed in 10% of the entire dataset. The six types of VF defects include central, hemianopia, normal, quadrantanopia, superior, and tunnel defect.

Figure 3a,b demonstrate the performance of VGGNet after enhanced BO has been applied. Figure 3a shows that the VGG-16 model classified superior, central, and hemianopia defects with 100% accuracy. As for quadrantanopia, the obtained precision is 93%, with 5% tunnel vision and 1% hemianopia misclassification. Normal vision achieved 98% precision with 2% quadrantanopia misclassification, while tunnel vision achieved 96% precision with 3% central scotoma and 1% quadrantanopia misclassification. The overall precision obtained from six classes of visual field defects in VGG-16 is 97.83% precision.

In Figure 3b, VGG-19 achieved a precision of 100% for central scotoma, superior, and hemianopia, 96% for quadrantanopia with 4% misclassified as tunnel vision, 99% for normal with 1% misclassified as superior, and 95% for tunnel vision with 5% misclassified as a central scotoma. The overall testing precision obtained from the six classes of visual field defects in VGG-16 is 98.33%.

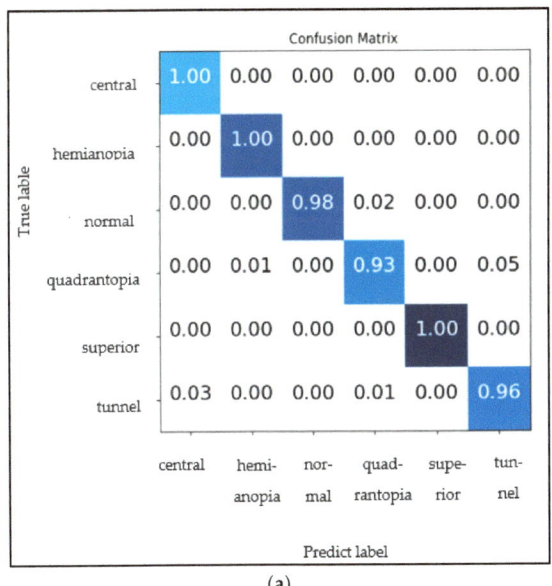 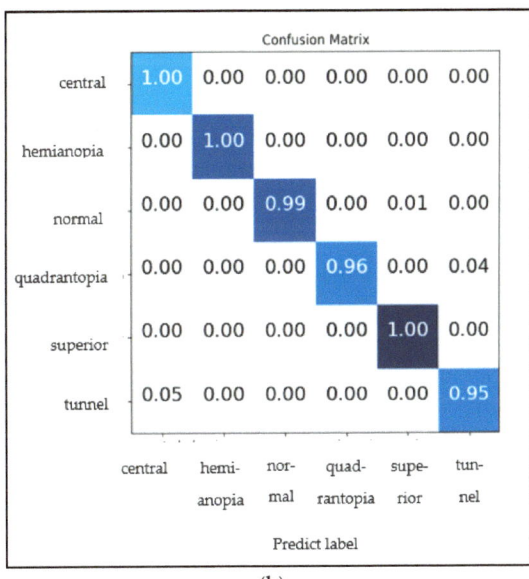

Figure 3. Confusion matrix for VGGNet; (**a**) VGG-16; (**b**) VGG-19.

Table 4. Comparison of performance accuracy of enhanced BO and existing methods.

Acquisition Function	Transfer Learning Model	Mean Accuracy (%)	Max Accuracy (%)	Min Accuracy (%)
CMA-ES [12]	VGG-16	20.10	20.55	15.67
	VGG-19	39.87	97.03	17.58
EI	VGG-16	34.03	97.92	18.81
	VGG-19	19.86	20.55	17.37
EI-PSO	VGG-16	38.35	97.80	17.16
	VGG-19	33.62	95.64	17.54
EI-ABC	VGG-16	36.76	97.84	14.41
	VGG-19	47.48	97.63	20.55

Table 4. *Cont.*

Acquisition Function	Transfer Learning Model	Mean Accuracy (%)	Max Accuracy (%)	Min Accuracy (%)
EI-HHO	VGG-16	41.46	98.26	19.36
	VGG-19	26.97	92.88	19.41
EI-SFO	**VGG-16**	**43.63**	**98.60**	**16.65**
	VGG-19	**47.40**	**98.34**	**15.51**
PI	VGG-16	33.54	96.23	15.68
	VGG-19	43.97	97.66	18.98
UCB	VGG-16	30.59	97.88	16.18
	VGG-19	26.40	93.64	15.47
LCB	VGG-16	47.17	98.26	16.91
	VGG-19	28.37	98.81	18.18

4. Conclusions

In conclusion, the acquisition function plays a crucial role in the BO process as it determines the next set of hyperparameters to be evaluated based on the trade-off between exploration and exploitation. EI is the default acquisition function for BO, which searches for the global optimum of the objective function within the given search space. Global search algorithms can be used as an initialization strategy to sample a diverse set of points in the search space. Then, the acquisition function is used to guide the search towards more promising regions around the initial points. This helps to balance the exploration-exploitation trade-off in the search for optimal hyperparameters. In other words, the performance of the acquisition function can have a significant impact on the efficiency and effectiveness of the optimization process.

Therefore, this work proposes combining swarm-based metaheuristic methods (PSO, ABC, HHO, and SFO) with the EI acquisition function. The aim of the proposed method is to examine how the metaheuristics approach can be utilized to optimize the exploration and exploitation of EI in BO to obtain a more optimum set of hyperparameters and fine-tuned layers. The effectiveness of the proposed method was observed in a multi-class classification task which involved six different types of VF defect images. Then, a comprehensive investigation and analysis of the classification performance were conducted to determine how effectively BO optimizes the objective function in VGGNet models following the improvement of the acquisition function. These include the analyses of the validation and testing performance of the model in the VF defect classification task.

Based on the experimental result, the metaheuristic methods boost the algorithm to explore new regions of the hyperparameter and fine-tuning layers search space while searching for the optimum set of hyperparameter and fine-tuned layers to obtain a set of hyperparameter that have improved the classification accuracy. The hyperparameter tuning and fine-tuning applied shows that the feature or knowledge learned by the pre-trained model can be effectively learned by the source model by choosing the specific task features for the visual field defect pattern. The enhanced optimization processes have improved the model's ability to identify accurate low-level features such as edges, corners and textures, as well as higher-level features such as shapes, objects, and scenes of visual field defects.

One of the proposed methods, EI-SFO, demonstrates a promising result by obtaining high accuracy in the classification task. In comparison to other metaheuristic methods, the EI-SFO-based OB produces the highest mean accuracy for VGG-19 at 47.40%. When EI is combined with the SFO method in BO, the most significant improvement is observed when the mean accuracy for the VGG-16 model increases from 34.03% to 43.63% percent and when it increases from 19.86% to 47.40% percent for the VGG-19 model. EI-SFO-based BO is capable of producing the highest accuracy for VGG-16 and VGG-19, which is

98.60% and 98.34%, respectively. The enhanced BO of transfer learning can significantly impact medical image classification in medical diagnosis by improving model performance, enabling data-efficient model training, boosting model robustness, and saving time and resources during the hyperparameter tuning process. This can lead to more accurate and reliable classification models for medical images, which can aid in the early and accurate diagnosis of medical conditions.

Due to the constraints of our computing resources, the number of BO iterations is limited to only 11. Hence, in future, more experiments will be conducted to further analyze the performance of the acquisition function in a more significant number of BO iterations in exploring better solutions. Besides that, the combination of metaheuristics and BO to a deep learning algorithm incurs high computational complexity. Therefore, improving the algorithm's efficiency is desirable for future investigation. In addition to the four algorithms (PSO, ABC, HHO, and SFO), more available metaheuristics algorithms such as Simulated Annealing, Ant Colony Optimization (ACO), and Flower Pollination Algorithm (FPA) can be combined with the EI acquisition function to observe their performance.

Author Contributions: Conceptualization, M.A., A.A. and N.A.H.Z.; methodology, M.A., A.A. and N.A.H.Z.; software, M.A. and M.I.I.; validation, M.A., A.A. and N.A.H.Z.; formal analysis, M.A.; investigation, M.A., A.A. and N.A.H.Z.; resources, M.A.; data curation, A.Y.; writing—original draft preparation, M.A.; writing—review and editing, N.A.H.Z. and A.A.; visualization, M.A., A.A. and N.A.H.Z.; supervision, N.A.H.Z. and A.A.; project administration, N.A.H.Z.; funding acquisition, F.F. and Y.S. All authors have read and agreed to the published version of the manuscript.

Funding: This research was funded by JSPS KAKENSHI grant number 22K12146.

Institutional Review Board Statement: Not applicable.

Informed Consent Statement: Not applicable.

Data Availability Statement: In this study, we used publicly available VF defect images, the Rotterdam ophthalmic Data Repository [http://www.rodrep.com/longitudinal-glaucomatous-vf-data{-}{-}-description.html (accessed on 23 September 2021)], S1-Dataset, Github dataset [https://github.com/serifeseda/early-glaucoma-identification (accessed on 29 September 2021)], and 10-2 Humphrey SITA dataset [https://datasetsearch.research.google.com/ (accessed on 23 September 2021)]. Universiti Sains Malaysia Visual Field Defect dataset. The VF defects can be made available for reasonable requests by contacting the corresponding authors.

Conflicts of Interest: The authors declare no conflict of interest. The funders had no role in the design of the study, as well as in the collection, analysis, or interpretation of data, in the writing of the manuscript, or in the decision to publish the results.

References

1. Ian, G.; Bengio, Y.; Courville, A. *Deep Learning Book Review*; MIT Press: Cambridge, MA, USA, 2016.
2. Pan, S.J.; Yang, Q. A Survey on Transfer Learning. *IEEE Trans. Knowl. Data Eng.* **2010**, *22*, 1345–1359. [CrossRef]
3. Bai, T.; Li, Y.; Shen, Y.; Zhang, X.; Zhang, W.; Cui, B. Transfer Learning for Bayesian Optimization: A Survey. *J. ACM* **2023**, *1*, 1–35. Available online: http://arxiv.org/abs/2302.05927 (accessed on 16 February 2023).
4. Zhuang, F.; Qi, Z.; Duan, K.; Xi, D.; Zhu, Y.; Zhu, H.; Xiong, H.; He, Q. A Comprehensive Survey on Transfer Learning. *Proc. IEEE* **2021**, *109*, 43–76. [CrossRef]
5. Li, Y.; Zhang, Y.; Zhou, G.; Gong, Y. Bayesian Optimization with Particle Swarm. In Proceedings of the 2021 International Joint Conference on Neural Networks, Shenzhen, China, 18–22 July 2021. [CrossRef]
6. Dewancker, I.; McCourt, M.; Clark, S. Bayesian Optimization Primer. 2018. Available online: https://static.sigopt.com/b/20a144d208ef255d3b981ce419667ec25d8412e2/static/pdf/SigOpt_Bayesian_Optimization_Primer.pdf (accessed on 11 January 2021).
7. Frazier, P.I. A Tutorial on Bayesian Optimization. *arXiv* **2018**, arXiv:1807.02811. Available online: http://arxiv.org/abs/1807.02811 (accessed on 17 November 2022).
8. He, C.; Wang, D.; Yu, Y.; Cai, Z. A Hybrid Deep Learning Model for Link Dynamic Vehicle Count Forecasting with Bayesian Optimization. *J. Adv. Transp.* **2023**, *2023*, 5070504. [CrossRef]
9. Tran-The, S.V.H.; Gupta, S.; Rana, S.; Tran-Thanh, L. Expected Improvement-based Contextual Bandits. 2022, pp. 1–23. Available online: https://openreview.net/forum?id=GIBm-_kax6 (accessed on 13 January 2023).
10. Shankar, K.; Zhang, Y.; Liu, Y.; Wu, L.; Chen, C.H. Hyperparameter Tuning Deep Learning for Diabetic Retinopathy Fundus Image Classification. *IEEE Access* **2020**, *8*, 118164–118173. [CrossRef]

11. Abu, M.; Zahri, N.A.H.; Amir, A.; Ismail, M.I.; Yaakub, A.; Anwar, S.A.; Ahmad, M.I. A Comprehensive Performance Analysis of Transfer Learning Optimization in Visual Field Defect Classification. *Diagnostics* **2022**, *12*, 1258. [CrossRef]
12. Loshchilov, I.; Hutter, F. CMA-ES for Hyperparameter Optimization of Deep Neural Networks. 2016. Available online: http://arxiv.org/abs/1604.07269 (accessed on 6 March 2023).
13. Alamri, N.M.H.; Packianather, M.; Bigot, S. Deep Learning: Parameter Optimization Using Proposed Novel Hybrid Bees Bayesian Convolutional Neural Network. *Appl. Artif. Intell.* **2022**, *36*, 2031815. [CrossRef]
14. Mukesh, M.; Sarkar, K.; Singh, U.K. The joint application of metaheuristic algorithm and Bayesian Statistics approach for uncertainty and stability assessment of nonlinear Magnetotelluric data. *Nonlinear Process. Geophys.* **2023**, *2023*.
15. Reddy, K.; Saha, A.K. A review of swarm-based metaheuristic optimization techniques and their application to doubly fed induction generator. *Heliyon* **2022**, *8*, e10956. [CrossRef]
16. Bhattacharyya, T.; Chatterjee, B.; Singh, P.K.; Yoon, J.H.; Geem, Z.W.; Sarkar, R. Mayfly in Harmony: A new hybrid meta-heuristic feature selection algorithm. *IEEE Access* **2020**, *8*, 195929–195945. [CrossRef]
17. He, J.; Zhu, Q.; Zhang, K.; Yu, P.; Tang, J. An evolvable adversarial network with gradient penalty for COVID-19 infection segmentation. *Appl. Soft Comput.* **2021**, *113*, 107947. [CrossRef]
18. Guilmeau, T.; Chouzenoux, E.; Elvira, V. Simulated Annealing: A Review and a New Scheme. *IEEE Work. Stat. Signal Process. Proc.* **2021**, *2021*, 101–105. [CrossRef]
19. Tameswar, K.; Suddul, G.; Dookhitram, K. A hybrid deep learning approach with genetic and coral reefs metaheuristics for enhanced defect detection in software. *Int. J. Inf. Manag. Data Insights* **2022**, *2*, 100795. [CrossRef]
20. Gundluru, N.; Rajput, D.S.; Lakshmanna, K.; Kaluri, R.; Shorfuzzaman, M.; Uddin, M.; Khan, M.A.R. Enhancement of Detection of Diabetic Retinopathy Using Harris Hawks Optimization with Deep Learning Model. *Comput. Intell. Neurosci.* **2022**, *2022*, 8512469. [CrossRef]
21. Cosma, G.; Brown, D.; Archer, M.; Khan, M.; Pockley, A.G. A Survey on Computational Intelligence Approaches for Predictive Modeling in Prostate Cancer. *Expert Syst. Appl.* **2017**, *70*, 1–19. [CrossRef]
22. Wang, C.; Shang, P.; Shen, P. An improved artificial bee colony algorithm based on Bayesian estimation. *Complex Intell. Syst.* **2022**, *8*, 4971–4991. [CrossRef]
23. Heidari, A.A.; Mirjalili, S.; Faris, H.; Aljarah, I.; Mafarja, M.; Chen, H. Harris hawks optimization: Algorithm and applications. *Futur. Gener. Comput. Syst.* **2019**, *97*, 849–872. [CrossRef]
24. Shadravan, S.; Naji, H.; Bardsiri, V. The Sailfish Optimizer: A novel nature-inspired metaheuristic algorithm for solving constrained engineering optimization problems. *Eng. Appl. Artif. Intell.* **2019**, *80*, 20–34. [CrossRef]
25. Hussain, K.; Salleh, M.N.M.; Cheng, S.; Shi, Y. Comparative analysis of swarm-based metaheuristic algorithms on benchmark functions. *Lect. Notes Comput. Sci.* **2017**, *10385*, 3–11. [CrossRef]
26. Google. Dataset Search. 2023. Available online: https://datasetsearch.research.google.com/ (accessed on 23 September 2021).
27. Gessesse, G.W.; Tamrat, L.; Damji, K.F. 10-2 Humphrey SITA standard visual field test and white on black amsler grid test results among 200 eyes. *PLoS ONE* **2020**, *15*, e0230017. [CrossRef]
28. Bryan, S.; Colen, T.; Jaakke, S.; Koolwijk, L.; Lemij, H.; Mai, T.; Nic, R.; Josine, S.; Gijs, T.; Mieke, T.; et al. Longitudinal Glaucomatous Visual Field Data. *Rotterdam Ophthalmic Data Repos.* 2014. Available online: http://www.rodrep.com/longitudinal-glaucomatous-vf-data{-}{-}description.html (accessed on 23 September 2021).
29. Erler, N.S.; Bryan, S.R.; Eilers, P.H.C.; Lesaffre, E.M.E.H.; Lemij, H.G.; Vermeer, K.A. Optimizing Structure-function Relationship by Maximizing Correspondence between Glaucomatous Visual Fields and Mathematical Retinal Nerve Fiber Models. *Investig. Ophthalmol. Vis. Sci.* **2014**, *55*, 2350–2357. [CrossRef] [PubMed]
30. Kucur, Ş.S.; Holló, G.; Sznitman, R. A Deep Learning Approach to Automatic Detection of Early Glaucoma from Visual Fields. *PLoS ONE* **2018**, *13*, e0206081. [CrossRef] [PubMed]
31. Kucur, Ş.S. Early Glaucoma Identification. GitHub. 2018. Available online: https://github.com/serifeseda/early-glaucoma-identification (accessed on 23 September 2021).
32. Simonyan, K.; Zisserman, A. Very deep convolutional networks for large-scale image recognition. In Proceedings of the 3rd International Conference on Learning Representations, ICLR 2015—Conference Track Proceedings, San Diego, CA, USA, 7–9 May 2015; pp. 1–14.
33. KHe, K.; Zhang, X.; Ren, S.; Sun, J. Deep residual learning for image recognition. In Proceedings of the IEEE Computer Society Conference on Computer Vision and Pattern Recognition, Las Vegas, NV, USA, 27–30 June 2016; pp. 770–778. [CrossRef]
34. Howard, A.G.; Zhu, M.; Chen, B.; Kalenichenko, D.; Wang, W.; Weyand, T.; Andreetto, M.; Adam, H. MobileNets: Efficient Convolutional Neural Networks for Mobile Vision Applications. 2017. Available online: http://arxiv.org/abs/1704.04861 (accessed on 6 March 2023).
35. Sandler, M.; Howard, A.; Zhu, M.; Zhmoginov, A.; Chen, L. MobileNetV2: Inverted Residuals and Linear Bottlenecks. In Proceedings of the IEEE/CVF Conference on Computer Vision and Pattern Recognition, Salt Lake City, UT, USA, 18–23 June 2018; pp. 4510–4520. [CrossRef]
36. Huang, G.; Liu, Z.; Van Der Maaten, L.; Weinberger, K.Q. Densely connected convolutional networks. In Proceedings of the 2017 IEEE Conference on Computer Vision and Pattern Recognition, Honolulu, HI, USA, 21–26 July 2017; pp. 2261–2269. [CrossRef]
37. Garnett, R. Bayesian Optimization. 2015. Available online: https://www.cse.wustl.edu/~garnett/cse515t/spring_2015/files/lecture_notes/12.pdf (accessed on 17 August 2022).

38. Koehrsen, W. A conceptual explanation of bayesian hyperparameter optimization for machine learning. *Towar. Data Sci.* **2018**, *5*. Available online: https://towardsdatascience.com/a-conceptual-explanation-of-bayesian-model-based-hyperparameter-optimization-for-machine-learning-b8172278050f (accessed on 14 February 2021).
39. Atteia, G.; Alhussan, A.A.; Samee, N.A. BO-ALLCNN: Bayesian-Based Optimized CNN for Acute Lymphoblastic Leukemia Detection in Microscopic Blood Smear Images. *Sensor* **2022**, *22*, 5520. [CrossRef]
40. Noè, U.; Husmeier, D. On a New Improvement-Based Acquisition Function for Bayesian Optimization. 2018. Available online: http://arxiv.org/abs/1808.06918 (accessed on 11 February 2023).
41. Wang, H.; van Stein, B.; Emmerich, M.; Back, T. A new acquisition function for Bayesian optimization based on the moment-generating function. In Proceedings of the IEEE International Conference on Systems, Man and Cybernetics, Banff, AB, Canada, 5–8 October 2017; pp. 507–512. [CrossRef]
42. Shahriari, B.; Swersky, K.; Wang, Z.; Adams, R.P.; De Freitas, N. Taking the Human Out of the Loop: A Review of Bayesian Optimization. *Proc. IEEE* **2016**, *104*, 148–175. [CrossRef]
43. Zuhal, L.R.; Palar, P.S.; Shimoyama, K. A comparative study of multi-objective expected improvement for aerodynamic design. *Aerosp. Sci. Technol.* **2019**, *91*, 548–560. [CrossRef]

Disclaimer/Publisher's Note: The statements, opinions and data contained in all publications are solely those of the individual author(s) and contributor(s) and not of MDPI and/or the editor(s). MDPI and/or the editor(s) disclaim responsibility for any injury to people or property resulting from any ideas, methods, instructions or products referred to in the content.

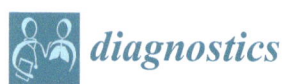

Article

Real-World Driver Stress Recognition and Diagnosis Based on Multimodal Deep Learning and Fuzzy EDAS Approaches

Muhammad Amin [1,2], Khalil Ullah [3,*], Muhammad Asif [1], Habib Shah [4], Arshad Mehmood [5] and Muhammad Attique Khan [6]

1 Department of Electronics, University of Peshawar, Peshawar 25120, Pakistan
2 Department of Computer Science, Iqra National University, Peshawar 25000, Pakistan
3 Department of Software Engineering, University of Malakand, Dir Lower, Chakdara 23050, Pakistan
4 Department of Computer Science, King Khalid University, Abha 61421, Saudi Arabia
5 Department of Mechanical Engineering, University of Engineering & Technology, Peshawar 25120, Pakistan
6 Department of Computer Science, HITEC University, Taxila 47080, Pakistan
* Correspondence: khalil.ullah@uom.edu.pk

Citation: Amin, M.; Ullah, K.; Asif, M.; Shah, H.; Mehmood, A.; Khan, M.A. Real-World Driver Stress Recognition and Diagnosis Based on Multimodal Deep Learning and Fuzzy EDAS Approaches. *Diagnostics* 2023, 13, 1897. https://doi.org/10.3390/diagnostics13111897

Academic Editors: Wan Azani Mustafa and Hiam Alquran

Received: 6 March 2023
Revised: 4 April 2023
Accepted: 13 May 2023
Published: 29 May 2023

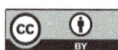

Copyright: © 2023 by the authors. Licensee MDPI, Basel, Switzerland. This article is an open access article distributed under the terms and conditions of the Creative Commons Attribution (CC BY) license (https://creativecommons.org/licenses/by/4.0/).

Abstract: Mental stress is known as a prime factor in road crashes. The devastation of these crashes often results in damage to humans, vehicles, and infrastructure. Likewise, persistent mental stress could lead to the development of mental, cardiovascular, and abdominal disorders. Preceding research in this domain mostly focuses on feature engineering and conventional machine learning approaches. These approaches recognize different levels of stress based on handcrafted features extracted from various modalities including physiological, physical, and contextual data. Acquiring good quality features from these modalities using feature engineering is often a difficult job. Recent developments in the form of deep learning (DL) algorithms have relieved feature engineering by automatically extracting and learning resilient features. This paper proposes different CNN and CNN-LSTSM-based fusion models using physiological signals (SRAD dataset) and multimodal data (AffectiveROAD dataset) for the driver's two and three stress levels. The fuzzy EDAS (evaluation based on distance from average solution) approach is used to evaluate the performance of the proposed models based on different classification metrics (accuracy, recall, precision, F-score, and specificity). Fuzzy EDAS performance estimation shows that the proposed CNN and hybrid CNN-LSTM models achieved the first ranks based on the fusion of BH, E4-Left (E4-L), and E4-Right (E4-R). Results showed the significance of multimodal data for designing an accurate and trustworthy stress recognition diagnosing model for real-world driving conditions. The proposed model can also be used for the diagnosis of the stress level of a subject during other daily life activities.

Keywords: driver stress recognition; multimodal data; deep learning; CNN; LSTM; fuzzy EDAS

1. Introduction

Successful driving activities always require both mental and physical skills [1–3]. Acute stress reduces the driver's ability to fix hazardous situations, which causes significant damage to humans and vehicles every year [4–8]. Dangerous driving situations are triggered due to human errors, individual factors, and ambiance conditions [9]. According to the National Motor Vehicle Crash Causation Survey (NMVCCS) in the United States (US), human errors caused 94% of crashes alone, while vehicle defects, ambiance conditions, and other factors collectively caused 6% of crashes during 2005–2007 [10]. Human errors are linked to the driver's perceptual conditions, so a complete understanding of these conditions is crucial for preventing traffic accidents.

To detect and diagnose drivers' different stress levels, physiological, physical, and contextual information are widely utilized [11]. Moreover, different traditional machine learning models based on handcrafted feature extraction methods are utilized for the classification of stress. Extracting the best features using these approaches is always a challenging task, as the quality of extracted features has a significant effect on the classification performance [12]. These approaches are laborious, ad hoc, less robust to noise, and need thorough skill [13]. To come through these challenges, deep learning models have been utilized to automatically produce complex nonlinear features reliably [14–16]. In addition to automatic feature extraction from raw data, these models offer noise robustness and better classification accuracy [17–19]. Different deep learning algorithms are used in recent research, e.g., CNN, RNN, DNN, and LSTM.

The models proposed in the current work are based on 1D CNN and hybrid 1D CNN-LSTM networks. The proposed models are separately trained using multiple physiological signals (SRAD) and multimodal data (AffectiveROAD) including physiological signals and other information about the vehicle, driver, and ambiance. Multimodal fusion of data based on deep learning approaches can be used to develop a precise driver stress level recognition model with improved performance and reliability.

Contributions of this research study include: (1) proposing 1D CNN and hybrid 1D CNN-LSTM-based real-world driver stress level recognition models using fused physiological signals (SRAD dataset) and fused multimodal data (AffectiveROAD dataset) and (2) ranking the assessment of the proposed models for the two and three levels of stress based on the fuzzy EDAS approach.

The organization of this research article is given below. Analysis of the existing stress recognition models is presented in Section 2. The proposed methodology is elaborated in Section 3 in terms of datasets, data pre-processing, architectures of the proposed CNN and hybrid CNN-LSTM models, and the fuzzy EDAS approach. Performance evaluation of the proposed models is conducted in Section 4. A fuzzy EDAS-based rank estimation of the proposed models for the driver's two and three levels of stress is also presented in this section. Section 5 gives a detailed assessment of the proposed and existing stress recognition schemes. Finally, Section 6 concludes the paper and gives future directions to further explore this research area.

2. Related Work

This section provides a review of the existing work in the driver's stress analysis domain and underscores the current contribution. Several driver stress level recognition schemes exist in the literature based on simulated and real-world driving environments. These schemes can be broadly categorized as conventional machine learning or deep learning models.

Several machine learning approaches have been proposed for real-world driver mental stress recognition based on different physiological signals. Dalmeida and Masala [20], Vargas-Lopez et al. [21], Khowaja et al. [8], Lopez-Martinez et al. [22], Haouij et al. [23], Chen et al. [4], Ghaderi et al. [24], Zhang et al. [25], and Healey and Picard [26] propose conventional machine models based on physiological signals obtained from the PhysioNet SRAD public database [27]. Unlike the previous studies, Rigas et al. [28] presented a real-world binary stress recognition model based on multimodal data, including physical and contextual data, in addition to physiological signals. On the other hand, Zontone et al. [29], Bianco et al. [30], Lee et al. [31], Lanatà et al. [32], and Gao et al. [33] proposed conventional machine learning models for driver stress recognition based on simulated driving situations. Lanatà et al. [32] and Lee et al. [31] presented driver stress recognition models based on multimodal data. Contrary to previous studies, Šalkevicius et al. [34], Rodríguez-Arce et al. [35], Can et al. [36], Al abdi et al. [37], Betti et al. [38], Siramprakas et al. [39], de Vries et al. [40], and Sun et al. [41] proposed stress recognition models during controlled, lab, semi-lab, and physical (such as sitting, standing, and walking) environments. Recent development in deep learning and machine learning models have shown good results in various applied domains that can be applied in driver stress detection [42,43].

All the mentioned studies are based on feature engineering techniques, and various conventional machine learning algorithms were employed to classify levels of stress. However, handcrafted features are less robust to noise and subjective changes, and need a considerable amount of time and hard work [8,13,19,34,35,44]. Moreover, capturing the features' sequential nature is difficult due to the absence of explicit features and high dimensionality despite using complex feature selection methods. Likewise, the dependence of the model on past observations would make it impractical to process all the information due to the growing complexity. The feature-level multimodal fusion models proposed by Chen et al. [4], Healey and Picard [26], Haouij et al. [23], Lee et al. [31], Bianco et al. [30], Sun et al. [41], and Can et al. [36] mainly concentrate on pattern learning in individual signals instead of multiple simultaneous signals [18]. Thus, these models are inappropriate to obtain the nonlinear correlation across multiple signals appearing simultaneously. Various linear and non-linear methods employed in these conventional machine learning models have not been able to perform the vigorous investigation of such manifold time series signals [19].

To address the issues faced by conventional machine learning models, deep learning methods have been introduced. Deep learning models are developed based on signal preprocessing (noise filtering), designing a particular deep neural network based on the area of interest, network training, and model testing. Deep learning models learn and classify raw data using multilayer deep neural networks [45]. The last fully connected (FC) layers are utilized to obtain the final output. Contrary to feature engineering techniques used in conventional machine learning approaches, deep learning models automatically produce steady features [14,15]. Moreover, deep learning models are more robust to noise and achieve improved classification accuracy [19]. Different deep learning algorithms are used in recent research, e.g., the recurrent neural network (RNN), deep aeural network (DNN), LSTM, and CNN. Rastgoo et al. [11], Zhang et al. [46], Kanjo et al. [17], Lim and Yang [47], Yan et al. [48], Hajinoroozi et al. [49], and Lee et al. [50] presented different deep learning models to identify different driver states. Rastgoo et al. [11], Kanjo et al. [17], Lim and Yang [47], and Yan et al. [48] proposed deep learning models based on multimodal data. On the other hand, the models proposed by Hajinoroozi et al. [49] and Lee et al. [50] are based on physiological signals only. The stress recognition model proposed by Zhang et al. [46] is based on facial images only. Apart from driving scenarios, Masood and Alghamdi [51], Cho et al. [52], Seo et al. [53], Hwang et al. [54], and He et al. [55] proposed stress recognition models based on deep learning techniques and physiological signals in academic, workplace, and lab settings. Most of these studies including [46,49,50,52–56] are based on two levels of stress only. Moreover, the schemes presented by [46,50,52,55,56] are based on images. Likewise, the schemes proposed by [49,52–56] are either based on physiological signals or a single modality. On the other hand, the model proposed by [11] is based on multimodal data collected during simulated driving.

The models proposed in this study are based on the fusion of multimodal data collected during real-world driving (SRAD and AffectiveROAD datasets). Moreover, these models are based on 1D CNN and 1D CNN-LSTM networks to detect driver's two (stressed and relaxed) and three levels (low, medium, and high). The fuzzy EDAS approach is also used to find the performance ranks of the proposed models based on different classification metrics.

3. Materials and Methods

The proposed unimodal and fusion models for real-world driver stress level recognition are based on physiological signals and deep learning approaches, such as CNN and hybrid CNN-LSTM. The proposed models are implemented in the latest MATLAB 2022a platform. The proposed stress recognition models are based on the fusion of ECG, HR, HGSR, FGSR, EMG, and RESP signals collected from the PhysioNet SRAD database, and breathing rate (BR), GSR, BVP, HR, TEMP, ACCEL, posture, and activity data are collected from AffectiveROAD database. Data input mechanisms used in this research are based on raw signals. These raw signals are preprocessed to obtain cleaned signals.

3.1. SRAD Dataset

The ECG, HR, GSR, EMG, and RESP signals analyzed in the current work belong to the SRAD PhysioNet public database [57]. Experiments were performed while driving a customized Volvo S70 series station wagon. Five different sensors were used to acquire physiological signals from the nine drivers during twenty-four drives. The sensors were connected to an embedded computer through an analog-to-digital converter (ADC). The ECG sensor was placed using a modified lead II configuration to decrease the motion artifacts. The EMG sensor was positioned on the shoulder near the trapezius muscle to record the emotional stress. Two GSR sensors were located on the driver's sole and palm of the left foot and hand. Expansion of the chest cavity was used to measure the RESP signals through an elastic Hall effect sensor fastened around the diaphragm.

All drives comprise rest, highway, and city driving phases on a specific route 31 km in length in Boston, US. These rest, highway, and city driving phases are assumed to trigger low, medium, and high levels of stress, respectively. Initially, the drivers are informed about the travel plan and compliance with certain guidelines regarding the speed limits and tuning out the radio. To avoid rush hours, all drives were performed in the midmorning and afternoon. Two rest intervals of 15 min in the parking area were added at the start and end of each drive to collect the driver's low-stress baseline. Due to stop-and-go traffic in the city area, drivers usually observe high-stress situations. After passing the toll booth, the city road then turns into the highway. Uninterrupted highway driving normally indicates medium-stress conditions. The trip completes after returning to the starting position using the same highway and city routes. The total length of all drives varies from 50 to 90 min, including two 15 min rest intervals.

The dataset contains information about 17 drives, but some drives have incomplete signals and markers. These incomplete drives are removed from the experiments. Figures 1–5 separately show the ECG, HR, GSR, EMG, and RESP waveforms for the three levels of stress. The figures show that all five signals have distinct waveforms for the three levels of stress.

3.2. AffectiveROAD Database

Experiments were performed using wireless sensors networked together inside different cars to collect physiological signals and additional information about the vehicle, driver, and ambiance. The Zephyr Bio-harness (BH) chest strap was placed on the driver's chest to collect HR, breathing rate (BR), posture, and activity information. Two Empatica E4-Left (E4-L) and E4-Right (E4-R) wearable devices were mounted on the driver's left and right arms to capture GSR, BVP, inter-beat interval (IBI), HR, TEMP, and ACCEL data. The Intel Edison developer kit-based environmental platform was placed in the car's rear seat for collecting luminosity, temperature, pressure, and humidity information. A sound meter and microphone were used to obtain sound amplitude and audio signal. Two cameras were placed on the windshield of the car to record inside and outside events. A real-time continuous subjective metric was prepared by an experimenter during each drive to monitor the driver's stress level. The stress metric along with two video recordings were then used by the drivers to correct and validate the experimenter's ratings.

All drives comprise rest, highway, and city driving phases on a fixed route 31 km in length in the Grand Tunis area. Fourteen driving experiments were performed by 10 experienced drivers with valid driver's licenses. Each drive included two 15 min rest periods at the start and end of the session. The whole experiment normally took about 86 min to travel through the zone, city1, highway, and city2, and then travel back in the opposite direction to reach the starting point. The rest, highway, and city drives were supposed to yield low, medium, and high levels of stress, respectively.

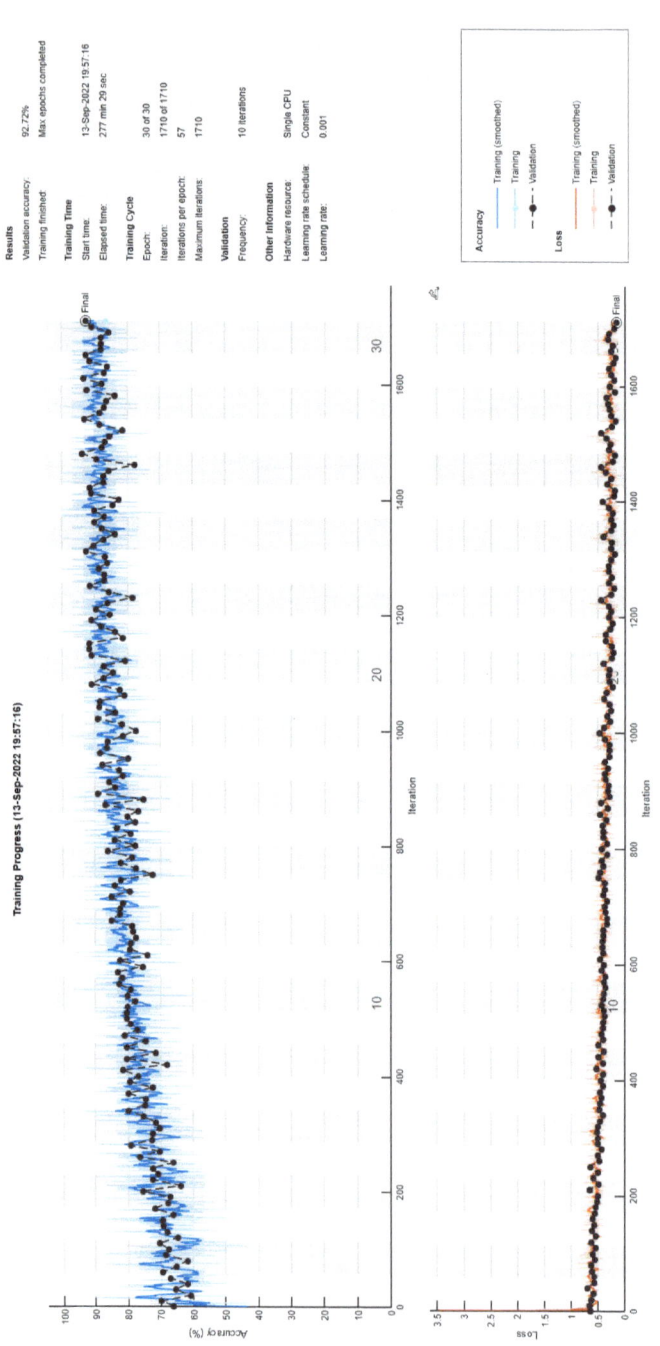

Figure 1. Training graph of the CNN model for the two-stress class based on the SRAD dataset.

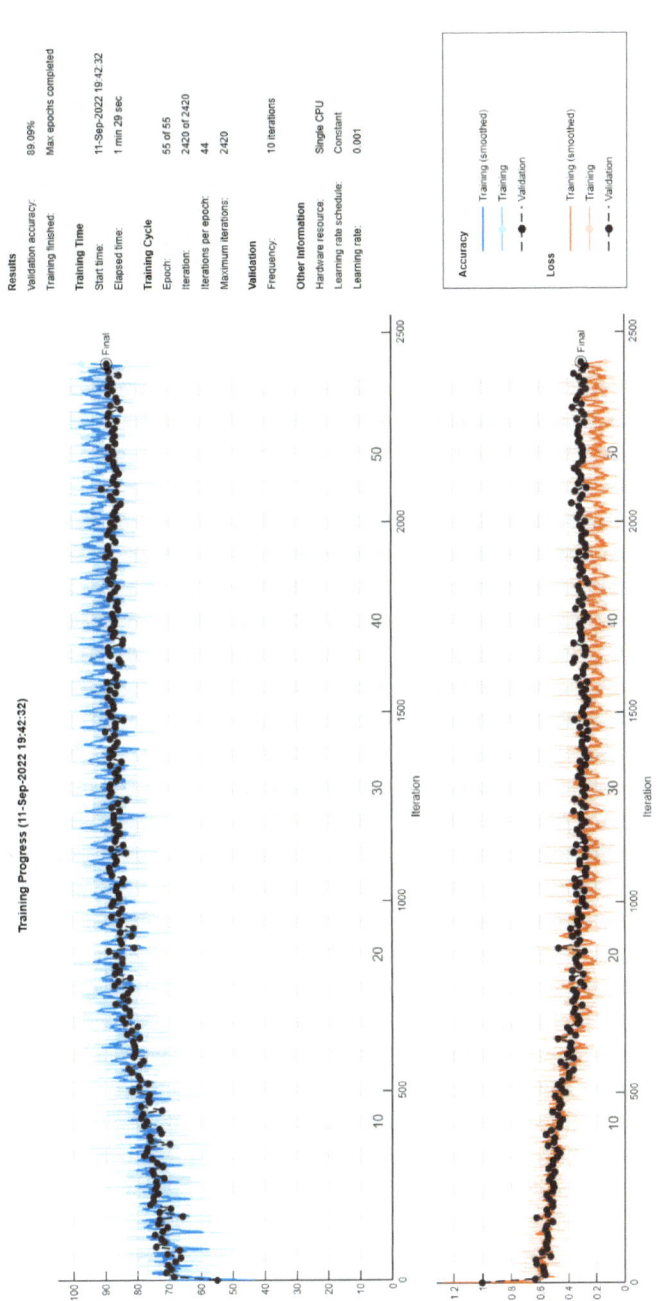

Figure 2. Training graph of the CNN model for the two-stress class based on the BH dataset.

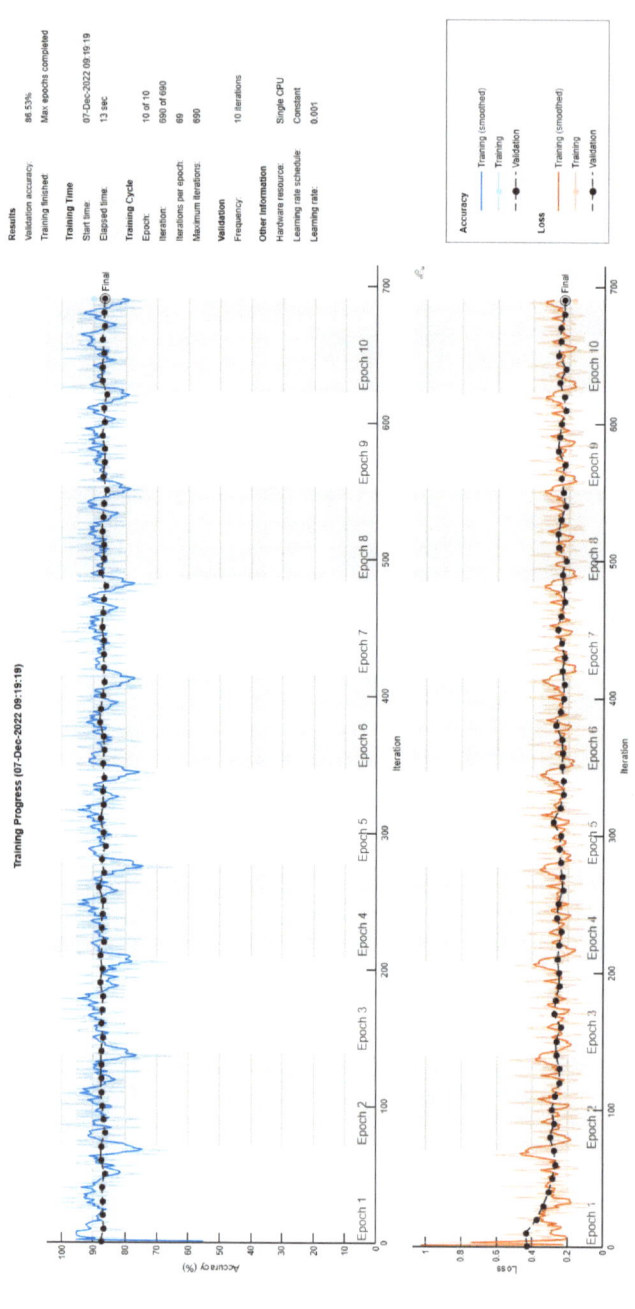

Figure 3. Training graph of the CNN model for the two-stress class based on the E4-L dataset.

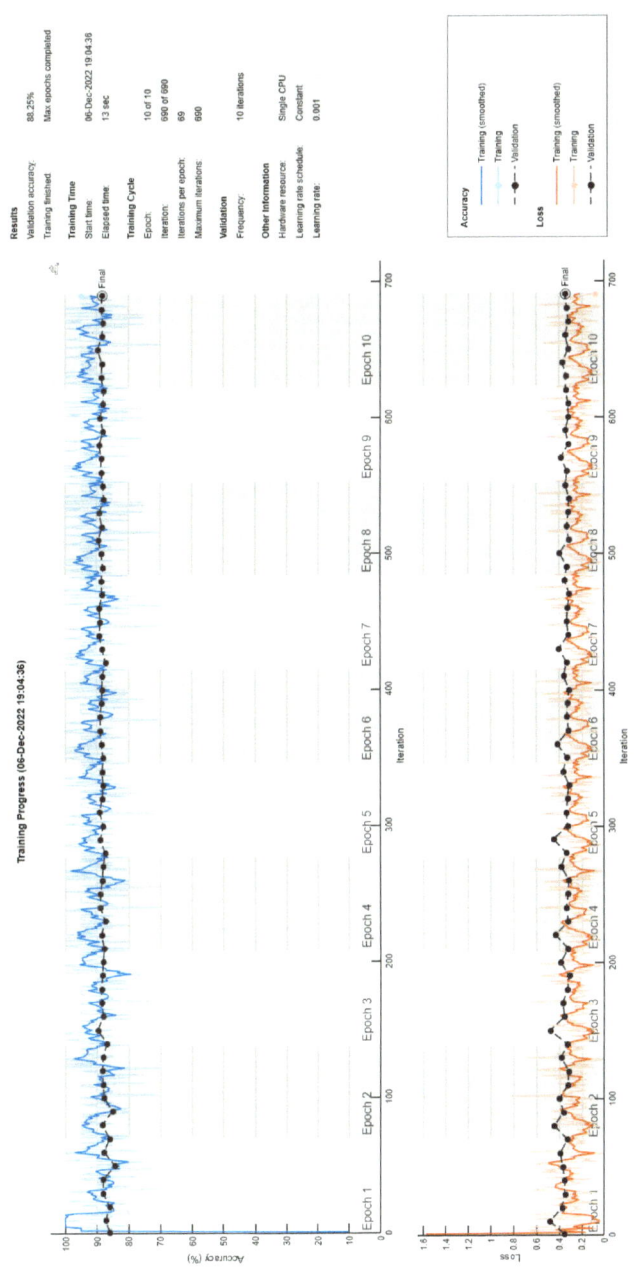

Figure 4. Training graph of the CNN model for the two-stress class based on the E4-R dataset.

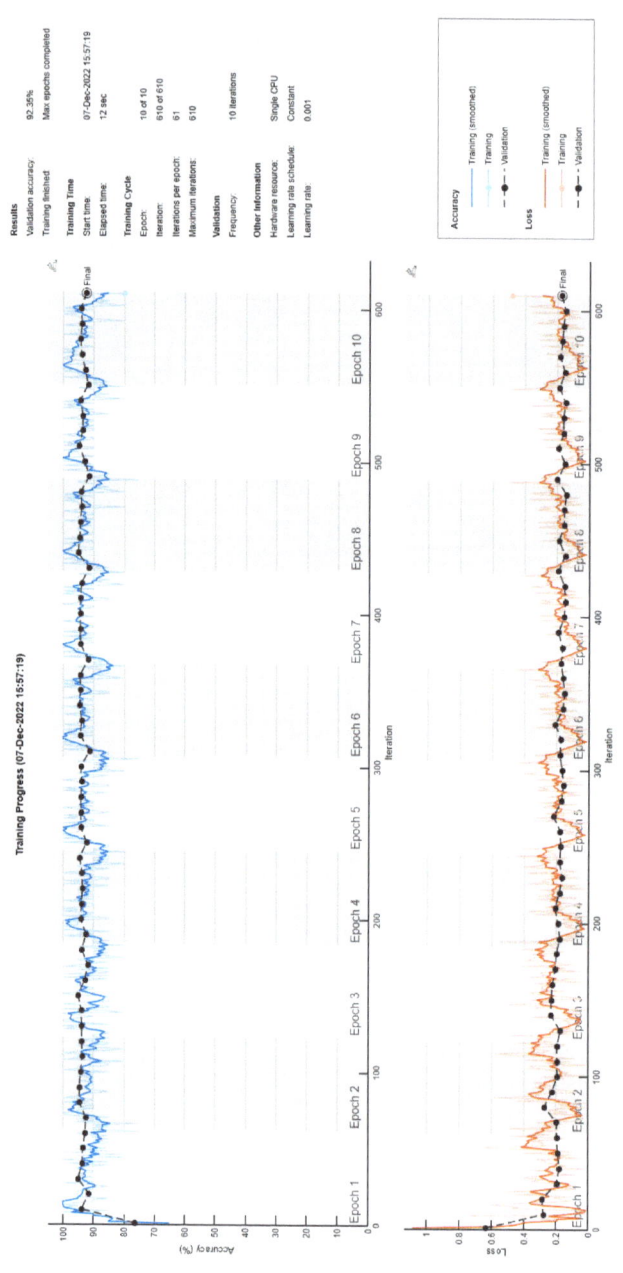

Figure 5. Training graph of the CNN model for the two-stress class based on the E4-(L+R) datasets.

3.3. Pre-Processing

Physiological data are normally derived from the human body in the form of low-amplitude signals with different frequency ranges. These signals are mostly polluted by different noises and artifacts. To model the driver's stress levels accurately, it is necessary to preprocess the ECG, HR, HGSR, FGSR, EMG, and RESP signals first.

ECG signals normally contain different unwanted components including baseline wander, powerline interference (PLI), and high-frequency EMG noise [58]. Moreover, the PLI adds 50–60 Hz noise components in ECG signals [59]. Likewise, high-frequency EMG noise components caused by muscle contractions contaminate the ECG signals [58]. HR signals are commonly derived from ECG signals, so they inherit some noise and artifacts from ECG signals. To remove the baseline wander and other artifacts form ECG signals, a band-pass Butterworth filter (5–15 Hz) was used to eliminate the baseline wander. Similarly, a finite impulse response (FIR), Notch filter (59–61 Hz), and FIR band-pass filter (1.5–150 Hz) were used for noise removal. The min–max normalization approach is then utilized to remove the subject-specific baseline and motion artifacts.

A GSR signal is an effective stress measure that is comparatively less susceptible to noise [60]. Yet, the authors of [61] used a low-pass filter (4 Hz) and a Gaussian filter for denoising the GSR signal. These filters are used in this study too to obtain cleaned GSR signals. The signals are also normalized to the maximum value.

The EMG signal is contaminated by several unwanted signals including motion artifacts, PLI, capacitive effects, and ECG artifact signals. In this work, a band-pass Butterworth filter (0.5–500 Hz) is used to remove the low- and high-frequency noises in the EMG signals. Likewise, PLI is eliminated using a 60 Hz Notch filter. The min–max normalization is performed to remove the subject-specific baseline and motion artifacts. EMG signals in the SRAD dataset were initially collected at a lower sampling frequency of 495 Hz. Although, the EMG signal contains information up to 450 Hz. As per the Nyquist theorem, at least a 900 Hz sampling frequency is required for the EMG signals.

The RESP signal is normally polluted by different undesirable signals including baseline wander, PLI, and motion artifacts. To remove high-frequency noise and baseline signal from the RESP signal, we applied Butterworth high-pass (0.05 Hz) and low-pass (0.70 Hz) filters, respectively.

3.4. 1D CNN Models

CNN-based models were originally developed to learn the internal representation of 2D images and then classify them into certain output classes. The same approach can be utilized for automatic feature learning and classification of time series sequenced data [62]. A 1D CNN uses several filters to perform 1D convolution (Conv1D) operations for constructing feature maps from such data. These networks can better match the 1D characteristic of different physiological signals. Increasing the convolutional layers can help CNN models to gradually extract unique and vigorous higher-level features. The 1D CNN models used in this research are based on the signal fusion of the SRAD and AffectiveROAD datasets for both two-stress and three-stress classes. Thus, all signals in the SRAD dataset are combinedly trained using the 1D CNN model. The AffectiveROAD dataset consists of multimodal data collected using BH, E4-L, and E4-R devices. So, different 1D CNN models are trained using the BH, E4-L, E4-R, E4-(Left+Right) (E4-(L+R)), and BH+E4-(L+R) datasets. A sliding window approach is used to convert each cleaned signal into equal size segments. These segments are then fed to a 1D CNN as new training data. The CNN-based driver stress recognition performs both feature learning and classification tasks.

A 1D CNN architecture is defined using multiple Conv1D blocks each containing convolution, ReLU, and layer normalization (LN) layers. One-dimensional CNN architectures based on SRAD, E4-L, E4-R, E4-(L+R), BH, and BH+E4-(L+R) datasets are shown in Table 1. The convolution layer utilizes trainable filters (kernels) to convolve the low-level features of each segment or the previous layer's output to produce a feature map. The number of filters in each convolutional block is set differently depending on the dataset. Causal padding is used in all convolutional layers to produce outputs with the same length. It pads the layer's input with zeros to predict the values of early time steps in the frame. The convolutional layer is followed by the ReLU layer, which is based on a piecewise linear function. This function returns output for positive inputs and is zero otherwise, thus alleviating the vanishing gradient problem [63]. Moreover, the function adds nonlinearity to the model to learn complex patterns in the data. A GAP layer is added after the four convolutional blocks to produce a single vector output. This layer finds the average output of each feature map generated by the convolutional layers and provides a substitute for the flattening block. The last three layers including FC, softmax, and classification layers perform the classification task. The vector output of the GAP layer is fed to the FC layer, which is also known as the hidden layer. The FC layer is used to map the output classes to a vector of probabilities. The output of the FC layer is utilized by the softmax layer to perform the final classification decision by allocating probabilities to low, medium, and high classes of stress. The final classification layer uses a cross-entropy loss function to evaluate the performance of the classification model. An increase in cross-entropy loss reflects the divergence of the predicted probability from the actual label and vice versa. The classification layer assumes the number of classes from the FC and softmax layers.

Table 1. One-dimensional CNN architectures and parameter settings.

Dataset	Filter Size	Padding	Feature Learning (1D CNN)		Training Options (1D CNN)				
			Layers		Optimization Algorithm (Feature Learning/ Classification)	No. of Epochs (Feature Learning/ Classification)	Mini-Batch size (Feature Learning/ Classification)	Validation Frequency	Training/ Validation Set
SRAD	03	Causal	1st Bloch: Conv1D (Filters: 8), ReLU, LN		Adam	20	30	10	80:20
E4-L			2nd: Bloch: Conv1D (Filters: 32), ReLU, LN 3rd Block: Conv1D (Filters: 64), ReLU, LN 4th Block: Conv1D (Filters: 128), ReLU, LN			30 20	20 10		
E4-R			Conv1D (Filters: 8) GAP; FC; Softmax; Classification			30 10	20 20		
E4-(L+R)			Sum of the layers of E4-L and E4-R			30 + 30 10	20 + 20 20		
BH			1st Bloch: Conv1D (Filters: 128), ReLU, LN 2nd: Bloch: Conv1D (Filters: 64), ReLU, LN 3rd Block: Conv1D (Filters: 32), ReLU, LN GAP; Softmax; FC; Classification			80 10	20 20		
BH+E4-(L+R)			Sum of the layers of BH, E4-L, and E4-R			80 + 30 + 30 10	20 + 20 + 20 20		

Network's Training

Before starting the training process, several parameters need to be settled. These pa-rameters include the training algorithm, mini-batch size, validation frequency, initial learning rate, and maximum epochs. Parameter settings for different 1D CNN models are shown in Table 1.

A training algorithm is used to reduce the loss function of a learning model iterative-ly based on a training dataset. Adaptive moment estimation (Adam) is used as a training algorithm. It combines the benefits of RMSProp and AdaGrad by calculating the individ-ual adaptive learning rates based on the parameters estimated for the first and second moments of gradients. The mini-batch represents a subset of segments used in a single training iteration. Min-batch size is set to a small value to ensure the uniform distribution and utilization of the full dataset during a single epoch. The validation frequency repre-sents the training iterations between evaluations of validation metrics, while training iter-ation is a single step performed by an optimization algorithm to reduce the loss function for a mini-batch. The network's validation frequency is set to 10. The epoch represents the maximum iterations completed by the optimization algorithm to reduce the loss function for the entire dataset. All datasets are divided into 80% for training data and 20% for vali-dation data.

3.5. Hybrid 1D CNN-LSTM Models

The LSTM is a particular type of RNN developed by Hochreiter and Schmidhuber [64]. It is useful to discover and remember long sequences of data efficiently. Generally, the LSTM is a chain of repeating cells of neural networks, such as a RNN, but both have different cell structures. The RNN's cell consists of a single neural network based on tangent hyperbolic function, while LSTM's cell has four interacting neural network layers based on sigmoid functions and pointwise multiplication operations. The LSTM has several cells connected to each other horizontally. Information can be added or removed from the cell state using four different gates. Each LSTM cell consists of an input gate, cell state gate, forget gate, and output gate. The forget gate is based on the sigmoid function, which determines which information needs to be forgotten from the cell state. The information is removed if the gate generates zero output and it is retained if the gate produces one output. The cell state gate determines the cell state based on the new information. First, the input gate based on the sigmoid function determines the values to be updated. Next, a vector is created for the new candidate values by the tangent hyperbolic activation function. The cell state is updated by combining the results of the two functions. To generate the output of a cell, the output gate first applies the sigmoid function to the part of a cell state. Next, a tangent hyperbolic function is applied to the cell state and the resulting value is multiplied by the output of the sigmoid function.

The hybrid CNN-LSTM model utilizes both 1D CNN and LSTM networks to classify sequenced data. In such a model, the CNN is used as a front end to extract features from physiological data followed by the LSTM layers to perform learning and classification tasks. The hybrid CNN-LSTM model has a similar architecture to the CNN model with additional LSTM cells after the FC layers. The architecture of the CNN model is already discussed in the previous section. The hybrid 1D CNN-LSTM architectures based on the SRAD, BH, E4-L, E4-R, E4-(L+R), and BH+E4-(L+R) datasets are shown in Table 2. Moreover, parameter settings for the proposed models are also shown in the same table.

3.6. Fuzzy EDAS Approach

The fuzzy EDAS approach is used to evaluate the performance of the proposed real-world driver stress level detection models based on different modalities. This approach performs the rank estimation of the proposed models in terms of accuracy, recall, precision, F-score, and specificity. Fuzzy EDAS is an eight-step process where each step performs some sort of calculations, which in turn is used by the coming steps, as elaborated below:

Step 1: First, the "solution of the average value (ψ)" is calculated for all matrices, as shown mathematically in the equation below:

$$(\psi) = [\psi_\beta]_{1 \times \delta} \quad (1)$$

where:

$$(\psi_\beta) = \frac{\sum_{i=1}^{x} X_{\alpha\beta}}{x} \quad (2)$$

The aggregate solution of Equations (1) and (2) can be found as the average value (ψ) against every criterion's estimated quantity for each performance metric.

Table 2. One-dimensional CNN-LSTM architectures and parameter settings.

Dataset	Filter Size	Padding	Features Learning (1D CNN)			Training Options (1D CNN-LSTM)					
			Layers	Hidden Layers	Dropout	Optimization Algorithm (Feature Learning/Classification)	Epochs (Feature Learning/Classification)	Mini-Batch Size (Feature Learning/Classification)	Validation Frequency	Training/Validation Set
SRAD	03	Causal	1st Bloch: Conv1D (Filters: 8), ReLU, LN; 2nd: Bloch: Conv1D (Filters: 32), ReLU, LN; 3rd Block: Conv1D (Filters: 64), ReLU, LN; 4th Block: Conv1D (Filters: 128), ReLU, LN; Conv1D (8 Filters); GAP; FC; Softmax; Classification	250	0.4	Adam	20 / 20	30	10	80:20
E4-L				300	0.5		30 / 10	20 / 20		
E4-R				200	0.5		30 / 10	20 / 20		
E4-(L+R)			Sum of the layers of E4-L and E4-R	200	0.5		30 + 30 / 10	20 + 20 / 20		
BH			1st Bloch: Conv1D (Filters: 128), ReLU, LN; 2nd: Bloch: Conv1D (Filters: 64), ReLU, LN; 3rd Block: Conv1D (Filters: 32), ReLU, LN; GAP; Softmax; FC; Classification	200	0.5		80 / 20	20 / 20		
BH+E4-(L+R)			Sum of the layers of BH, E4-L, and E4-R	200	0.5		80 + 30 + 30 / 15	20 + 20 + 20 / 20		

Step 2: The positive distances from the average (P_J) of each signal for the driver's each stress level is calculated using the following equation:

$$P_J = [(P_J)_{\alpha\beta}]_{\delta \times \delta} \quad (3)$$

The $(P_J)_{\alpha\beta}$ in Equation (3) is the positive distance of β_{th} model from the average value for the α_{th} parameter. It can be found using either of two ways. If β_{th} criterion is more favorable, then it is calculated using the equation below:

$$(P_J)_{\alpha\beta} = \frac{Maximum(0, (A_{V_\beta} - X_{\alpha\beta}))}{A_{V_\beta}} \quad (4)$$

On the other hand, if the β_{th} criterion is not favorable, it is calculated by the following equation:

$$(P_J)_{\alpha\beta} = \frac{Maximum(0, (X_{\alpha\beta} - A_{V_\beta}))}{A_{V_\beta}} \quad (5)$$

Step 3: The negative distances from the average (N_J) of each signal for the driver's stress level is calculated using the following equation:

$$(N_J) = [(N_J)_{\alpha\beta}]_{\delta \times \delta} \quad (6)$$

The $(N_J)_{\alpha\beta}$ in Equation (6) is the negative distance of the β_{th} model from the average value for the α_{th} parameter. It can be found using either of two ways. If the β_{th} criterion is more favorable, then it is calculated using the equation below:

$$(N_J)_{\alpha\beta} = \frac{Maximum(0, (A_{V_\beta} - X_{\alpha\beta}))}{A_{V_\beta}} \quad (7)$$

On the other hand, if the β_{th} criterion is not favorable, it is calculated by the following equation:

$$(N_{\mathfrak{I}})_{\alpha\beta} = \frac{Maximum(0, (X_{\alpha\beta} - A_{V_\beta}))}{A_{V_\beta}} \tag{8}$$

Step 4: The weighted sum of $(P_{\mathfrak{I}})_{\alpha\beta}$ is calculated using the following equation:

$$(SP_{\mathfrak{I}})_\alpha = \sum_{\beta=1}^{x} y_\beta (P_{\mathfrak{I}})_{\alpha\beta} \tag{9}$$

The aggregate $(P_{\mathfrak{I}})$ is estimated for each signal evaluated using the proposed model for each stress level.

Step 5: The weighted sum of $(N_{\mathfrak{I}})_{\alpha\beta}$ is calculated using the following equation:

$$(SN_{\mathfrak{I}})_\alpha = \sum_{\beta=1}^{x} y_\beta (N_{\mathfrak{I}})_{\alpha\beta} \tag{10}$$

The aggregate $(N_{\mathfrak{I}})$ is estimated for each signal evaluated using the proposed model for each stress level.

Step 6: The normalized values of $(SP_{\mathfrak{I}})_\alpha$ and $(SN_{\mathfrak{I}})_\alpha$ of each signal for the driver's stress level are found using the following two equations:

$$N(SP_{\mathfrak{I}})_\alpha = \frac{(SP_{\mathfrak{I}})_\alpha}{maximum_\alpha((SP_{\mathfrak{I}})_\alpha)} \tag{11}$$

$$N(SN_{\mathfrak{I}})_\alpha = 1 - \frac{(SN_{\mathfrak{I}})_\alpha}{maximum_\alpha((SN_{\mathfrak{I}})_\alpha)} \tag{12}$$

Step 7: The appraisal score (λ) of each signal for the driver's stress level is calculated using the equation given below:

$$\lambda_\alpha = \frac{1}{2}(N(SP_{\mathfrak{I}})_\alpha - N(SP_{\mathfrak{I}})_\alpha) \tag{13}$$

The appraisal score (λ_α) lies are given as $0 \leq \lambda_\alpha \leq 1$.

Step 8: Each signal for the driver's stress level is ranked according to the decreasing values of the appraisal score (λ_α). Thus, the signal with the lowest appraisal score (λ_α) for a particular stress level has the highest performance among the other signals.

4. Results

The SRAD and AffectiveROAD datasets are randomly distributed into two groups, with 85% and 15% for training and validation, respectively. Results are acquired for the 1D CNN and 1D CNN-LSTM models trained using the SRAD, BH, E4-L, E4-R, and BH+E4-(L+R) datasets. A performance assessment of the proposed driver stress recognition models for the low, medium, and high classes of stress is carried out using different classification metrics. These performance metrics include accuracy (ACC), recall (RCL), precision (PRC), F-score (F1), and specificity (SPC).

4.1. Models' Evaluation for the Two-Stress Class

Results of the proposed driver stress recognition models for the two-stress class are shown in Table 3. These results are based on the training data obtained from the SRAD and AffectiveROAD datasets for real-world driving. The training graphs of the proposed CNN models are shown in Figures 1–6. Similarly, the training graphs of the proposed hybrid CNN-LSTM models are shown in Figures 7–12. Results show that the BH+E4-(L+R)-based CNN model outperformed other models based on the SRAD, Bio BH, E4-L, E4-R, and E4-(L+R) datasets by 2.9%, 6.5%, 9.1%, 7.3%, and 3.25%, respectively, with an overall validation accuracy of 95.6% for the two-stress class. The proposed BH+E4-(L+R)-based hybrid CNN-LSTM model outperformed other models based on SRAD, BH, E4-L, E4-R, and E4-(L+R) datasets by 4.79%, 1.1%, 7.76%, 5.94%, and 1.94%, respectively, with an overall validation accuracy of 96.59% for the two-stress class.

Confusion matrices of the proposed CNN and hybrid CNN-LSTM models are shown in Figures 13 and 14. In Figure 13f, 214 relaxed instances are predicted correctly, while 5 relaxed instances are incorrectly predicted as stressed by the model. Thus, the total correct prediction for the relaxed class is 97.7%. Similarly, for the stressed class, 291 out of 309 instances are correctly predicted, which amounts to a total accuracy of 94.2% for the stressed class. In Figure 14f, 233 relaxed instances are predicted correctly, while 15 relaxed instances are incorrectly predicted as stressed by the model. Thus, the total correct prediction for the relaxed class is 94%. Similarly, for the stressed class, 277 out of 280 instances are correctly predicted, which amounts to a total accuracy of 98.9% for the stressed class.

Table 3. Performance analysis of the proposed fusion models for the two-stress class.

Deep Learning Model	Dataset	Driver's Stress Level	Performance Measure					Overall ACC
			ACC	RCL	PRC	F1	SPC	
1D CNN	SRAD	Relaxed	0.9271	0.8774	0.9118	0.8942	0.9541	92.7%
		Stressed	0.9271	0.9541	0.9350	0.9444	0.8774	
	BH	Relaxed	0.8909	0.9278	0.8267	0.8743	0.8654	89.1%
		Stressed	0.8909	0.8654	0.9454	0.9036	0.9278	
	E4-L	Relaxed	0.8653	0.8072	0.9394	0.8683	0.9363	86.53%
		Stressed	0.8653	0.9363	0.7989	0.8622	0.8073	
	E4-R	Relaxed	0.8825	0.8636	0.8693	0.8664	0.8974	88.3%
		Stressed	0.8825	0.8974	0.8929	0.8951	0.8636	
	E4-(L+R)	Relaxed	0.9235	0.9776	0.8617	0.916	0.8833	92.35%
		Stressed	0.9235	0.8833	0.9815	0.9298	0.9776	
	BH+E4-(L+R)	Relaxed	0.9564	0.9772	0.9224	0.949	0.9417	95.6%
		Stressed	0.9564	0.9417	0.9831	0.962	0.9772	
1D CNN-LSTM	SRAD	Relaxed	0.9180	0.9041	0.8742	0.8889	0.9261	91.8%
		Stressed	0.9181	0.9261	0.9444	0.9352	0.9041	
	BH	Relaxed	0.9545	0.9857	0.9079	0.9452	0.9340	95.5%
		Stressed	0.9545	0.9340	0.9900	0.9612	0.9857	
	E4-L	Relaxed	0.8882	0.9007	0.85	0.8746	0.8788	88.83%
		Stressed	0.8882	0.8788	0.9206	0.8992	0.9007	
	E4-R	Relaxed	0.9065	0.9099	0.8649	0.8868	0.9041	90.65%
		Stressed	0.9065	0.9041	0.9371	0.9203	0.9099	
	E4-(L+R)	Relaxed	0.9465	0.9555	0.9328	0.944	0.9384	94.65%
		Stressed	0.9465	0.9384	0.9593	0.9487	0.9555	
	BH+E4-(L+R)	Relaxed	0.9659	0.9395	0.9873	0.9628	0.9893	96.59%
		Stressed	0.9659	0.9893	0.9486	0.9685	0.9395	

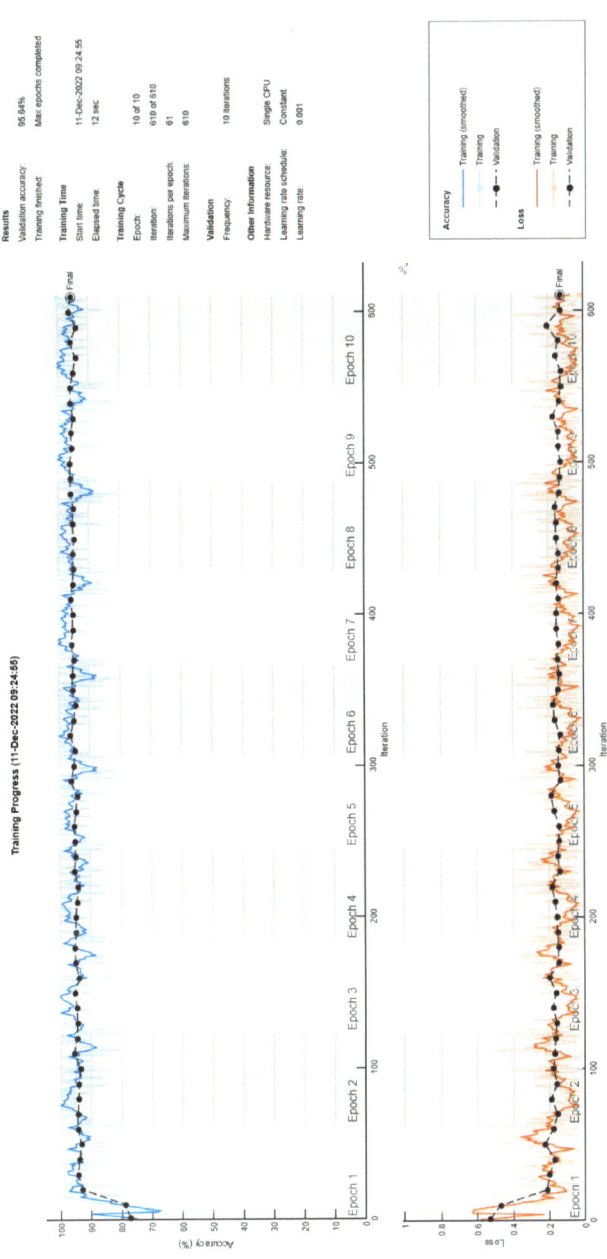

Figure 6. Training graph of the CNN model for the two-stress class based on the BH+E4-(L+R) datasets.

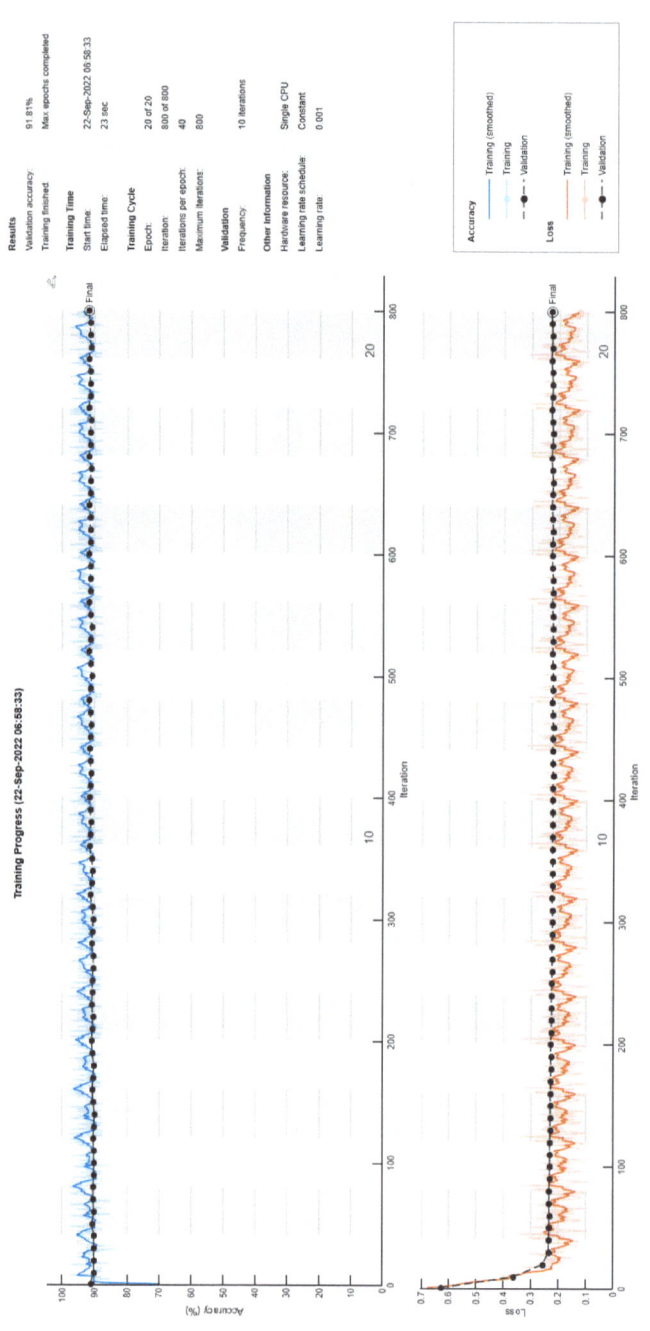

Figure 7. Training graph of the hybrid CNN-LSTM model for the two-stress class based on the SRAD dataset.

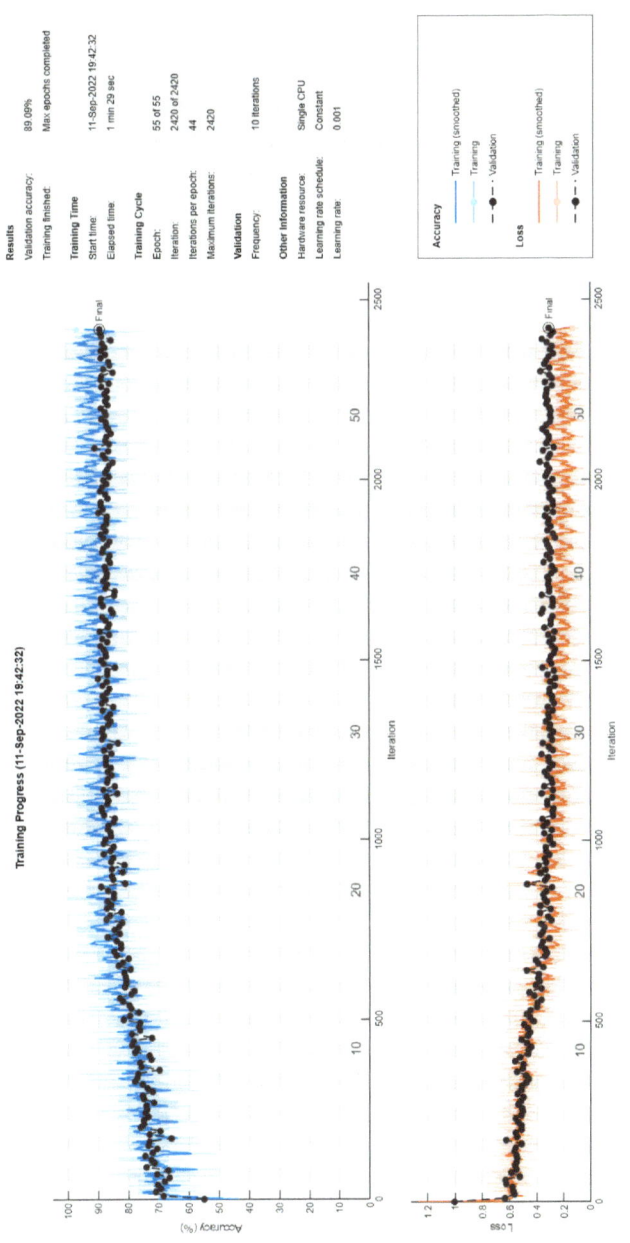

Figure 8. Training graph of the hybrid CNN-LSTM model for the two-stress class based on the BH dataset.

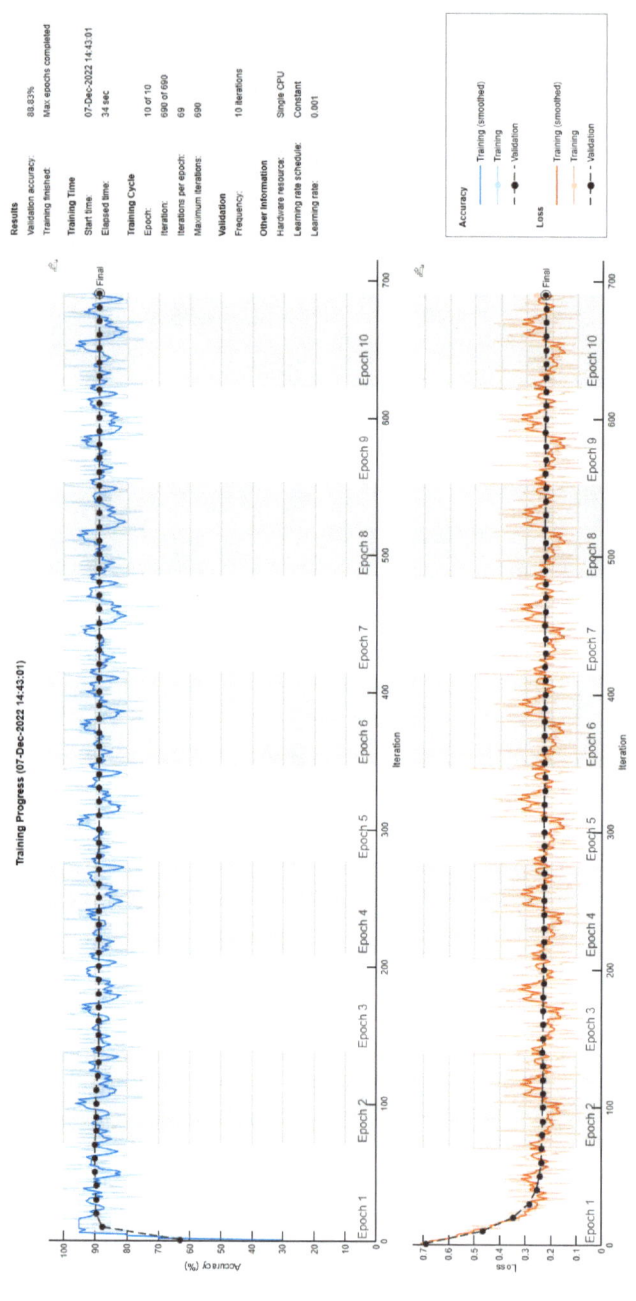

Figure 9. Training graph of the hybrid CNN-LSTM model for the two-stress class based on the E4-L dataset.

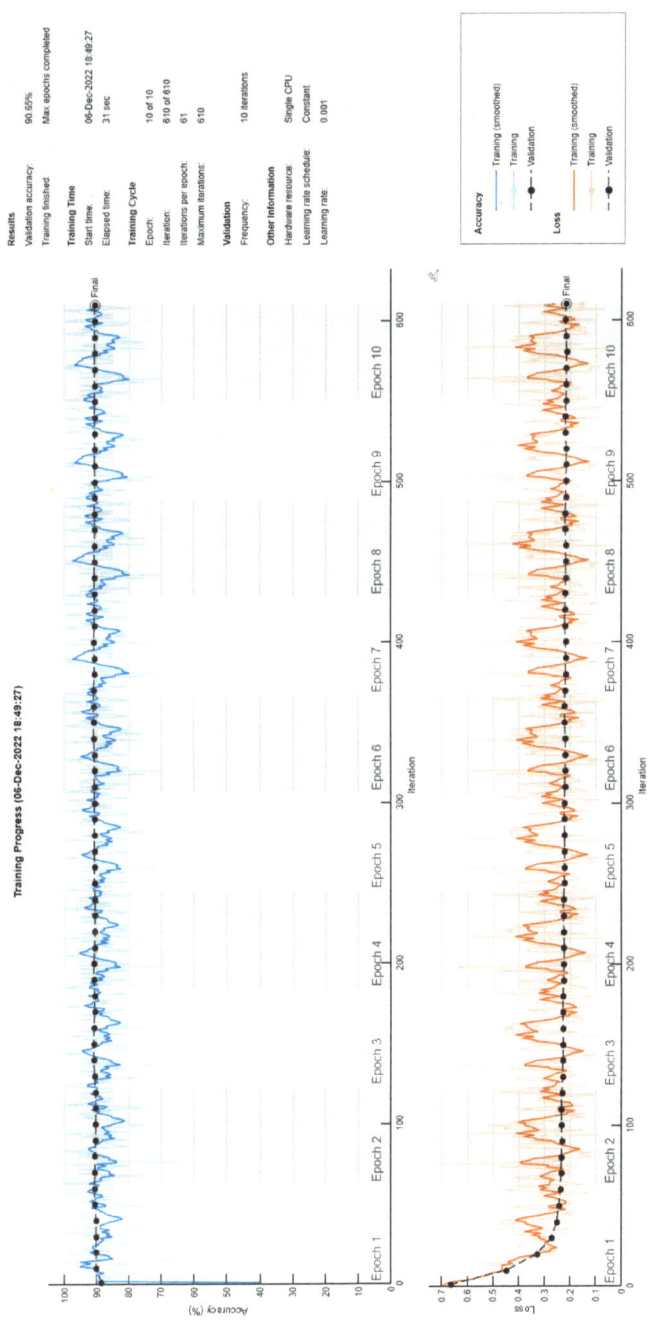

Figure 10. Training graph of the hybrid CNN-LSTM model for the two-stress class based on the E4-R dataset.

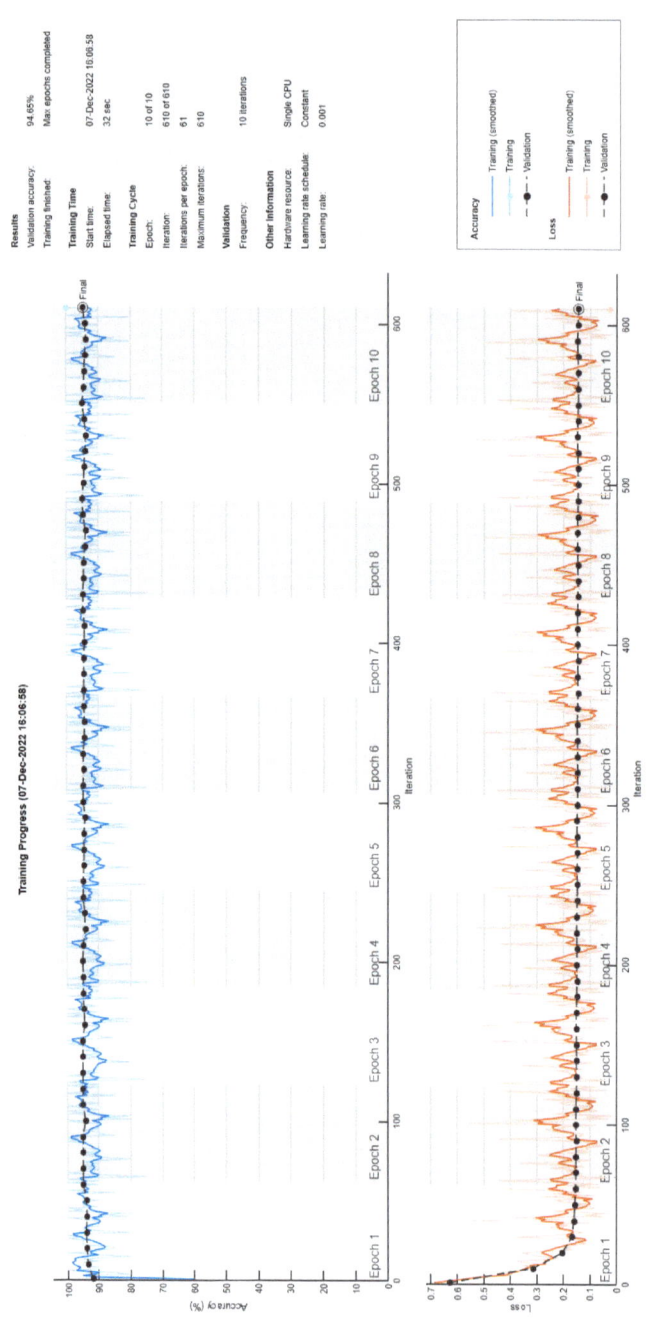

Figure 11. Training graph of the hybrid CNN-LSTM model for the two-stress class based on the E4-(L+R) datasets.

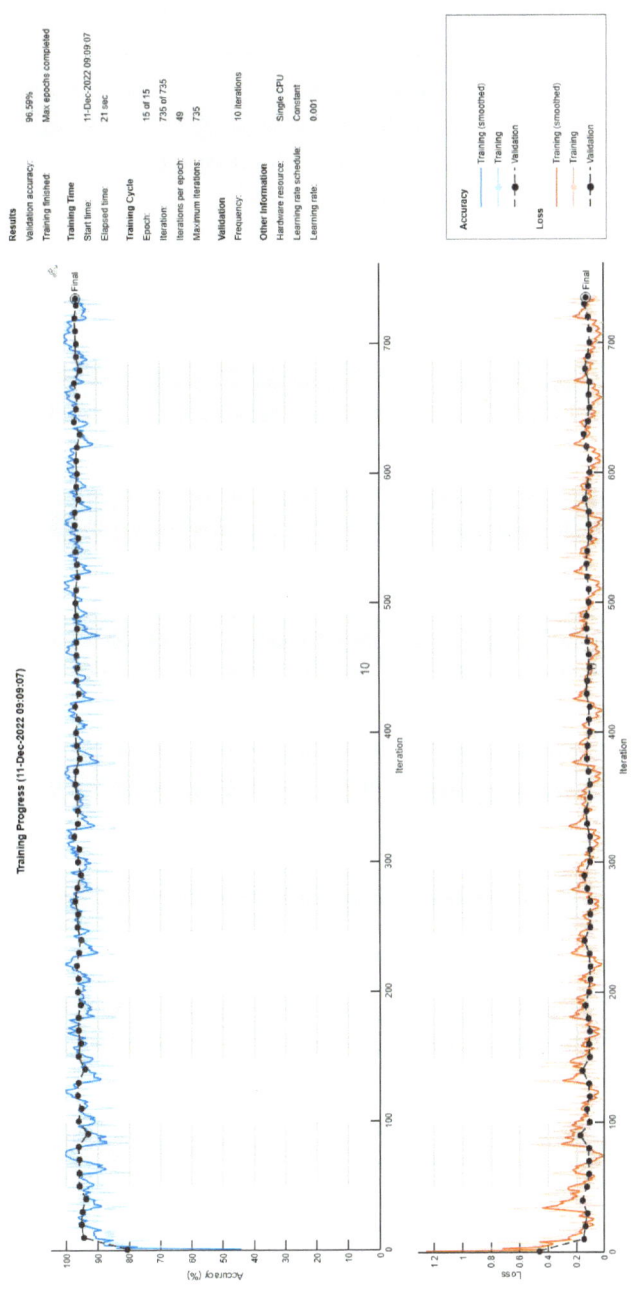

Figure 12. Training graph of the hybrid CNN-LSTM model for the two-stress class based on the BH+E4-(L+R) datasets.

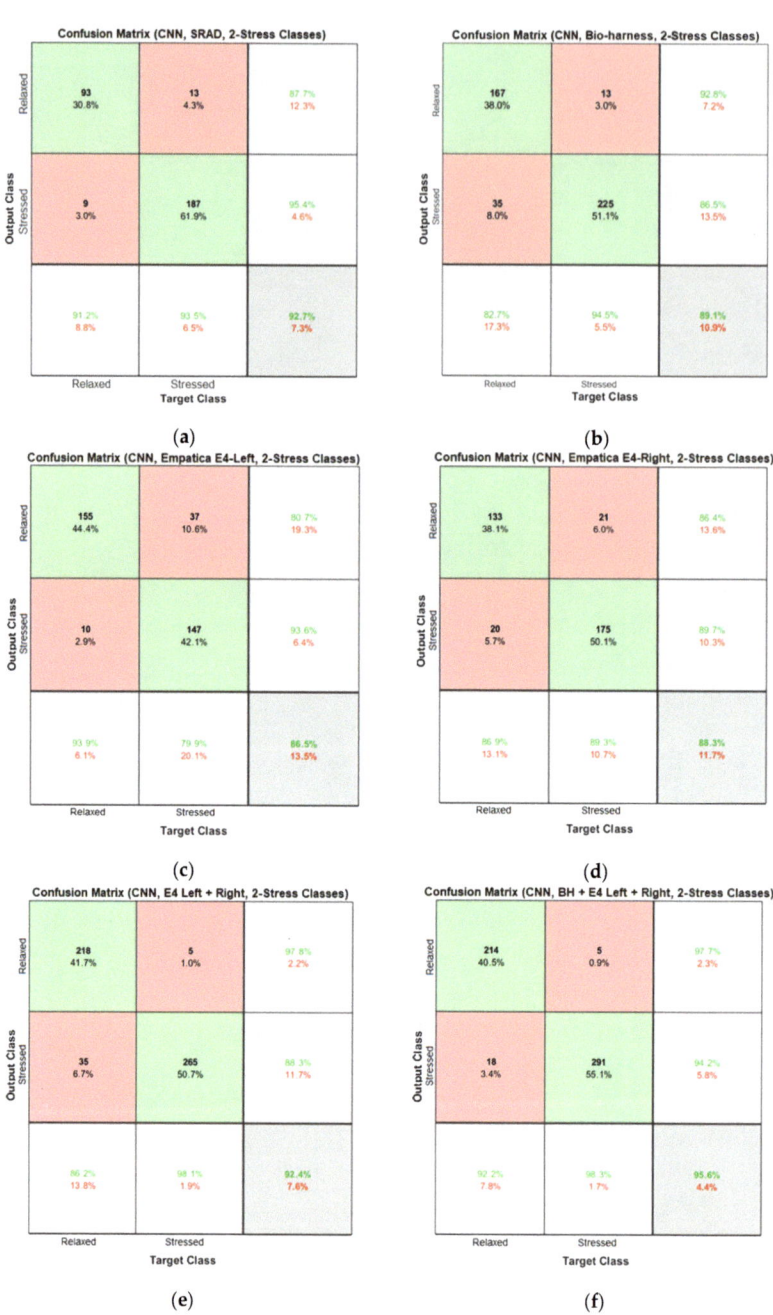

Figure 13. Confusion matrices of the CNN models for the two-stress class based on: (**a**) the SRAD dataset; (**b**) BH dataset; (**c**) E4-L dataset; (**d**) E4-R dataset; (**e**) E4-(L+R) datasets; (**f**) BH+E4-(L+R) datasets.

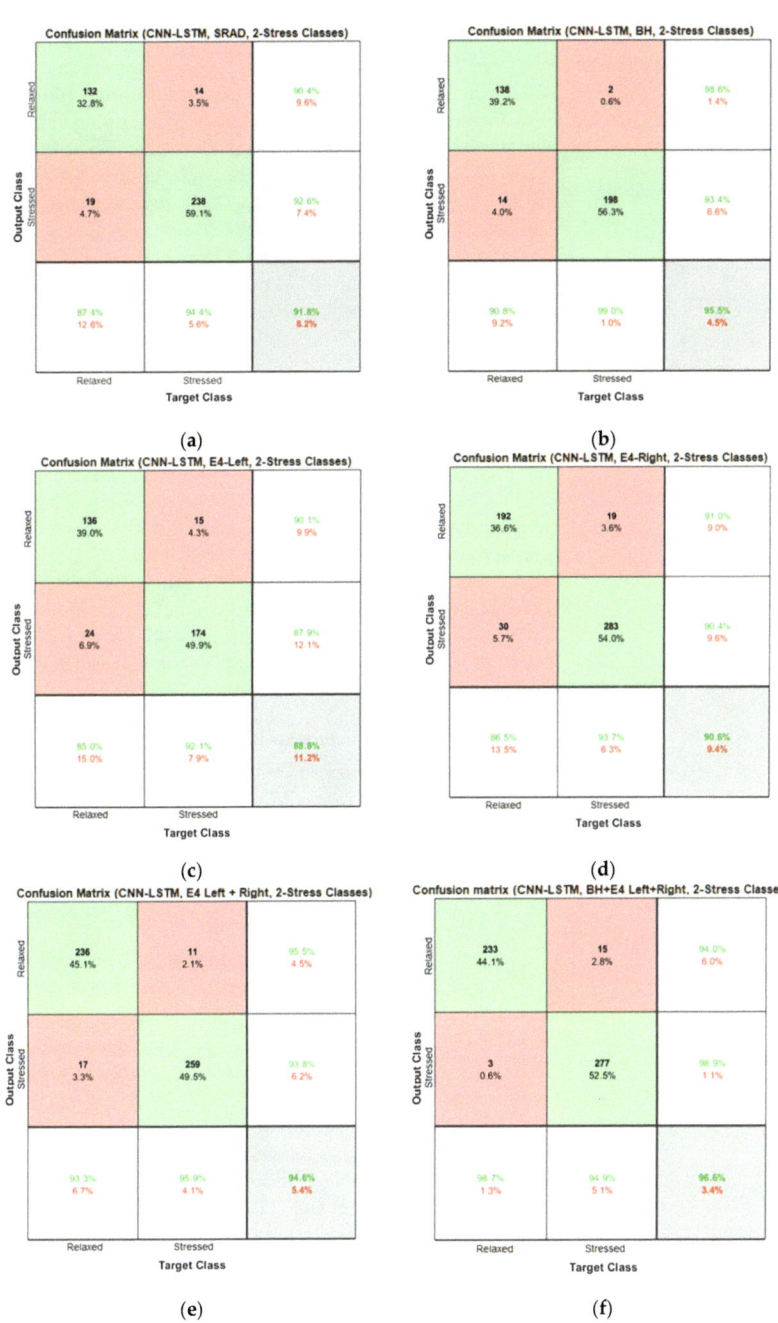

Figure 14. Confusion matrices of the hybrid CNN-LSTM models for the two-stress class based on: (**a**) the SRAD dataset; (**b**) BH dataset; (**c**) E4-L dataset; (**d**) E4-R dataset; (**e**) E4-(L+R) datasets; (**f**) BH+E4-(L+R) datasets.

4.2. Models' Evaluation for the Three-Stress Class

Results of the proposed driver stress recognition models for the three-stress class are shown in Table 4. These results are based on the training data obtained for the SRAD and AffectiveROAD datasets for real-world driving. The training graphs of the proposed CNN models are shown in Figures 15–20. Similarly, the training graphs of the proposed hybrid CNN-LSTM models are shown in Figures 21–26. Results show that the proposed CNN model based on the BH+E4-(L+R) datasets outperform the other models based on the SRAD, BH, E4-L, E4-R, and E4-(L+R) datasets significantly by 6.16%, 6.76%, 9.16%, 8.87%, and 1.72%, respectively, with an overall validation accuracy of 85.66%. Similarly, the proposed hybrid CNN-LSTM model based on the BH+E4-(L+R) datasets outperform the other models based on the SRAD, BH, E4-L, E4-R, and E4-(L+R) datasets significantly by 2.15%, 0.15%, 11.22%, 5.89%, and 3.82%, respectively, with an overall validation accuracy of 87.95%.

Confusion matrices for the proposed CNN and hybrid CNN-LSTM models are shown in Figures 27 and 28. In Figure 27f, 190 low instances are predicted correctly, while 3 and 6 low instances are incorrectly predicted as medium and high by the CNN model. So, the total correct prediction for the high-stress class is 95.5%. Likewise, for the medium- and high-stress classes, 34 out of 50 and 224 out of 274 instances were correctly predicted, which amounts to total accuracies of 68% and 81.8% for medium- and high-stress classes, respectively. Similarly, in Figure 28f, 214 low instances are predicted correctly, while 3 and 8 low instances are incorrectly predicted as medium and high by the CNN-LSTM model. Therefore, the total correct prediction for the low-stress class is 95.1%. Similarly, for the medium- and high-stress classes, 47 out of 61 and 199 out of 237 instances were correctly predicted, which amounts to total accuracies of 77% and 84% for the medium- and high-stress classes, respectively.

4.3. Rank-Based Performance Evaluation

The eight-step fuzzy EDAS procedure [65] defined in Section 3.6 is utilized here to evaluate the ranks of the SRAD, BH, E4-L, E4-R, E4-(L+R), and BH+E4-(L+R)-based CNN and hybrid CNN-LSTM models for the two-stress and three-stress classes. This procedure is separately followed for each the driver's stress level. The classification metrics calculated in Tables 3 and 4 are regarded as a criterion for the proposed CNN and hybrid CNN-LSTM driver stress level classification models for the two-stress and three-stress classes.

4.3.1. Rank Estimation of the CNN Models for Two Levels of Stress

A rank estimation of the CNN models for the two-stress class (relaxed state) is performed in a series of steps. The results of each step are shown in Tables 5–10. The first step determines the cross-efficient values (ψ_β) using Equations (1) and (2), as shown in Table 5. In the next two steps, the positive distance (P_J) and negative distance (N_J) are separately determined based by Equations (5) and (8), as given in Tables 6 and 7. In the fourth and fifth steps, the weighted sum of (P_J) and (N_J) are separately calculated with the help of Equations (9) and (10), as shown in Tables 8 and 9. The sixth step normalizes the weighted sums $(SP_J)_\alpha$ and $(SN_J)_\alpha$ independently to obtain the aggregate scores of the models based on Equations (11) and (12), as indicated in Table 10. Finally, the appraisal score (λ_α) is determined based on the aggregate scores $N(SP_J)_\alpha$ and $N(SN_J)_\alpha$ in the seventh step with the help of Equation (13), as given in Table 10. The eighth step uses the appraisal scores (λ_α) to determine the ranks of the proposed CNN models based on the BH, E4-L, E4-R, E4-(L+R), and BH+E4-(L+R) datasets. The model with the lowest appraisal score (λ_α) has the highest performance among the candidate models. Table 10 shows that the proposed BH+E4-(L+R), E4-L, E4-R, SRAD, E4-(L+R), and BH-based CNN models achieved first, second, third, fourth, fifth, and fifth positions for the relaxed state. Likewise, the same eight-step procedure is utilized for the stressed state, and the resulting ranks of each CNN model are given in Table 11. Table 11 shows that the proposed BH+E4-(L+R), SRAD, E4-L,

E4-R, E4-(L+R), and BH-based CNN models achieved first, second, third, fourth, fifth, and fifth positions for the stressed state.

Table 4. Performance analysis of the proposed fusion models for the three-stress class.

Deep Learning Model	Dataset	Driver's Stress Level	Performance Measure					Overall ACC
			ACC	RCL	PRC	F1	SPC	
1D CNN	SRAD	Low	0.9338	0.8596	0.9607	0.9074	0.9787	79.5%
		Medium	0.8377	0.5921	0.7143	0.6475	0.9203	
		High	0.8377	0.8661	0.708	0.7791	0.7895	
	BH	High	0.8659	0.8461	0.8959	0.8703	0.8883	78.9%
		Medium	0.8886	0.6216	0.3965	0.4842	0.9131	
		Low	0.8227	0.7456	0.7826	0.7636	0.8708	
	E4-L	Low	0.8911	0.8514	0.9255	0.8869	0.931	76.5%
		Medium	0.8567	0.6667	0.1132	0.1935	0.8618	
		High	0.7822	0.6788	0.8296	0.7467	0.875	
	E4-R	Low	0.8997	0.8687	0.9085	0.8882	0.9259	76.79%
		Medium	0.8481	0.493	0.6731	0.5691	0.9388	
		High	0.788	0.7966	0.6528	0.7176	0.7835	
	E4-(L+R)	Low	0.9312	0.9159	0.9241	0.9200	0.9428	83.94%
		Medium	0.893	0.7600	0.4634	0.5758	0.907	
		High	0.8547	0.7854	0.894	0.8362	0.9167	
	BH+E4-(L+R)	Low	0.9541	0.9548	0.9268	0.9406	0.9537	85.66%
		Medium	0.8929	0.6800	0.4595	0.5484	0.9154	
		High	0.8662	0.8175	0.918	0.8649	0.9197	
1D CNN-LSTM	SRAD	Low	0.9454	0.9388	0.9139	0.9262	0.9492	85.6%
		Medium	0.9032	0.8033	0.6447	0.7153	0.9210	
		High	0.8635	0.8103	0.8977	0.8517	0.9135	
	BH	Low	0.9574	0.9245	0.9800	0.9515	0.9845	87.8%
		Medium	0.9204	0.9130	0.4468	0.6000	0.9210	
		High	0.8778	0.8294	0.9097	0.8677	0.9231	
	E4-L	Low	0.8596	0.8415	0.8571	0.8492	0.8757	76.22%
		Medium	0.8768	0.6552	0.3654	0.4691	0.8969	
		High	0.788	0.6987	0.8015	0.7466	0.8601	
	E4-R	Low	0.9027	0.9021	0.8833	0.8926	0.9031	82.06%
		Medium	0.9046	0.62	0.5	0.5536	0.9346	
		High	0.834	0.7824	0.8423	0.8113	0.8772	
	E4-(L+R)	Low	0.9235	0.9395	0.8821	0.9099	0.9123	84.13%
		Medium	0.9082	0.7857	0.4583	0.5789	0.9189	
		High	0.8509	0.7707	0.9234	0.8402	0.9338	
	BH+E4-(L+R)	Low	0.9522	0.9511	0.9386	0.9448	0.953	87.95%
		Medium	0.9178	0.7705	0.6184	0.6861	0.9372	
		High	0.8891	0.8397	0.9087	0.8728	0.9301	

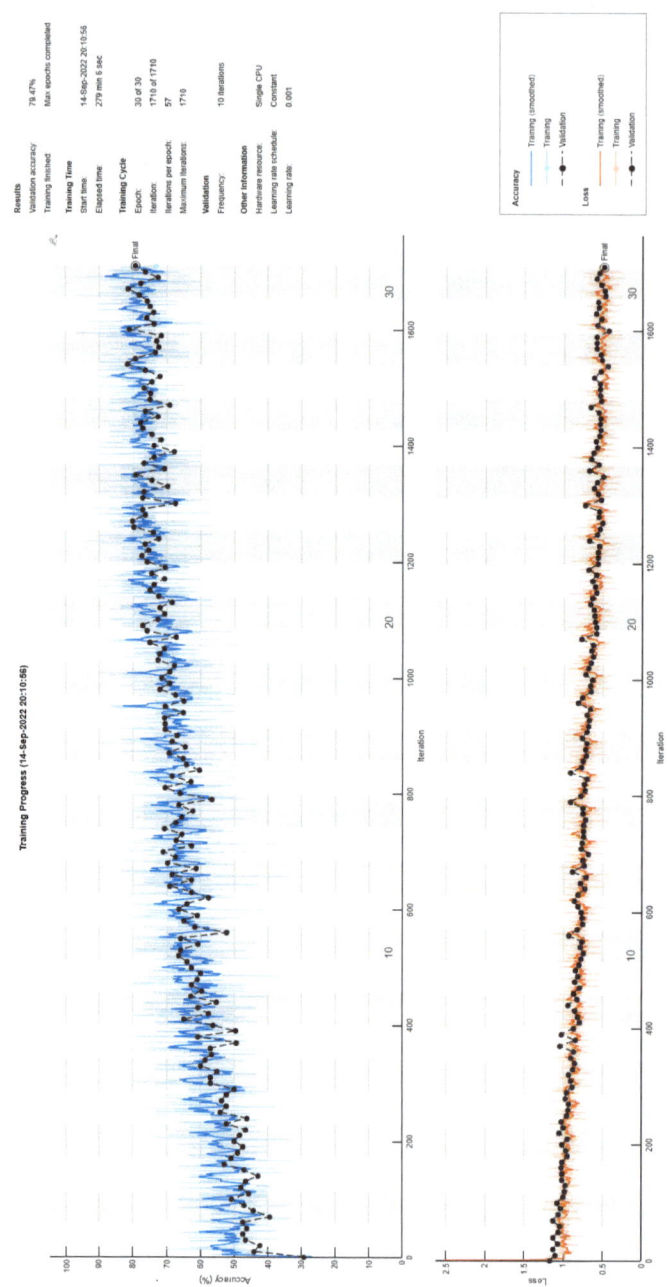

Figure 15. Training graph of the CNN model for the three-stress class based on the SRAD dataset.

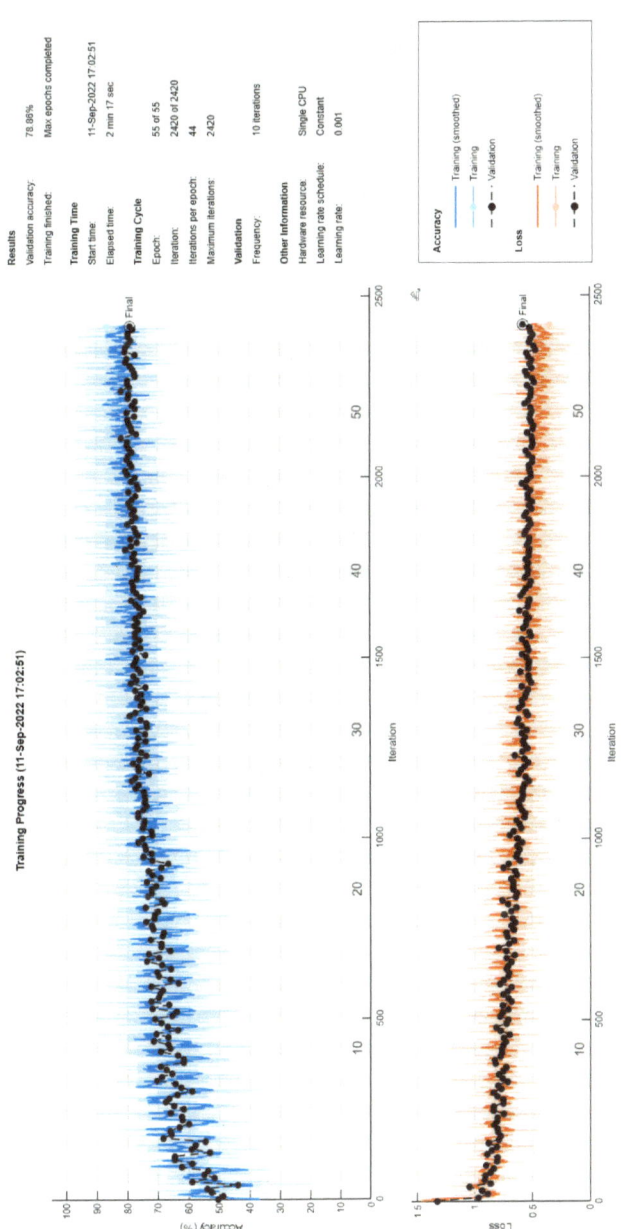

Figure 16. Training graph of the CNN model for the three-stress class based on the BH dataset.

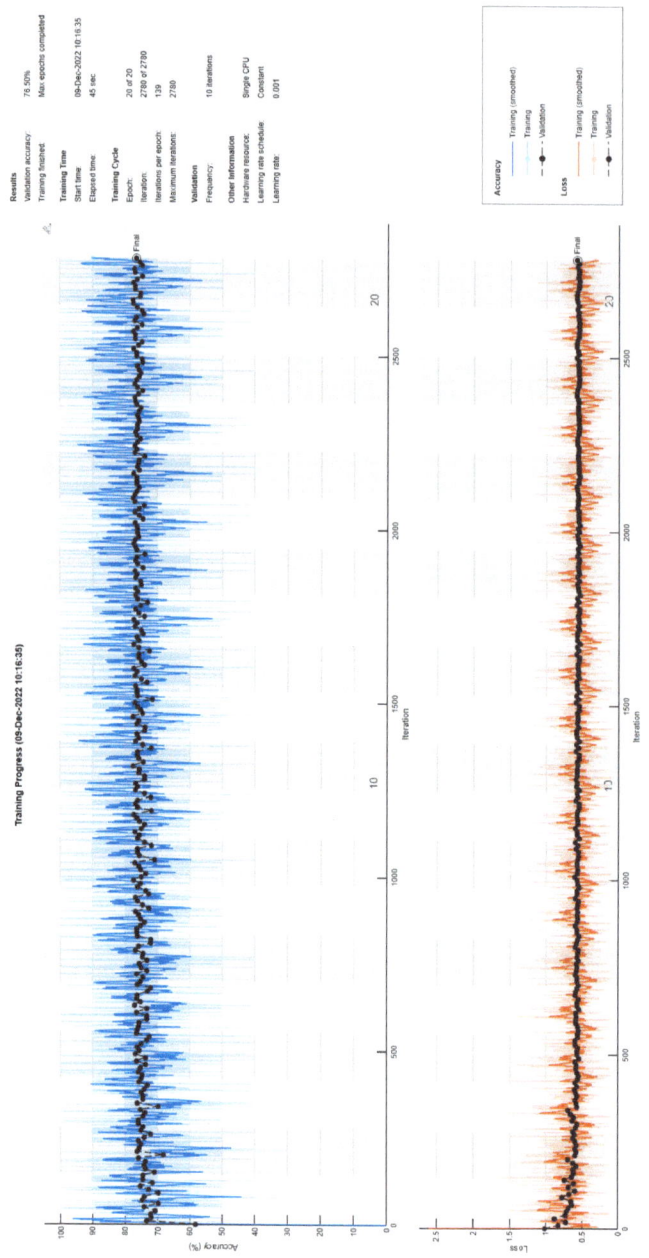

Figure 17. Training graph of the CNN model for the three-stress class based on the E4-L dataset.

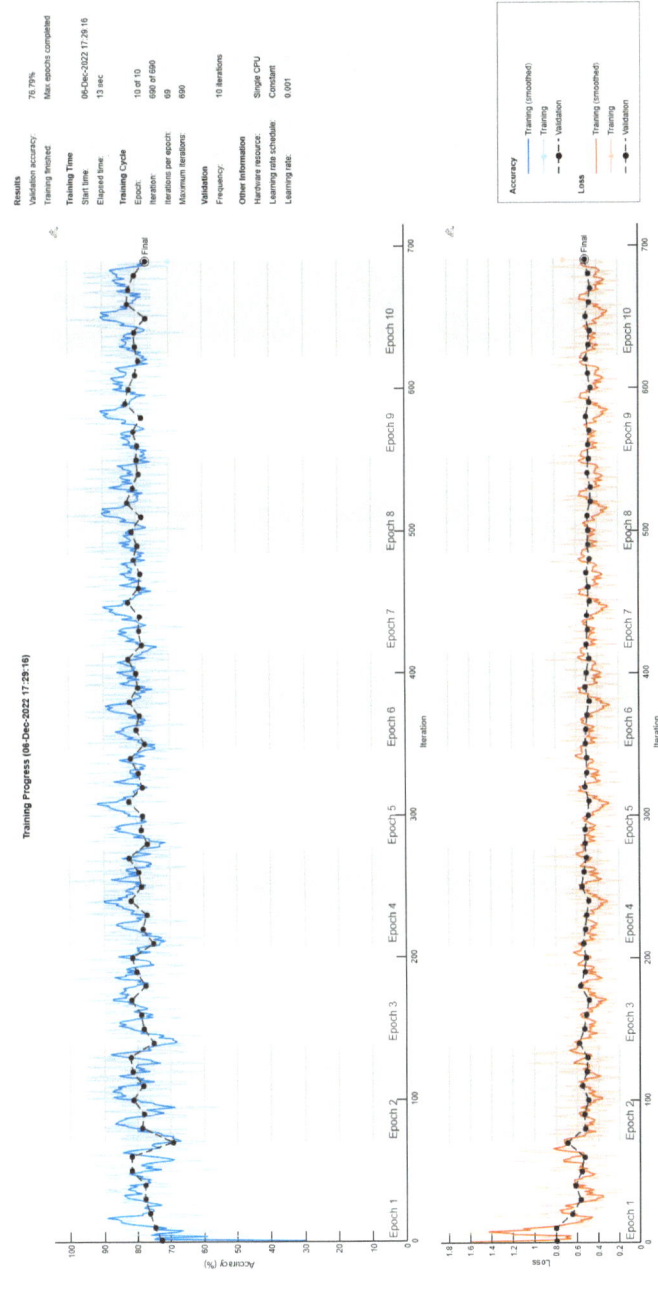

Figure 18. Training graph of the CNN model for the three-stress class based on the E4-R dataset.

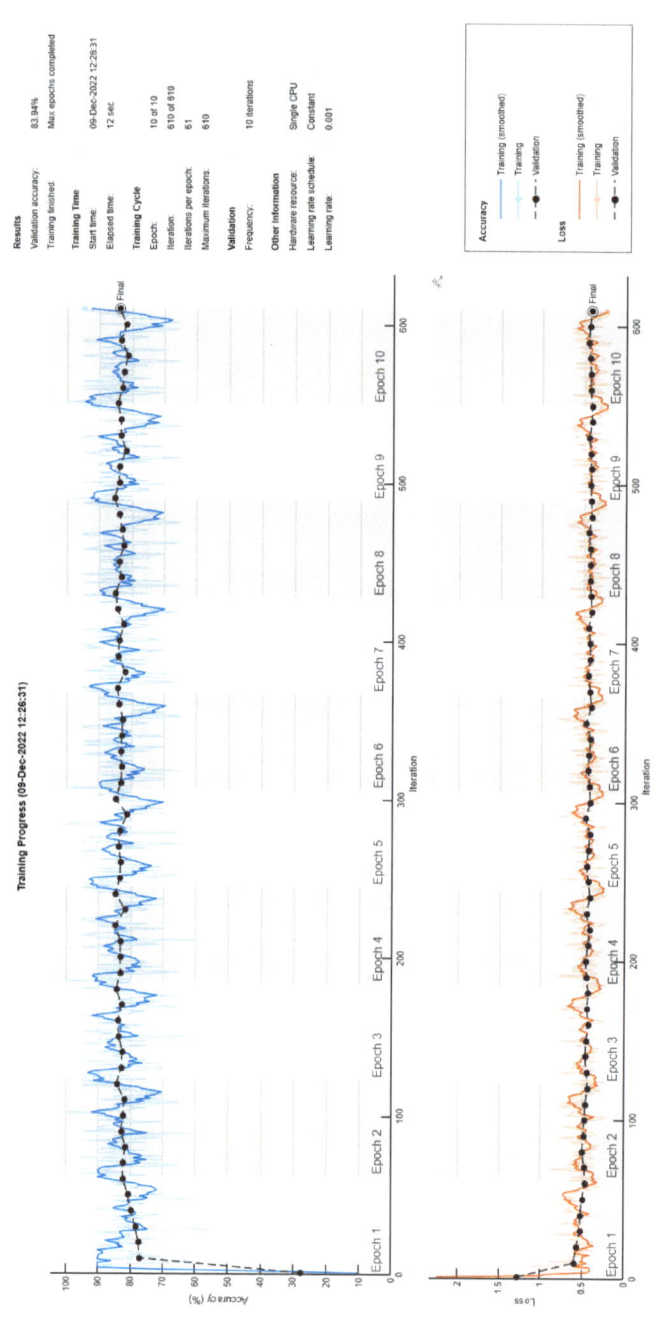

Figure 19. Training graph of the CNN model for the three-stress class based on the E4-(L+R) datasets.

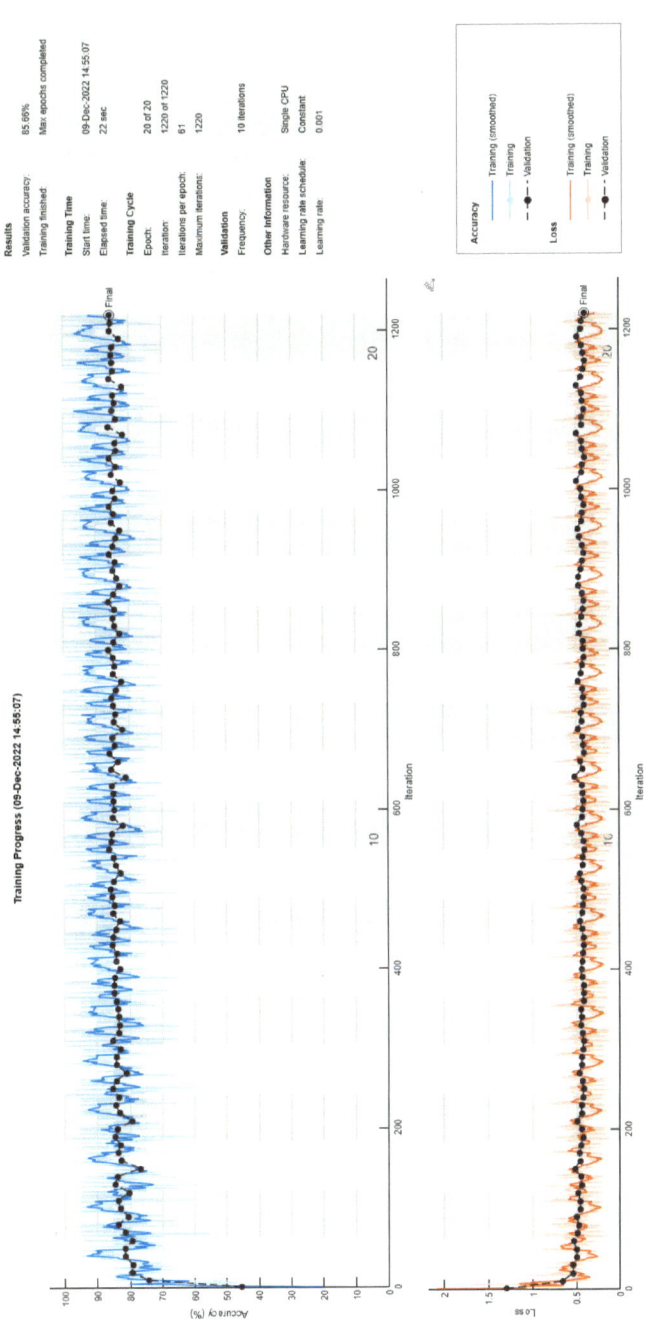

Figure 20. Training graph of the CNN model for the three-stress class based on the BH+E4+(L+R) datasets.

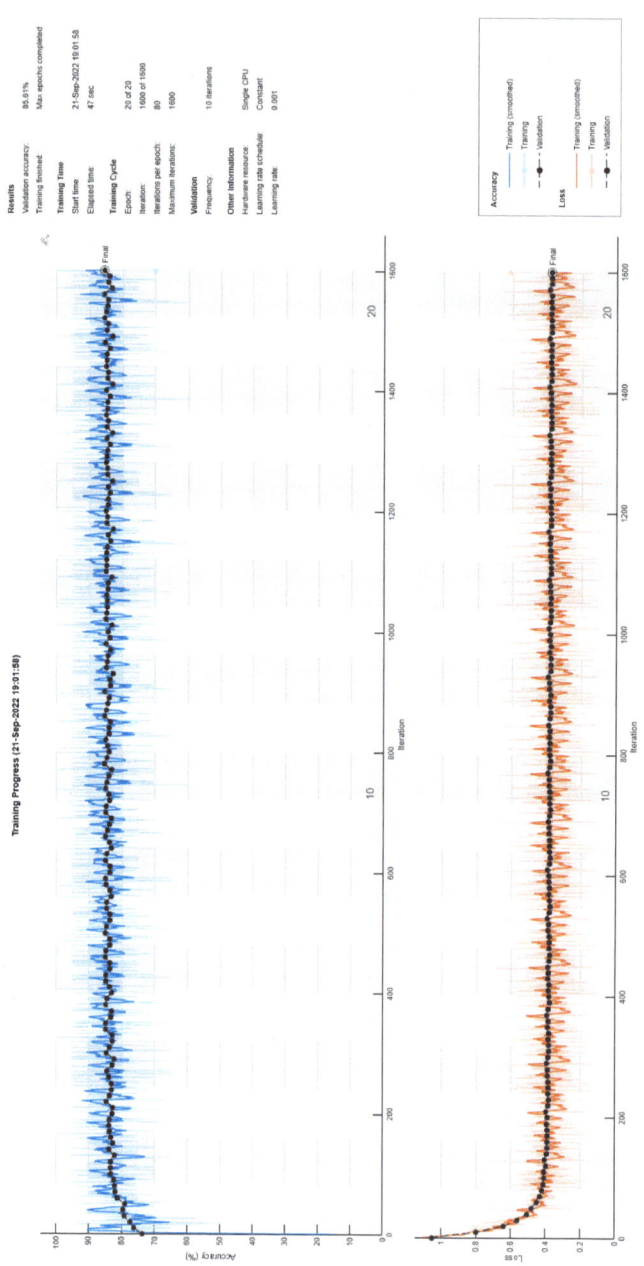

Figure 21. Training graph of the hybrid CNN-LSTM model for the three-stress class based on the SRAD dataset.

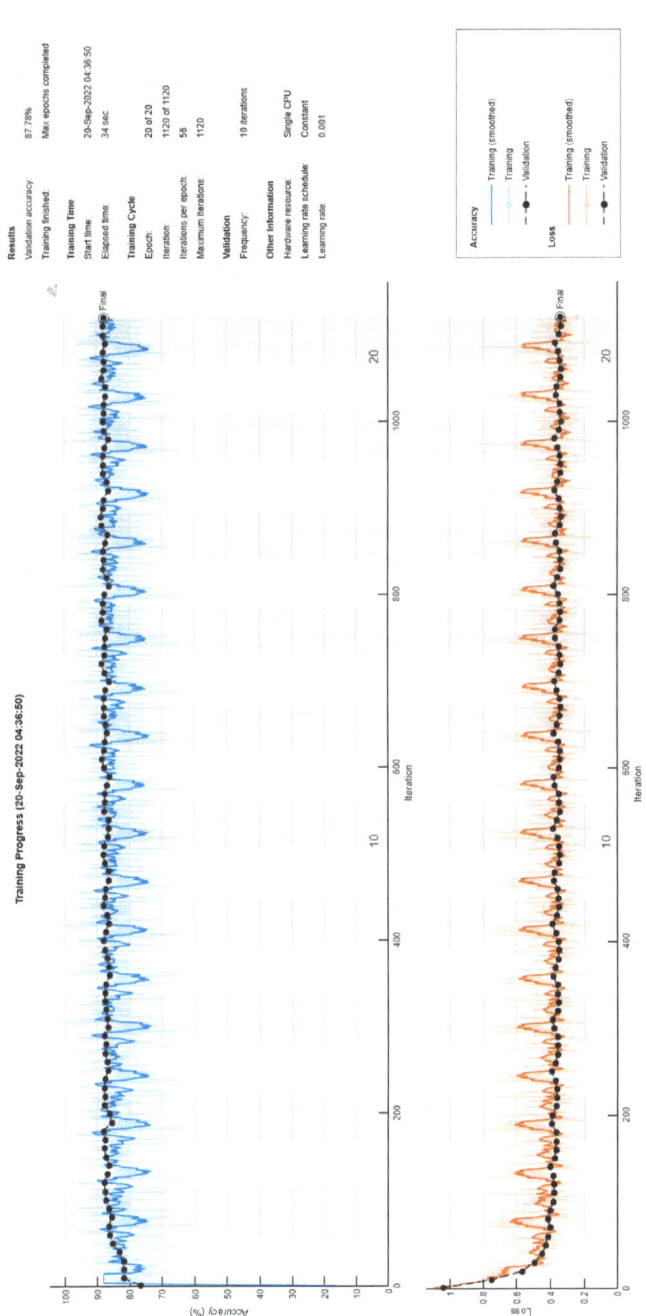

Figure 22. Training graph of the hybrid CNN-LSTM model for the three-stress class based on the BH dataset.

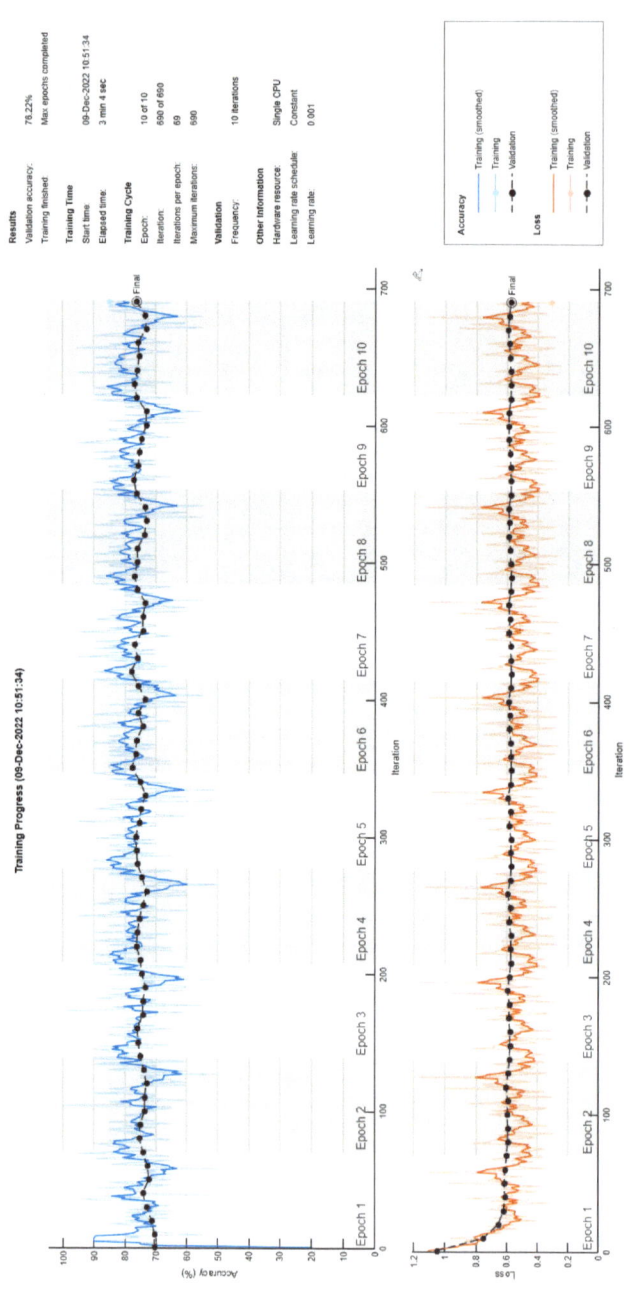

Figure 23. Training graph of the hybrid CNN-LSTM model for the three-stress class based on the E4-L dataset.

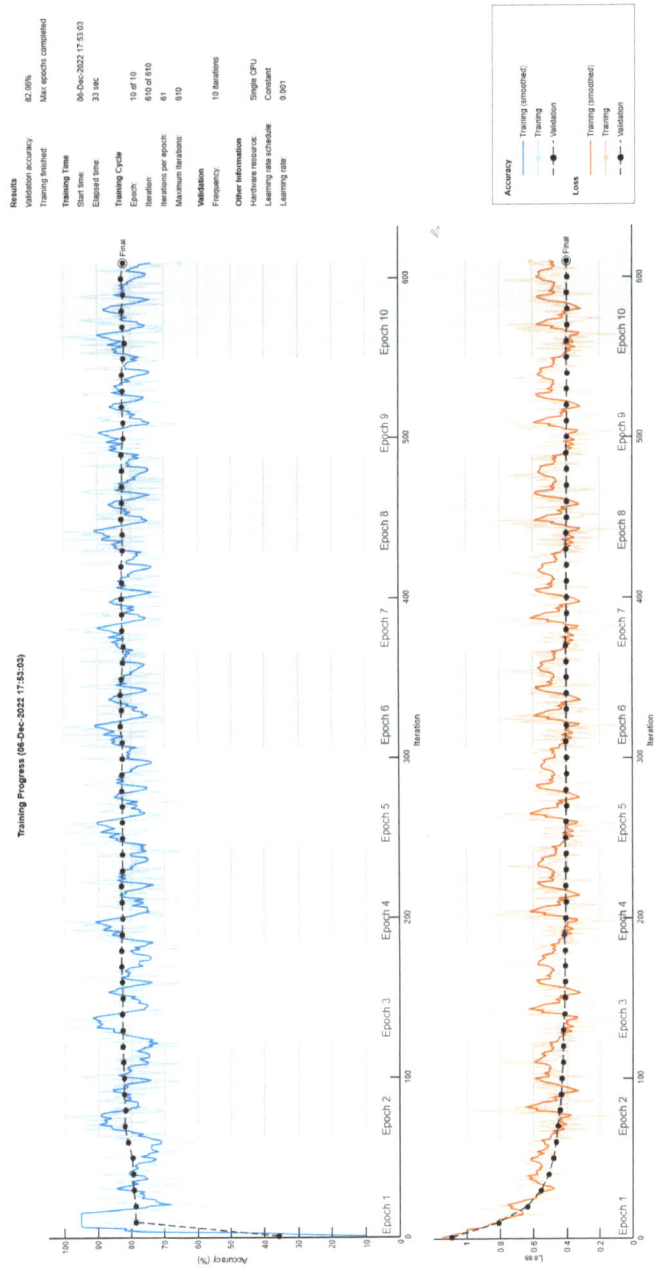

Figure 24. Training graph of the hybrid CNN-LSTM model for the three-stress class based on the E4-R dataset.

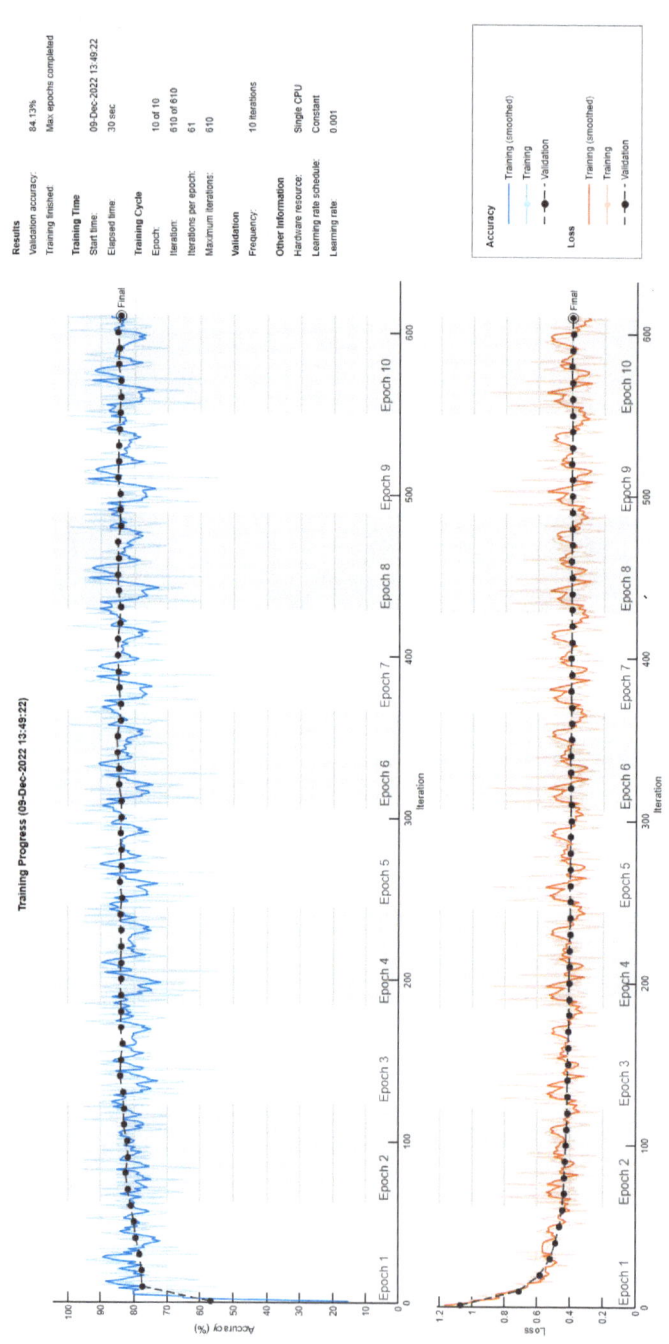

Figure 25. Training graph of the hybrid CNN-LSTM model for the three-stress class based on the E4-(L+R) datasets.

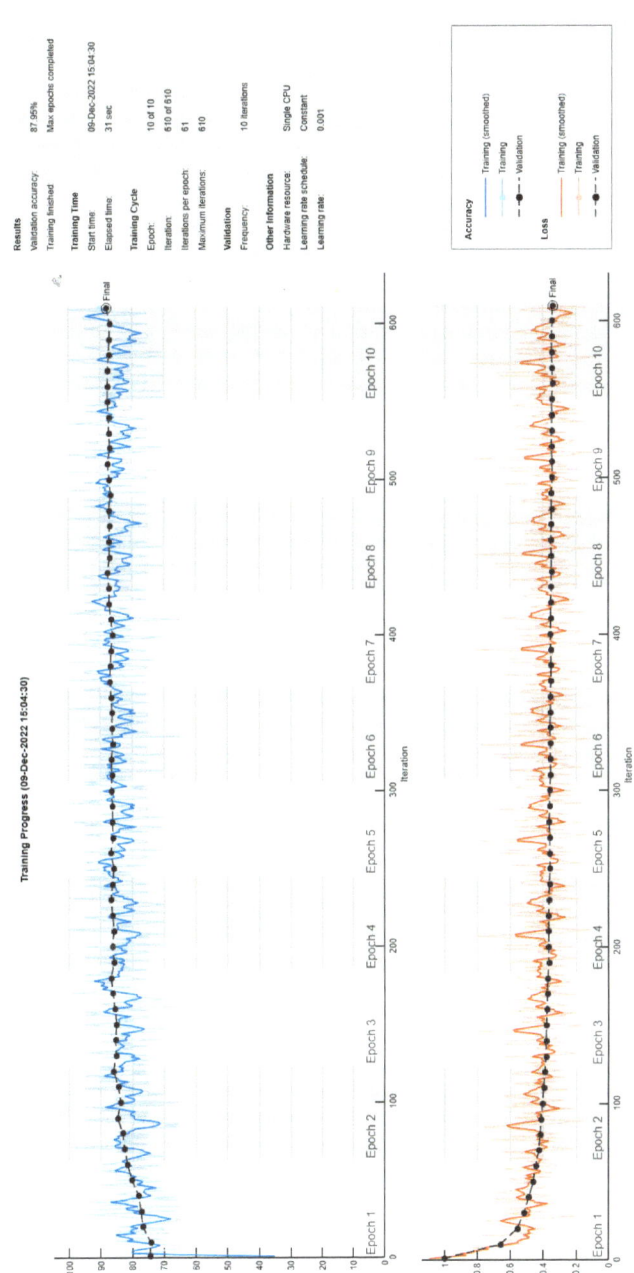

Figure 26. Training graph of the hybrid CNN-LSTM model for the three-stress class based on the BH+E4-(L+R) datasets.

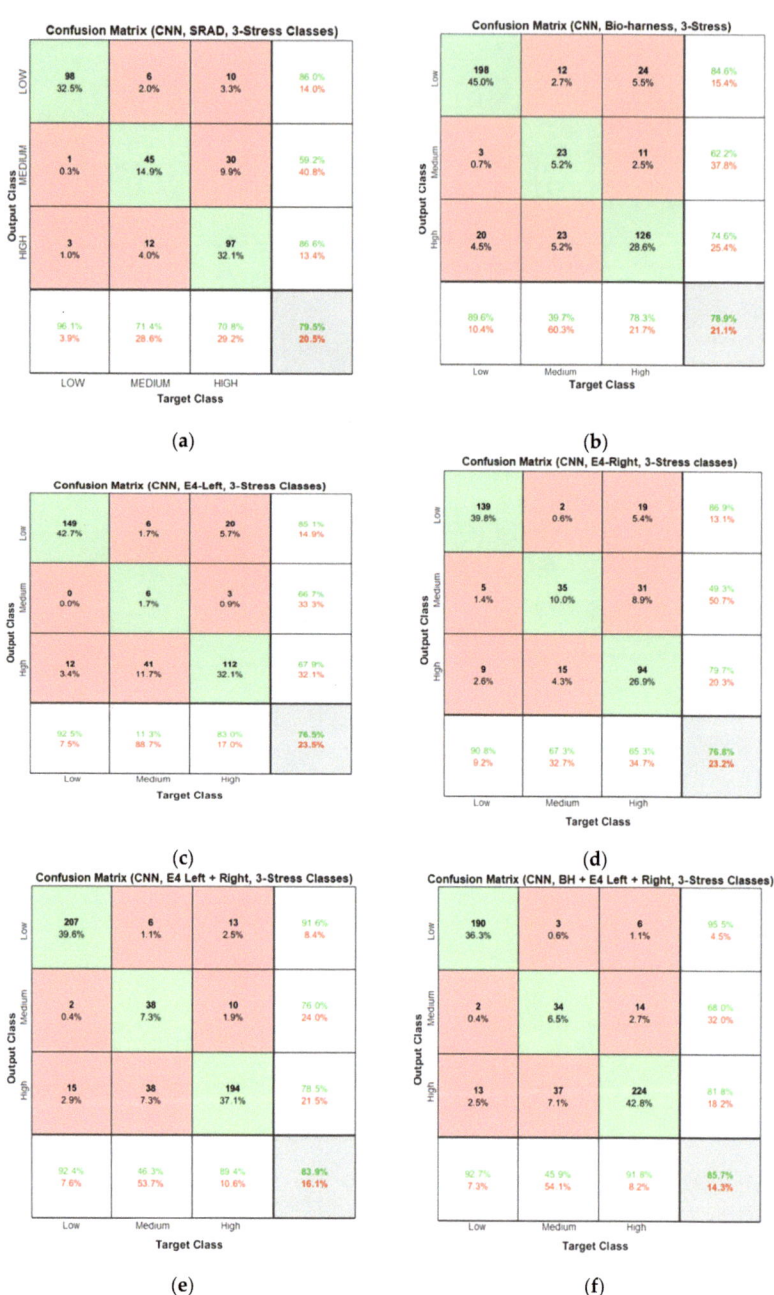

Figure 27. Confusion matrices of the CNN models for the three-stress class based on: (**a**) the SRAD dataset; (**b**) BH dataset; (**c**) E4-L dataset; (**d**) E4-R dataset; (**e**) E4-(L+R) datasets; (**f**) BH+E4-(L+R) datasets.

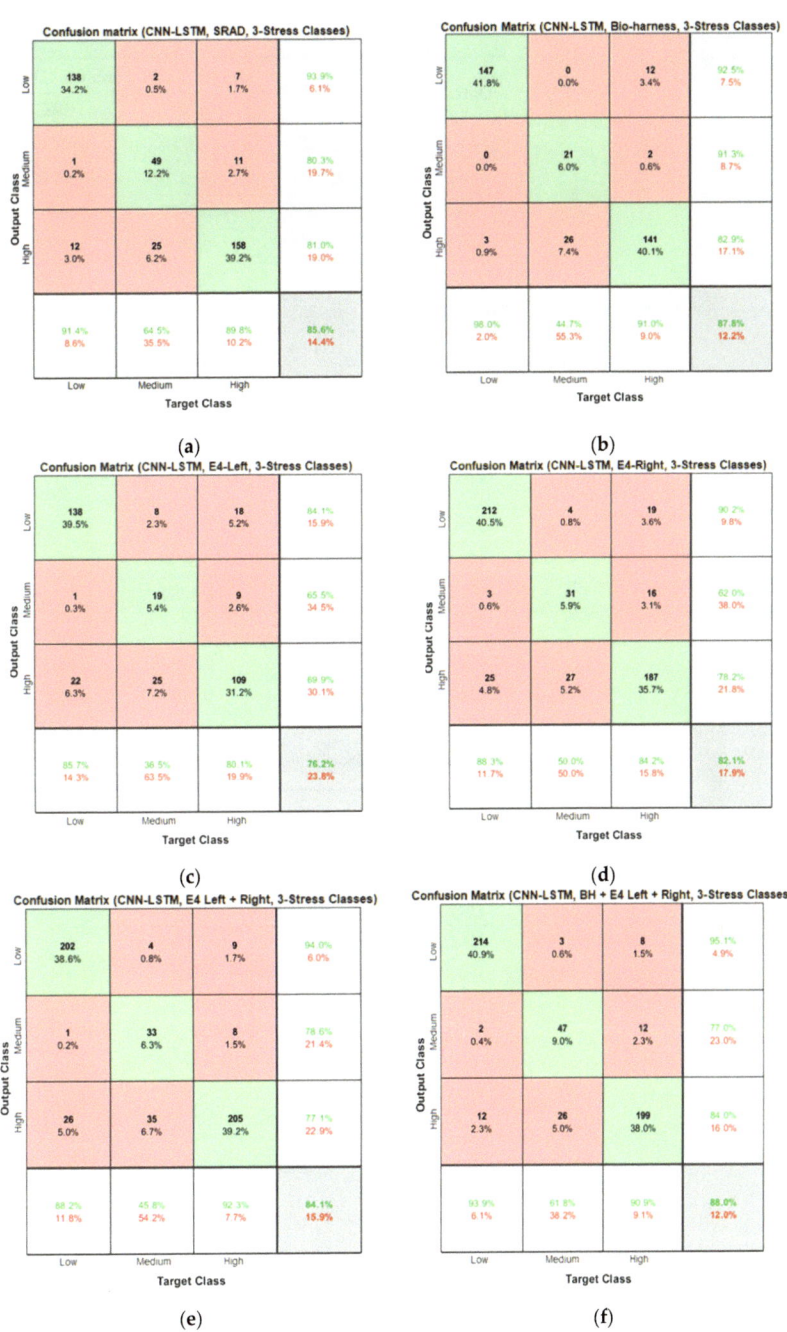

Figure 28. Confusion matrices of the hybrid CNN-LSTM models for the three-stress class based on: (**a**) the SRAD dataset; (**b**) BH dataset; (**c**) E4-L dataset; (**d**) E4-R dataset; (**e**) E4-(L+R) datasets; (**f**) BH+E4-(L+R) datasets.

Table 5. Cross-efficient values of the CNN models for the relaxed state.

Dataset	Performance Measure (Driver's Relaxed State)				
	ACC	RCL	PRC	F1	SPC
SRAD	0.9271	0.8774	0.9118	0.8942	0.9541
BH	0.8909	0.9278	0.8267	0.8743	0.8654
E4-L	0.8653	0.8072	0.9394	0.8683	0.9363
E4-R	0.8825	0.8636	0.8693	0.8664	0.8974
E4-(L+R)	0.9235	0.9776	0.8617	0.916	0.8833
BH+E4-(L+R)	0.9564	0.9772	0.9224	0.949	0.9417
ψ_β	0.9076	0.9051	0.8886	0.8947	0.9130

Table 6. Analysis results of the average $(P_\jmath)$ of the CNN models for the relaxed state.

Dataset	Performance Measure (Driver's Relaxed State)				
	ACC	RCL	PRC	F1	SPC
SRAD	0.0000	0.0306	0.0000	0.0006	0.0000
BH	0.0184	0.0000	0.0696	0.0228	0.0522
E4-L	0.0466	0.1082	0.0000	0.0295	0.0000
E4-R	0.0277	0.0459	0.0217	0.0249	0.0171
E4-(L+R)	0.0000	0.0000	0.0302	0.0000	0.0326
BH+E4-(L+R)	0.0000	0.0000	0.0000	0.0000	0.0000

Table 7. Analysis results of the average $(N_\jmath)$ of the CNN models for the relaxed state.

Dataset	Performance Measure (Driver's Relaxed State)				
	ACC	RCL	PRC	F1	SPC
SRAD	0.0000	0.0000	0.0262	0.0000	0.0450
BH	0.0000	0.0250	0.0000	0.0000	0.0000
E4-L	0.0000	0.0000	0.0572	0.0000	0.0255
E4-R	0.0000	0.0000	0.0000	0.0000	0.0000
E4-(L+R)	0.0175	0.0801	0.0000	0.0238	0.0000
BH+E4-(L+R)	0.0537	0.0796	0.0191	0.0607	0.0314

Table 8. Analysis results of the aggregate $(P_\jmath)$ of the CNN models for the relaxed state.

Weight of Criteria	0.4176	0.2850	0.14533	0.0844	0.0676	
Dataset	Performance Measure (Driver's Relaxed State)					
	ACC	RCL	PRC	F1	SPC	$(SP_\jmath)_\alpha$
SRAD	0.0000	0.0087	0.0000	0.0005	0.0000	0.0088
BH	0.0077	0.0000	0.0100	0.0019	0.0035	0.0233
E4-L	0.0000	0.0000	0.0000	0.0000	0.0000	0.0000
E4-R	0.0116	0.0000	0.0031	0.0027	0.0012	0.0185
E4-(L+R)	0.0000	0.0000	0.0044	0.0000	0.0022	0.0066
BH+E4-(L+R)	0.0000	0.0000	0.0000	0.0000	0.0000	0.0000

Table 9. Analysis results of the aggregate $(N_{\mathcal{I}})$ of the CNN models for the relaxed state.

Weight of Criteria	0.4176	0.2850	0.1453	0.0844	0.0676	
Dataset	Performance Measure (Driver's Relaxed State)					
	ACC	RCL	PRC	F1	SPC	$(SN_{\mathcal{I}})_\alpha$
SRAD	0.0090	0.0000	0.0038	0.0000	0.0030	0.0158
BH	0.0000	0.0071	0.0000	0.0000	0.0000	0.0071
E4-L	0.0000	0.0000	0.0083	0.0000	0.0017	0.0100
E4-R	0.0000	0.0000	0.0000	0.0000	0.0000	0.0000
E4-(L+R)	0.0073	0.0228	0.0000	0.0020	0.0000	0.0321
BH+E4-(L+R)	0.0224	0.0227	0.0055	0.0051	0.0021	0.0579

Table 10. Analysis results of the CNN models for the relaxed state.

Dataset	$(SP_{\mathcal{I}})_\alpha$	$(SN_{\mathcal{I}})_\alpha$	$N(SP_{\mathcal{I}})_\alpha$	$N(SN_{\mathcal{I}})_\alpha$	λ_α	Ranks
SRAD	0.0088	0.0158	0.3774	0.7270	0.5522	4
BH	0.0233	0.0071	1.0000	0.8768	0.9384	6
E4-L	0.0000	0.0100	0.0000	0.8267	0.4133	2
E4-R	0.0000	0.0000	0.0000	1.0000	0.5000	3
E4-(L+R)	0.0185	0.0321	0.7968	0.4452	0.6210	5
BH+E4-(L+R)	0.0066	0.0579	0.2835	0.0000	0.1417	1

Table 11. Analysis results of the CNN models for the stressed state.

Dataset	$(SP_{\mathcal{I}})_\alpha$	$(SN_{\mathcal{I}})_\alpha$	$N(SP_{\mathcal{I}})_\alpha$	$N(SN_{\mathcal{I}})_\alpha$	λ_α	Ranks
SRAD	0.0021	0.0263	0.0874	0.4791	0.2832	2
BH	0.0237	0.0052	1.0000	0.8960	0.9480	6
E4-L	0.0000	0.0073	0.0000	0.8562	0.4280	3
E4-R	0.0000	0.0000	0.0000	1.0000	0.5000	4
E4-(L+R)	0.0213	0.0232	0.8985	0.5401	0.7193	5
BH+E4-(L+R)	0.0093	0.0505	0.3913	0.0000	0.1956	1

4.3.2. Rank Estimation of the CNN-LSTM Models for Two Levels of Stress

For the rank estimation of the SRAD, BH, E4-L, E4-R, E4-(L+R), and BH+E4-(L+R)-based hybrid CNN-LSTM models, the same eight-step procedure is utilized for the relaxed state and stressed state, and the resulting ranks are given in Tables 12 and 13, respectively. Table 12 shows that the proposed BH+E4-(L+R), BH, E4-L, E4-R, E4-(L+R), and SRAD-based CNN-LSTM models achieved first, second, third, third, fourth, and fifth positions for the relaxed state. Similarly, Table 13 shows that the proposed fused BH+E4-(L+R), BH, E4-L, E4-R, SRAD, and E4-(L+R)-based CNN-LSTM models achieved first, second, third, third, fourth, and fifth positions for the stressed state.

4.3.3. Rank Estimation of the CNN Models for Three Levels of Stress

The eight-step fuzzy EDAS procedure is also utilized for the three levels of stress (low, medium, and high) and the resulting ranks of the SRAD, BH, E4-L, E4-R, E4-(L+R), and BH+E4-(L+R)-based CNN models are shown in Tables 14–16, respectively. For the low-stress level, BH+E4-(L+R), SRAD, E4-(L+R), E4-L, E4-R, and BH-based CNN models achieved first, second, third, fourth, fifth, and fifth positions, as shown in Table 14. For the medium-stress level, E4-R, E4-(L+R), BH+E4-(L+R), E4-L, SRAD and BH-based CNN models achieved first, second, third, fourth, fifth, and fifth positions, as shown in Table 15. Likewise, Table 16 shows that the proposed BH+E4-(L+R), SRAD, E4-L, E4-R, BH, and E4-(L+R)-based CNN models achieved first, second, third, fourth, fifth, and fifth positions for the high-stress level.

Table 12. Analysis results of the CNN-LSTM models for the relaxed state.

Dataset	$(SP_J)_\alpha$	$(SN_J)_\alpha$	$N(SP_J)_\alpha$	$N(SN_J)_\alpha$	λ_α	Ranks
SRAD	0.0214	0.0000	1.0000	1.0000	1.0000	5
BH	0.0000	0.0311	0.0000	0.2328	0.1164	2
E4-L	0.0000	0.0000	0.0000	1.0000	0.5000	3
E4-R	0.0000	0.0000	0.0000	1.0000	0.5000	3
E4-(L+R)	0.0212	0.0225	0.9887	0.4452	0.7169	4
BH+E4-(L+R)	0.0000	0.0405	0.0000	0.0000	0.0000	1

Table 13. Analysis results of the CNN-LSTM models for the stressed state.

Dataset	$(SP_J)_\alpha$	$(SN_J)_\alpha$	$N(SP_J)_\alpha$	$N(SN_J)_\alpha$	λ_α	Ranks
SRAD	0.0093	0.0000	0.5875	1.0000	0.7938	4
BH	0.0000	0.0247	0.0000	0.3496	0.1748	2
E4-L	0.0000	0.0000	0.0000	1.0000	0.5000	3
E4-R	0.0000	0.0000	0.0000	1.0000	0.5000	3
E4-(L+R)	0.0158	0.0145	1.0000	0.6195	0.8097	5
BH+E4-(L+R)	0.0000	0.0380	0.0000	0.0000	0.0000	1

Table 14. Analysis results of the CNN models for the low-stress level.

Dataset	$(SP_J)_\alpha$	$(SN_J)_\alpha$	$N(SP_J)_\alpha$	$N(SN_J)_\alpha$	λ_α	Ranks
SRAD	0.0075	0.0190	0.1696	0.5996	0.3846	2
BH	0.0441	0.0000	1.0000	1.0000	1.0000	6
E4-L	0.0000	0.0003	0.0000	0.9937	0.4968	4
E4-R	0.0000	0.0000	0.0000	1.0000	0.5000	5
E4-(L+R)	0.0104	0.0214	0.2357	0.5504	0.3931	3
BH+E4-(L+R)	0.0000	0.0476	0.0000	0.0000	0.0000	1

Table 15. Analysis results of the CNN models for the medium-stress level.

Dataset	$(SP_J)_\alpha$	$(SN_J)_\alpha$	$N(SP_J)_\alpha$	$N(SN_J)_\alpha$	λ_α	Ranks
SRAD	0.0348	0.1006	1.0000	0.0000	0.5000	5
BH	0.0322	0.0094	0.9250	0.9061	0.9155	6
E4-L	0.0000	0.0140	0.0000	0.8240	0.4120	4
E4-R	0.0000	0.0761	0.0000	0.2438	0.1219	1
E4-(L+R)	0.0103	0.0793	0.2956	0.2117	0.2537	2
BH+E4-(L+R)	0.0022	0.0392	0.0638	0.6101	0.3370	3

Table 16. Analysis results of the CNN models for the high-stress level.

Dataset	$(SP_\Im)_\alpha$	$(SN_\Im)_\alpha$	$N(SP_\Im)_\alpha$	$N(SN_\Im)_\alpha$	λ_α	Ranks
SRAD	0.0224	0.0371	0.3835	0.4636	0.4236	2
BH	0.0194	0.0009	0.3326	0.9868	0.6597	5
E4-L	0.0000	0.0071	0.0000	0.8974	0.4487	3
E4-R	0.0000	0.0054	0.0000	0.9212	0.4606	4
E4-(L+R)	0.0584	0.0439	1.0000	0.3648	0.6824	6
BH+E4-(L+R)	0.0000	0.0691	0.0000	0.0000	0.0000	1

4.3.4. Rank Estimation of the CNN-LSTM Models for Three Levels of Stress

For the rank estimation of the SRAD, BH, E4-L, E4-R, E4-(L+R), and BH+E4-(L+R)-based hybrid CNN-LSTM models, the same eight-step procedure is utilized for low-stress, medium-stress, and high-stress, and the resulting ranks are given in Tables 17–19, respectively. Table 17 shows that the proposed BH+F4-(L+R), BH, E4-L, E4-R, SRAD, and E4-(L+R)-based CNN-LSTM models achieved first, second, third, third, fourth, and fifth positions for the low-stress level. Moreover, Table 18 shows that the proposed, SRAD, E4-R, E4-L, BH, and BH+E4-(L+R)-based CNN-LSTM models achieved first, second, third, third, fourth, and fifth positions for the medium-stress level. For the high-stress level, BH, BH+E4-(L+R), SRAD, E4-L, E4-R, and E4-(L+R)-based CNN models achieved first, second, third, third, fourth, and fifth positions, as shown in Table 19.

Table 17. Analysis results of the CNN-LSTM models for the low-stress level.

Dataset	$(SP_\Im)_\alpha$	$(SN_\Im)_\alpha$	$N(SP_\Im)_\alpha$	$N(SN_\Im)_\alpha$	λ_α	Ranks
SRAD	0.0000	0.0204	0.0000	0.4467	0.2233	4
BH	0.0000	0.0368	0.0000	0.0000	0.0000	2
E4-L	0.0000	0.0000	0.0000	1.0000	0.5000	3
E4-R	0.0000	0.0000	0.0000	1.0000	0.5000	3
E4-(L+R)	0.0173	0.0072	1.0000	0.8034	0.9017	5
BH+E4-(L+R)	0.0058	0.0332	0.3365	0.0981	0.2173	1

Table 18. Analysis results of the CNN-LSTM models for the medium-stress level.

Dataset	$(SP_\Im)_\alpha$	$(SN_\Im)_\alpha$	$N(SP_\Im)_\alpha$	$N(SN_\Im)_\alpha$	λ_α	Ranks
SRAD	0.0009	0.0732	0.0559	0.0000	0.0280	1
BH	0.0170	0.0653	1.0000	0.1072	0.5536	4
E4-L	0.0000	0.0000	0.0000	1.0000	0.5000	3
E4-R	0.0000	0.0009	0.0000	0.9870	0.4935	2
E4-(L+R)	0.0085	0.0118	0.4974	0.8383	0.6678	6
BH+E4-(L+R)	0.0168	0.0561	0.9891	0.2327	0.6109	5

Table 19. Analysis results of the CNN-LSTM models for the high-stress level.

Dataset	$(SP_\mathfrak{I})_\alpha$	$(SN_\mathfrak{I})_\alpha$	$N(SP_\mathfrak{I})_\alpha$	$N(SN_\mathfrak{I})_\alpha$	λ_α	Ranks
SRAD	0.0000	0.0196	0.0000	0.5913	0.2956	3
BH	0.0000	0.0379	0.0000	0.2113	0.1057	1
E4-L	0.0000	0.0000	0.0000	1.0000	0.5000	4
E4-R	0.0000	0.0000	0.0000	1.0000	0.5000	4
E4-(L+R)	0.0187	0.0102	1.0000	0.7884	0.8942	5
BH+E4-(L+R)	0.0064	0.0480	0.3450	0.0000	0.1725	2

4.4. Comparison of the Proposed 1D CNN and 1D CNN-LSTM Models

Comparisons of the proposed 1D CNN and 1D CNN-LSTM models for two and three levels of stress based on training time, accuracy, and fuzzy EDAS ranking are shown in Tables 20–23. Execution environments for all proposed models are based on a single CPU. The fuzzy EDAS approach performs a comprehensive rank estimation of the proposed models in terms of accuracy, recall, precision, F-score, and specificity. The model with the lowest appraisal score (λ_α) has the highest performance among the candidate models.

A comparison shows that there is a tradeoff between the training time and performance of various models, with the exception of the SRAD dataset. For example, Table 20 shows that the proposed BH+E4-(L+R)-based 1D CNN model achieved the best EDAS ranks at the cost of a maximum training time of 72 min and 42 s. On the other hand, the BH-based 1D CNN model has the worst EDAS rank with the lowest training time of 3 min and 15 s. The performance of the SRAD-based model is somehow in between with the highest computational cost of 277 min and 29 s. Similarly, Table 21 reveals that the proposed BH+E4-(L+R)-based 1D CNN-LSTM model secured the top EDAS ranks at the cost of a maximum training time of 72 min and 42 s. Moreover, the BH-based 1D CNN model has the worst EDAS rank with the lowest training time of 3 min and 15 s. However, the SRAD-based model achieved average performance, with a maximum computational cost of 167 min and 56 s.

Table 20. Comparison of the proposed CNN models for the two-stress class.

Dataset	Execution Environment	Training Time 1D CNN		Performance				
				Accuracy (%)			Fuzzy EDAS Rank	
		Feature Learning	Classification	Relaxed State	Stressed State	Overall	Relaxed State	Stressed State
SRAD	Single CPU	277 min 29 s		92.71	92.71	92.72	4	2
E4-L		35 min, 18 s	13 s	86.53	86.53	86.53	2	3
E4-R		35 min, 26 s	13 s	88.25	88.25	88.25	3	4
E4-(L+R)		70 min, 26 s	12 s	92.35	92.35	92.35	5	5
BH		1 min, 46 s	1 min, 29 s	89.09	89.09	89.09	6	6
BH+E4-(L+R)		72 min, 30 s	12 s	95.64	9564	95.64	1	1

Table 21. Comparison of the proposed CNN-LSTM models for the two-stress class.

Dataset	Execution Environment	Training Time 1D CNN-LSTM		Performance					
				Accuracy (%)			Fuzzy EDAS Rank		
		Feature Learning	Classification	Relaxed State	Stressed State	Overall	Relaxed State	Stressed State	
SRAD	Single CPU	167 min 33 s	23 s	91.80	91.80	91.81	5	4	
E4-L		35 min 18 s	34 s	88.82	88.82	88.83	3	3	
E4-R		35 min 26 s	31 s	90.65	90.65	90.65	3	3	
E4-(L+R)		70 min 26 s	32 s	94.65	94.65	94.65	4	5	
BH		1 min 46 s	33 s	95.45	95.45	95.45	2	2	
BH+E4-(L+R)		72 min 30 s	21 s	96.59	96.59	96.59	1	1	

Table 22. Comparison of the proposed CNN models for the three-stress class.

Dataset	Execution Environment	Training Time 1D CNN		Performance						
				Accuracy (%)				Fuzzy EDAS Rank		
		Feature Learning	Classification	Low-stress State	Medium-Stress State	High-Stress State	Overall	Low-Stress State	Medium-Stress State	High-Stress State
SRAD	Single CPU	279 min, 6 s		93.38	83.77	83.77	79.47	2	5	2
E4-L		35 min, 20 s	45 s	89.11	85.67	78.22	76.50	4	4	3
E4-R		35 min, 19 s	13 s	89.97	84.81	78.80	76.79	5	1	4
E4-(L+R)		70 min, 39 s	12 s	93.12	89.30	85.47	83.94	3	2	6
BH		1 min, 28 s	2 min, 17 s	86.59	88.86	82.27	78.86	6	6	5
BH+E4-(L+R)		72 min, 7 s	22 s	95.41	89.29	86.62	85.66	1	3	1

Table 23. Comparison of the proposed CNN-LSTM models for the three-stress class.

Dataset	Execution Environment	Training Time 1D CNN-LSTM		Performance						
				Accuracy (%)				Fuzzy EDAS Rank		
		Feature Learning	Classification	Low-Stress State	Medium-Stress State	High-Stress State	Overall	Low-Stress State	Medium-Stress State	High-Stress State
SRAD	Single CPU	170 min, 44 s	47 s	94.54	90.32	86.35	85.61	4	1	1
E4-L		35 min, 20 s	3 min, 4 s	85.96	87.68	78.80	76.22	3	3	3
E4-R		35 min, 19 s	33 s	90.27	90.46	83.40	82.06	3	2	2
E4-(L+R)		70 min, 39 s	30 s	92.35	90.82	85.09	84.13	5	6	6
BH		1 min, 28 s	34 s	95.74	92.04	87.78	87.78	2	4	4
BH+E4-(L+R)		72 min, 7 s	31 s	95.22	91.78	88.91	87.95	1	5	5

Table 22 shows the comparison of the 1D CNN model for the three-stress class. As usual, the proposed BH+E4-(L+R) secured the best EDAS ranks at a maximum cost of 72 min and 51 s. On the other hand, the BH-based model has the worst EDAS rank for a minimum computational cost of 3 min and 45 s. However, the SRAD-based model has average performance with the highest training time of 279 min and 6 s. Similarly, Table 23 reveals that the proposed SRAD-based 1D CNN-LSTM model secured the top EDAS rank at the cost of a maximum training time of 171 min and 31 s. The BH-based 1D CNN-LSTM model achieved an average EDAS rank with the lowest training time of 2 min and 2 s. However, the E4-(L+R)-based model has the worst EDAS rank despite the high training time of 71 min and 9 s. The proposed models have a high training time due to the usage of a single CPU. Utilizing GPUs may reduce the training time of the proposed algorithms.

5. Discussion

The proposed CNN and hybrid CNN-LSTM models are analyzed using the SRAD and AffectiveROAD datasets in the previous section. AffectiveROAD is based on the BH, Empatica E4-L, Empatica E4-R, and E4-(L+R) datasets. Both BH and Empatica E4 datasets are individually and combinedly used to train the proposed models for the two-stress and three-stress classes. It is evident from the previous tables that the models trained on multimodal data (AffectiveROAD) achieved the maximum performance compared to SRAD data. This shows the importance of physiological, physical, and contextual information in the domain of stress recognition. Moreover, it is also clear that the hybrid 1D CNN-LSTM models achieved better performance than the 1D CNN models. The fuzzy EDAS procedure also shows that the proposed CNN and hybrid CNN-LSTM models achieved the first rank based on the fused AffectiveROAD BH+E4-(L+R) datasets. The achieved performance of the proposed real-world driver stress recognition models is greatly enhanced compared to the existing schemes. A comparison of the proposed driver stress recognition models with the existing schemes is shown in Table 24. It is clear from the table that the proposed models achieved the highest performance for both two and three levels of stress compared to the existing schemes. Rastgoo et al. [11] achieved a higher performance than the proposed models for the three-stress class but their study was based on simulated driving conditions, while the proposed models were based on real-world driving conditions.

Table 24. Comparison of the proposed stress recognition models with existing schemes.

Article / Year	Signal(s) / Modalities	Environment	No. of Subjects	Data I/P Mechanism	Deep Learning Approach	Stress Levels	ACC (%)	RCL	PRC	F1	SPC
Proposed Models	HR, BR, Posture, Activity, TEMP, IBI, GSR, ACCL	Real-World Driving	10	1D Signal	CNN-LSTM	2	96.6	96.4	96.8	96.6	96.4
						3	88	85.4	82.2	83.5	94
[50]/2021	HR, GSR		9	Continues RPs	CNN	2	95.7	95.7	95.9	95.7	-
[46]/2019	Facial Images		123	Images	Pre-Trained MTCNN	2	97.3	-	-	-	-
[11]/2019	ECG, VDD, EP	Simulated Driving	27	1D Signal	CNN-LSTM	3	92.8	94.1	95	-	97.4
[49]/2016	EEG		37	1D Signal	CCNN	2	86.1	-	-	-	-
[53]/2019	RESP and ECG		18	1D Signal	CNN-LSTM	3	83.9	-	-	81.1	-
[56]/2021	EEG	Cognitive Tasks (Lab/Workplace)	32	Spectrogram	Pre-Trained AlexNet	2	84.8	85.2	-	-	84.3
[55]/2019	ECG		20		CNN	2	82.7	-	-	-	-
[54]/2018	ECG		13	1D Signal	1D CNN	2	80	-	-	-	-
[52]/2017	Thermographic Patterns of Breath		8	Spectrogram	CNN	2	84.6	-	-	-	-

6. Conclusions

This paper concludes that in addition to physiological signals, other information regarding the driver, vehicle, and ambiance has an important role in designing reliable and accurate driver stress recognition systems. It is also evident that the hybrid CNN-LSTM models have better performance than the CNN models. Moreover, the fusion of the AffectiveROAD datasets (BH, E4-L, and E4-R) achieved the best performance with the least computational cost compared to the SRAD dataset. This is due to several factors including the utilization of multimodal information (physiological signals and information regarding the driver, vehicle, and environment), quality of the hardware and software tools used for capturing the data, and accurate sampling of the signals. Thus, hybrid deep learning models and multimodal data have a key role in designing an accurate and reliable stress recognition model for real-world driving conditions.

The fusion models based on 1D CNN and hybrid 1D CNN-LSTM produced promising results, but these models may be further improved by utilizing more complex CNN and LSTM architectures. Moreover, a joint CNN-LSTM architecture may be used to further improve stress level recognition. The current study is based on the driver's stress level, thus in the future, these models may be utilized for drowsiness, cognitive workload, activity, fatigue, and feeling recognition. The AffectiveROAD and PhysioNet SRAD datasets used in this study are based on real-world driving conditions. Such datasets are usually contaminated by different noises and artifacts. Enhanced pre-processing techniques can further improve the performance of the models. Future work may also include stress recognition by training the proposed models using physiological signals acquired using non-contact sensors and smart watches.

Author Contributions: Methodology, M.A. (Muhammad Amin); Software, K.U.; Investigation, M.A. (Muhammad Asif); Resources, K.U. and A.M.; Data curation, M.A. (Muhammad Amin) and M.A.K.; Writing—original draft, M.A. (Muhammad Amin); Writing—review & editing, K.U. and M.A. (Muhammad Asif); Visualization, A.M.; Supervision, K.U. and M.A.K.; Project administration, H.S. and A.M.; Funding acquisition, H.S. All authors have read and agreed to the published version of the manuscript.

Funding: The authors extend their appreciation to the Deanship of Scientific Research at King Khalid University KSA for funding this work through Small Group: RGP.1/368/43.

Institutional Review Board Statement: Not applicable.

Informed Consent Statement: Not applicable.

Data Availability Statement: The data will be available on request.

Conflicts of Interest: The authors declare no conflict of interest.

References

1. Evans, G.W.; Carrère, S. Traffic Congestion, Perceived Control, and Psychophysiological Stress among Urban Bus Drivers. *J. Appl. Psychol.* **1991**, *76*, 658–663. [CrossRef]
2. Hanzlíková, I. Professional drivers: The sources of occupational stress. In Proceedings of the Young Researchers Seminar, The Hague, The Netherlands, 2005.
3. de Naurois, C.J.; Bourdin, C.; Stratulat, A.; Diaz, E.; Vercher, J.L. Detection and prediction of driver drowsiness using artificial neural network models. *Accid. Anal. Prev.* **2019**, *126*, 95–104. [CrossRef]
4. Chen, L.L.; Zhao, Y.; Ye, P.F.; Zhang, J.; Zou, J.Z. Detecting driving stress in physiological signals based on multimodal feature analysis and kernel classifiers. *Expert Syst. Appl.* **2017**, *85*, 279–291. [CrossRef]
5. Manseer, M.; Riener, A. Evaluation of driver stress while transiting road tunnels. In Proceedings of the 6th International Conference on Automotive User Interfaces and Interactive Vehicular Applications, Seattle, WA, USA, 17–19 September 2014; Association for Computing Machinery (ACM): New York, NY, USA, 2014; pp. 1–6.
6. Benlagha, N.; Charfeddine, L. Risk factors of road accident severity and the development of a new system for prevention: New insights from China. *Accid. Anal. Prev.* **2020**, *136*, 105411. [CrossRef] [PubMed]
7. American Psychological Association. *Stress in America: The State of our Nation. Stress in America Survey*; American Psychological Association: Washington, DC, USA, 2017.
8. Khowaja, S.A.; Prabono, A.G.; Setiawan, F.; Yahya, B.N.; Lee, S.L. Toward soft real-time stress detection using wrist-worn devices for human workspaces. *Soft Comput.* **2021**, *25*, 2793–2820. [CrossRef]
9. Shinar, D.; Compton, R. Aggressive driving: An observational study of driver, vehicle, and situational variables. *Accid. Anal. Prev.* **2004**, *36*, 429–437. [CrossRef]

10. Singh, S. Critical reasons for crashes investigated in the National Motor Vehicle Crash Causation Survey. *Natl. Highw. Traffic Saf. Adm.* **2015**, 1–2.
11. Rastgoo, M.N.; Nakisa, B.; Maire, F.; Rakotonirainy, A.; Chandran, V. Automatic driver stress level classification using multimodal deep learning. *Expert Syst. Appl.* **2019**, *138*, 112793. [CrossRef]
12. Nakisa, B.; Rastgoo, M.N.; Tjondronegoro, D.; Chandran, V. Evolutionary computation algorithms for feature selection of EEG-based emotion recognition using mobile sensors. *Expert Syst. Appl.* **2018**, *93*, 143–155. [CrossRef]
13. Pourbabaee, B.; Roshtkhari, M.J.; Khorasani, K. Deep Convolutional Neural Networks and Learning ECG Features for Screening Paroxysmal Atrial Fibrillation Patients. *IEEE Trans. Syst. Man Cybern. Syst.* **2018**, *48*, 2095–2104. [CrossRef]
14. Liu, Y.; Chen, X.; Peng, H.; Wang, Z. Multi-focus image fusion with a deep convolutional neural network. *Inf. Fusion* **2017**, *36*, 191–207. [CrossRef]
15. Zheng, Y.; Liu, Q.; Chen, E.; Ge, Y.; Zhao, J.L. Exploiting multi-channels deep convolutional neural networks for multivariate time series classification. *Front. Comput. Sci.* **2016**, *10*, 96–112. [CrossRef]
16. Zheng, Y.; Liu, Q.; Chen, E.; Ge, Y.; Zhao, J.L. Time series classification using multi-channels deep convolutional neural networks. In Proceedings of the Lecture Notes in Computer Science (Including Subseries Lecture Notes in Artificial Intelligence and Lecture Notes in Bioinformatics), Macau, China, 16–18 June 2014; Springer: Berlin/Heidelberg, Germany, 2014; Volume 8485, pp. 298–310.
17. Kanjo, E.; Younis, E.M.G.; Ang, C.S. Deep learning analysis of mobile physiological, environmental and location sensor data for emotion detection. *Inf. Fusion* **2019**, *49*, 46–56. [CrossRef]
18. Ngiam, J.; Khosla, A.; Kim, M.; Nam, J.; Lee, H.; Ng, A.Y. Multimodal deep learning. In Proceedings of the 28th International Conference on Machine Learning, ICML 2011, Bellevue, WA, USA, 28 June–2 July 2011; pp. 689–696.
19. Deng, L.; Yu, D. Deep learning: Methods and applications. *Found. Trends Signal Process.* **2013**, *7*, 197–387. [CrossRef]
20. Dalmeida, K.M.; Masala, G.L. Hrv features as viable physiological markers for stress detection using wearable devices. *Sensors* **2021**, *21*, 2873. [CrossRef] [PubMed]
21. Vargas-Lopez, O.; Perez-Ramirez, C.A.; Valtierra-Rodriguez, M.; Yanez-Borjas, J.J.; Amezquita-Sanchez, J.P. An explainable machine learning approach based on statistical indexes and svm for stress detection in automobile drivers using electromyographic signals. *Sensors* **2021**, *21*, 3155. [CrossRef]
22. Lopez-Martinez, D.; El-Haouij, N.; Picard, R. Detection of Real-World Driving-Induced Affective State Using Physiological Signals and Multi-View Multi-Task Machine Learning. In Proceedings of the 2019 8th International Conference on Affective Computing and Intelligent Interaction Workshops and Demos, ACIIW 2019, Cambridge, UK, 3–6 September 2019; pp. 356–361.
23. El Haouij, N.; Poggi, J.M.; Ghozi, R.; Sevestre-Ghalila, S.; Jaïdane, M. Random forest-based approach for physiological functional variable selection for driver's stress level classification. *Stat. Methods Appl.* **2019**, *28*, 157–185. [CrossRef]
24. Ghaderi, A.; Frounchi, J.; Farnam, A. Machine learning-based signal processing using physiological signals for stress detection. In Proceedings of the 2015 22nd Iranian Conference on Biomedical Engineering, ICBME 2015, Tehran, Iran, 25–27 November 2016; pp. 93–98.
25. Zhang, L.; Tamminedi, T.; Ganguli, A.; Yosiphon, G.; Yadegar, J. Hierarchical multiple sensor fusion using structurally learned Bayesian network. In Proceedings of the Proceedings—Wireless Health 2010, WH'10, San Diego, CA, USA, 5–7 October 2010; pp. 174–183.
26. Healey, J.A.; Picard, R.W. Detecting stress during real-world driving tasks using physiological sensors. *IEEE Trans. Intell. Transp. Syst.* **2005**, *6*, 156–166. [CrossRef]
27. PhysioNet. *Stress Recognition in Automobile Drivers, Version: 1.0.0*; PhysioNet (MIT Laboratory for Computational Physiology US): Cambridge, MA, USA, 2008. [CrossRef]
28. Rigas, G.; Goletsis, Y.; Bougia, P.; Fotiadis, D.I. Towards driver's state recognition on real driving conditions. *Int. J. Veh. Technol.* **2011**, *2011*, 617210. [CrossRef]
29. Zontone, P.; Affanni, A.; Bernardini, R.; Piras, A.; Rinaldo, R.; Formaggia, F.; Minen, D.; Minen, M.; Savorgnan, C. Car Driver's Sympathetic Reaction Detection through Electrodermal Activity and Electrocardiogram Measurements. *IEEE Trans. Biomed. Eng.* **2020**, *67*, 3413–3424. [CrossRef]
30. Bianco, S.; Napoletano, P.; Schettini, R. Multimodal car driver stress recognition. In Proceedings of the PervasiveHealth: Pervasive Computing Technologies for Healthcare, Trento, Italy, 20–23 May 2019; pp. 302–307.
31. Lee, D.S.; Chong, T.W.; Lee, B.G. Stress Events Detection of Driver by Wearable Glove System. *IEEE Sens. J.* **2017**, *17*, 194–204. [CrossRef]
32. Lanatà, A.; Valenza, G.; Greco, A.; Gentili, C.; Bartolozzi, R.; Bucchi, F.; Frendo, F.; Scilingo, E.P. How the Autonomic nervous system and driving style change with incremental stressing conditions during simulated driving. *IEEE Trans. Intell. Transp. Syst.* **2015**, *16*, 1505–1517. [CrossRef]
33. Gao, H.; Yuce, A.; Thiran, J.P. Detecting emotional stress from facial expressions for driving safety. In Proceedings of the 2014 IEEE International Conference on Image Processing, ICIP 2014, Paris, France, 27–30 October 2014; pp. 5961–5965.
34. Šalkevicius, J.; Damaševičius, R.; Maskeliunas, R.; Laukienė, I. Anxiety level recognition for virtual reality therapy system using physiological signals. *Electronics* **2019**, *8*, 1039. [CrossRef]
35. Rodríguez-Arce, J.; Lara-Flores, L.; Portillo-Rodríguez, O.; Martínez-Méndez, R. Towards an anxiety and stress recognition system for academic environments based on physiological features. *Comput. Methods Programs Biomed.* **2020**, *190*, 105408. [CrossRef]

36. Can, Y.S.; Chalabianloo, N.; Ekiz, D.; Ersoy, C. Continuous stress detection using wearable sensors in real life: Algorithmic programming contest case study. *Sensors* **2019**, *19*, 1849. [CrossRef]
37. Al abdi, R.M.; Alhitary, A.E.; Abdul Hay, E.W.; Al-bashir, A.K. Objective detection of chronic stress using physiological parameters. *Med. Biol. Eng. Comput.* **2018**, *56*, 2273–2286. [CrossRef] [PubMed]
38. Betti, S.; Lova, R.M.; Rovini, E.; Acerbi, G.; Santarelli, L.; Cabiati, M.; Del Ry, S.; Cavallo, F. Evaluation of an integrated system of wearable physiological sensors for stress monitoring in working environments by using biological markers. *IEEE Trans. Biomed. Eng.* **2018**, *65*, 1748–1758. [CrossRef] [PubMed]
39. Sriramprakash, S.; Prasanna, V.D.; Murthy, O.V.R. Stress Detection in Working People. In Proceedings of the Procedia Computer Science, Cochin, India, 22–24 August 2017; Volume 115, pp. 359–366.
40. de Vries, G.J.J.; Pauws, S.C.; Biehl, M. Insightful stress detection from physiology modalities using Learning Vector Quantization. *Neurocomputing* **2015**, *151*, 873–882. [CrossRef]
41. Sun, F.T.; Kuo, C.; Cheng, H.T.; Buthpitiya, S.; Collins, P.; Griss, M. Activity-aware mental stress detection using physiological sensors. In Proceedings of the Lecture Notes of the Institute for Computer Sciences, Social-Informatics and Telecommunications Engineering, LNICST, Santa Clara, CA, USA, 25–28 October 2012; Volume 76, pp. 282–301.
42. Anceschi, E.; Bonifazi, G.; De Donato, M.C.; Corradini, E.; Ursino, D.; Virgili, L. Savemenow.ai: A machine learning based wearable device for fall detection in a workplace. *Stud. Comput. Intell.* **2021**, *911*, 493–514. [CrossRef]
43. Bonifazi, G.; Corradini, E.; Ursino, D.; Virgili, L. Defining user spectra to classify Ethereum users based on their behavior. *J. Big Data* **2022**, *9*, 37. [CrossRef]
44. Zalabarria, U.; Irigoyen, E.; Martinez, R.; Larrea, M.; Salazar-Ramirez, A. A Low-Cost, Portable Solution for Stress and Relaxation Estimation Based on a Real-Time Fuzzy Algorithm. *IEEE Access* **2020**, *8*, 74118–74128. [CrossRef]
45. Lecun, Y.; Bengio, Y.; Hinton, G. Deep learning. *Nature* **2015**, *521*, 436–444. [CrossRef] [PubMed]
46. Zhang, J.; Mei, X.; Liu, H.; Yuan, S.; Qian, T. Detecting negative emotional stress based on facial expression in real time. In Proceedings of the 2019 IEEE 4th International Conference on Signal and Image Processing, ICSIP 2019, Wuxi, China, 19–21 July 2019; pp. 430–434.
47. Lim, S.; Yang, J.H. Driver state estimation by convolutional neural network using multimodal sensor data. *Electron. Lett.* **2016**, *52*, 1495–1497. [CrossRef]
48. Yan, S.; Teng, Y.; Smith, J.S.; Zhang, B. Driver behavior recognition based on deep convolutional neural networks. In Proceedings of the 2016 12th International Conference on Natural Computation, Fuzzy Systems and Knowledge Discovery, ICNC-FSKD 2016, Changsha, China, 13–15 August 2016; pp. 636–641.
49. Hajinoroozi, M.; Mao, Z.; Jung, T.P.; Lin, C.T.; Huang, Y. EEG-based prediction of driver's cognitive performance by deep convolutional neural network. *Signal Process. Image Commun.* **2016**, *47*, 549–555. [CrossRef]
50. Lee, J.; Lee, H.; Shin, M. Driving stress detection using multimodal convolutional neural networks with nonlinear representation of short-term physiological signals. *Sensors* **2021**, *21*, 2381. [CrossRef] [PubMed]
51. Masood, K.; Alghamdi, M.A. Modeling Mental Stress Using a Deep Learning Framework. *IEEE Access* **2019**, *7*, 68446–68454. [CrossRef]
52. Cho, Y.; Bianchi-Berthouze, N.; Julier, S.J. DeepBreath: Deep learning of breathing patterns for automatic stress recognition using low-cost thermal imaging in unconstrained settings. In Proceedings of the 2017 7th International Conference on Affective Computing and Intelligent Interaction, ACII 2017, San Antonio, TX, USA, 23–26 October 2017; Volume 2018, pp. 456–463.
53. Seo, W.; Kim, N.; Kim, S.; Lee, C.; Park, S.M. Deep ECG-respiration network (DeepER net) for recognizing mental stress. *Sensors* **2019**, *19*, 3021. [CrossRef]
54. Hwang, B.; You, J.; Vaessen, T.; Myin-Germeys, I.; Park, C.; Zhang, B.T. Deep ECGNet: An optimal deep learning framework for monitoring mental stress using ultra short-term ECG signals. *Telemed. E-Health* **2018**, *24*, 753–772. [CrossRef]
55. He, J.; Li, K.; Liao, X.; Zhang, P.; Jiang, N. Real-Time Detection of Acute Cognitive Stress Using a Convolutional Neural Network from Electrocardiographic Signal. *IEEE Access* **2019**, *7*, 42710–42717. [CrossRef]
56. Martínez-Rodrigo, A.; García-Martínez, B.; Huerta, Á.; Alcaraz, R. Detection of negative stress through spectral features of electroencephalographic recordings and a convolutional neural network. *Sensors* **2021**, *21*, 3050. [CrossRef]
57. Healey, J.A.; Picard, R.W. Stress Recognition in Automobile Drivers. *IEEE Trans. Intell. Transp. Syst.* **2005**.
58. Clifford, G.D.; Azuaje, F.; Mcsharry, P. ECG statistics, noise, artifacts, and missing data. *Adv. Methods Tools ECG Data Anal.* **2006**, *6*, 18.
59. Sörnmo, L.; Laguna, P. *Bioelectrical Signal Processing in Cardiac and Neurological Applications*; Academic Press: Cambridge, MA, USA, 2005; ISBN 9780124375529.
60. Rahman, J.S.; Gedeon, T.; Caldwell, S.; Jones, R.; Jin, Z. Towards Effective Music Therapy for Mental Health Care Using Machine Learning Tools: Human Affective Reasoning and Music Genres. *J. Artif. Intell. Soft Comput. Res.* **2021**, *11*, 5–20. [CrossRef]
61. Sánchez-Reolid, R.; López de la Rosa, F.; López, M.T.; Fernández-Caballero, A. One-dimensional convolutional neural networks for low/high arousal classification from electrodermal activity. *Biomed. Signal Process. Control* **2022**, *71*, 103203. [CrossRef]
62. Ordóñez, F.J.; Roggen, D. Deep convolutional and LSTM recurrent neural networks for multimodal wearable activity recognition. *Sensors* **2016**, *16*, 115. [CrossRef]
63. Zhao, G.; Zhang, Z.; Guan, H.; Tang, P.; Wang, J. Rethinking ReLU to Train Better CNNs. In Proceedings of the Proceedings—International Conference on Pattern Recognition, Beijing, China, 20–24 August 2018; Volume 2018, pp. 603–608.

64. Hochreiter, S.; Schmidhuber, J. Long short-term memory. *Neural Comput.* **1997**, *9*, 1735–1780. [CrossRef]
65. Amin, M.; Ullah, K.; Asif, M.; Waheed, A.; Haq, S.U.; Zareei, M.; Biswal, R.R. ECG-Based Driver's Stress Detection Using Deep Transfer Learning and Fuzzy Logic Approaches. *IEEE Access* **2022**, *10*, 29788–29809. [CrossRef]

Disclaimer/Publisher's Note: The statements, opinions and data contained in all publications are solely those of the individual author(s) and contributor(s) and not of MDPI and/or the editor(s). MDPI and/or the editor(s) disclaim responsibility for any injury to people or property resulting from any ideas, methods, instructions or products referred to in the content.

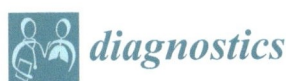

Article

Improving the Trustworthiness of Interactive Visualization Tools for Healthcare Data through a Medical Fuzzy Expert System

Abdullah M. Albarrak

College of Computer and Information Sciences, Imam Mohammad Ibn Saud Islamic University, Riyadh 13318, Saudi Arabia; amsbarrak@imamu.edu.sa

Abstract: Successful healthcare companies and illness diagnostics require data visualization. Healthcare and medical data analysis are needed to use compound information. Professionals often gather, evaluate, and monitor medical data to gauge risk, performance capability, tiredness, and adaptation to a medical diagnosis. Medical diagnosis data come from EMRs, software systems, hospital administration systems, laboratories, IoT devices, and billing and coding software. Interactive diagnosis data visualization tools enable healthcare professionals to identify trends and interpret data analytics results. Selecting the most trustworthy interactive visualization tool or application is crucial for the reliability of medical diagnosis data. Thus, this study examined the trustworthiness of interactive visualization tools for healthcare data analytics and medical diagnosis. The present study uses a scientific approach for evaluating the trustworthiness of interactive visualization tools for healthcare and medical diagnosis data and provides a novel idea and path for future healthcare experts. Our goal in this research was to make an idealness assessment of the trustworthiness impact of interactive visualization models under fuzzy conditions by using a medical fuzzy expert system based on an analytical network process and technique for ordering preference by similarity to ideal solutions. To eliminate the ambiguities that arose due to the multiple opinions of these experts and to externalize and organize information about the selection context of the interactive visualization models, the study used the proposed hybrid decision model. According to the results achieved through trustworthiness assessments of different visualization tools, BoldBI was found to be the most prioritized and trustworthy visualization tool among other alternatives. The suggested study would aid healthcare and medical professionals in interactive data visualization in identifying, selecting, prioritizing, and evaluating useful and trustworthy visualization-related characteristics, thereby leading to more accurate medical diagnosis profiles.

Keywords: interactive visualization; healthcare data; data visualization; trustworthiness assessment; decision making

Citation: Albarrak, A.M. Improving the Trustworthiness of Interactive Visualization Tools for Healthcare Data through a Medical Fuzzy Expert System. Diagnostics 2023, 13, 1733. https://doi.org/10.3390/diagnostics13101733

Academic Editors: Wan Azani Mustafa and Hiam Alquran

Received: 22 April 2023
Revised: 7 May 2023
Accepted: 12 May 2023
Published: 13 May 2023

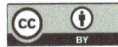

Copyright: © 2023 by the author. Licensee MDPI, Basel, Switzerland. This article is an open access article distributed under the terms and conditions of the Creative Commons Attribution (CC BY) license (https://creativecommons.org/licenses/by/4.0/).

1. Introduction

1.1. Overview

The fourth industrial revolution has completely rethought the way the medical industry has been organized in the past. A lot of the fight against the COVID-19 epidemic has been carried out with the help of Industry 4.0 and its more advanced information and communications technologies (ICTs) [1]. During this pandemic, information and communication technology have helped solve a number of problems and led to some promising solutions. Since the early days of CT scanners and MRIs, there has been a significant advancement in the field of medical diagnostics. The field of medical diagnostics has recently shifted its focus to interactive visualization. Emerging technologies, such as artificial intelligence and deep learning, are utilized, together with data sets from medical imaging, to assist in the creation of interactive visualization models. At the heart of the Industry 4.0 initiative is the idea of interactive visualization, which can be achieved with the help of different artificial intelligence (AI) and decision-making systems [2].

AI is widely used as a result of the Industrial Revolution and technology's significant advancements [3]. AI systems are widely used in a variety of industries, including healthcare, and have demonstrated tremendous effectiveness in the interpretation of complicated patterns [4]. Most people agree that AI systems are powerful tools in Industry 4.0, and they have been used a lot in the fight against this pandemic. The interactive visualization tools developed with the help of AI techniques have been used, for example, to analyze complicated medical diagnostics, lessen the effects of the epidemic, figure out the best treatment, and look for viruses by analyzing the symptoms of patients using medical imaging tools, such as CT scans and X-rays. Many examples of tasks where AI applications operate as well as or better than humans include the analysis of medical pictures and the correlation of symptoms and biomarkers from electronic medical records (EMRs) with the diagnosis and prognosis of the disease [5]. The real figures for the number of healthcare practitioners who are employing visualizations to clearly communicate data in medical diagnosis are presented in Figure 1.

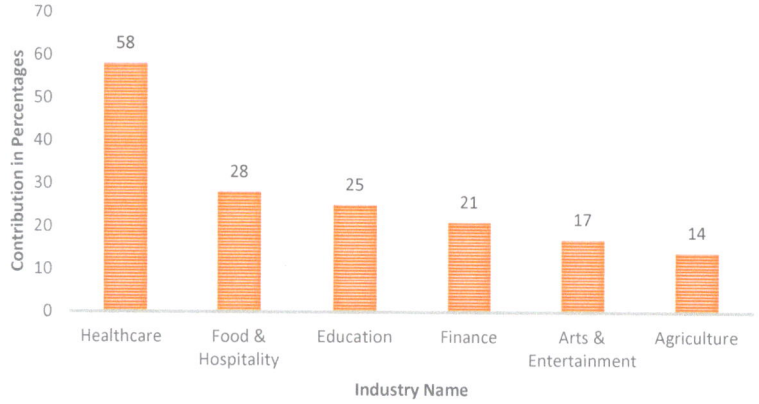

Figure 1. Statistics of data visualization markets in various industries.

According to Figure 1, about 58 percent of healthcare practitioners use interactive data visualizations for medical diagnosis and treatment of critical patients, which is more than in any other industry. Further, G. Stiglic et al. state that an AI system with a higher level of interpretability is one that end users will have an easier time understanding and in explaining future forecasts [6]. In addition, interpretable AI systems enable healthcare professionals to make decisions that are reasonable and driven by data, thereby providing personalized decisions that have the potential to ultimately lead to a higher quality of diagnosis service in the healthcare industry. The main goal of competitive health is to improve healthcare performance and eventually help people by providing them with good and speedy health services. This can be attained by pushing for higher standards of achievement, encouraging people to be active, and teaching people how to reach for good health services and deal with different services [1]. The information comes from patients as well as professionals working in the medical field, and their actions are at the heart of competitive health. These healthcare data used for medical diagnosis should be trustworthy to achieve a trustworthy visualization, which further becomes a deciding factor for multiple crucial medical treatments [7,8].

1.2. Background

Assessment of trustworthiness is moving away from mathematical methods and towards AI and decision-making methods right now because AI is good at extracting complex features without the help of humans [9]. There are many opportunities to start creative projects and scientific research in this area of research, which is growing all the time. For instance, predictive analysis carried out by AI may be utilized in the service of improving one's health [10]. Interactive healthcare data visualization tools have the ability to improve public health practice by addressing questions that were previously unanswerable in medical diagnosis. For instance, at Massachusetts General Hospital, they are utilizing 3D visualization of medical imaging in order to study the anatomical makeup of their patients. This procedure not only boosts the productivity of radiologists and ultrasonographers but also contributes to the successful outcome of efforts to save the lives of patients and improve healthcare data visualization tools [11].

Alfredo Vellido, in his work, states the problem of interpretability and visualization in AI systems for medical diagnostic purposes. He argued that medical experts should be integrated into the design of medical data analysis for the sake of good interpretation [12]. The health sector depends heavily on healthcare data, and trustworthy interactive data visualization can help doctors diagnose critical diseases, treat them, and make treatments more effective [11]. Healthcare and medical diagnostic data are essential components of the health industry. In addition to this, we are able to build better plans for healthcare thanks to big data. Trust management is a vital component of any healthcare business, whether the focus is on the health of individuals or teams. These techniques are dependent on the presence of professional healthcare teams in order to compete against their rivals. The modern approach to coaching makes use of enormous healthcare data sets in order to design effective strategies for both individuals and teams.

Dhillon et al. examined in one of their works the conceptual integration of traditional statistics and AI, with a primary emphasis on the research undertaken in the field of health. They found that researchers in the field of medicine might look at using AI to supplement traditional statistical methods of decision making in order to obtain additional trustworthy validation metrics [13]. In the healthcare industry, analyzing the trustworthiness of performance helps doctors and other professionals reach their goals by pointing out actions that can help guide decision making, improve performance, and get them started on the path to security and excellence.

Guangyue Zhang et al. emphasize in their work that technologies such as interactive healthcare data visualization and AI, along with decision making, have the potential to reduce the amount of information that management must process in the continuous monitoring of trustworthy healthcare software [14]. The process of visually representing healthcare data is the first step towards making sense of it. Users are able to tell stories through the use of data visualization by arranging data into a form that is simpler to comprehend, highlighting patterns, and drawing attention to outliers. An interactive healthcare data visualization should be able to tell a story in addition to filtering out irrelevant information and presenting the information that is important. To make an interactive healthcare data visualization, you need to find a good balance between how the tool looks and how it works. As a result of this, healthcare data analysts use a wide range of tools, such as graphs, diagrams, and maps, to understand and show healthcare data as well as the connections between them. Most of the time, the right method and how it is set up are needed to make healthcare data understandable.

1.3. Scope and Contributions

In addition, the evaluation of the trustworthiness of the interactive visualization achieved through fuzzy decision making in healthcare for medical diagnosis purposes is an ongoing process that is required to be carried out on a regular basis by industry professionals in order to test the security, effectiveness, and accuracy of these products. As a result, the goal of this research endeavor on our part is to evaluate the trustworthiness of interactive visualization achieved by means of fuzzy decision making in the medical field and to carry out an idealness evaluation while taking into account the constraints imposed by multi-criteria decision-making (MCDM) methodologies, since this problem is divided into different criteria [15,16]. For the purpose of this evaluation, the identification and selection of the pertinent characteristics are determined by the opinions of the specialists, which are provided in the second section of this paper.

The goal of this study is to comprehend how interactive healthcare data visualizations using a hybrid medical expert fuzzy system algorithm can be used in the healthcare industry to diagnose patterns. To perform rank analysis for various hybrid medical expert system classification algorithms employing decision-making analysis algorithms, such as fuzzy analytic network processing using TOPSIS, five different aspects of healthcare data visualization are used in this analysis [17–20]. Five alternatives to interactive visualization applications (SAS Visual Analytics, Tableau, QlikView, Bold BI, and DOMO BI) have been applied to the healthcare data in TOPSIS as alternatives in order to enhance the study's findings. Further, the author of this study determined the sensitivity of the results, compared the results of the proposed method with three other methods, and analyzed the statistical significance. The remainder of the research paper consists of an introduction to interactive visualization using a hybrid medical expert system, a description of the computational methodology adopted, the results, discussion, and a conclusion.

1.4. Organization of the Paper

This article's structure is as follows: The first section of the paper analyzes many trends and statistics from previous years to give the reader a summary and a sense of the relevance of the topic. As background, previous practitioners' relevant studies are examined, in which their trustworthy interactive visualization tools are presented. The paper's second portion discusses trustworthiness and interactive visualization tools. These components were given a network-like structure and ranked by impact probability. The fuzzy ANP-TOPSIS approach was used to analyze the suggested network problem numerically. The final section presents this study. In the fifth section, a discussion with a comparative study is given. The detailed debate and study limitations are summarized in a conclusion.

2. Materials and Methods

2.1. Trustworthy Interactive Visualization for Healthcare Data

Interactive data visualization in the healthcare sector is dependent on advanced current technology, which enables professionals from a variety of professions to effectively take decisions in medical diagnosis [21–24]. Interactive visualization tools help healthcare practitioners comprehend trends that have occurred in the past as well as those that are occurring in the present, in addition to helping them predict and anticipate future trends and directions. Interactive healthcare data visualization, in its broadest sense, refers to the practice of displaying information and healthcare data for medical diagnosis purposes in a variety of formats, including graphs, charts, diagrams, and photographs [25–28]. These interactive healthcare data visualization approaches can make it simple for healthcare providers to recognize and comprehend patterns, trends, and outliers in healthcare data [2].

Trustworthiness issues in interactive visualization techniques have become increasingly relevant in many areas of healthcare, particularly with regard to assisting medical professionals in the formulation of vitally important clinical choices for the health of patients and communities. A healthcare organization is able to transform raw healthcare data into graphs and then exhibit them in charts by utilizing a variety of approaches for healthcare data visualization [14]. This enables the organization to perform rapid analysis of trends and patterns.

A trustworthy tool or piece of software provides efficient and interactive visualization by utilizing systems associated with healthcare, examining threats, and responding to incidents swiftly and instinctively. To solve the many challenges that come with healthcare data visualization, specialists and researchers have brought a variety of assurance issues to light [17]. The overall level of trustworthiness of healthcare interactive visualization tools can be broken down into their component parts. The combination of these characteristics can vary depending on who is receiving treatment. For consumers, for instance, trustworthiness in healthcare visualization tools consists primarily of a perceived amount of control and privacy. On the other hand, for healthcare professionals, trustworthiness in visualization involves a far bigger and more diverse collection of concerns, such as reliability and a transparent healthcare data storage policy. When compared to the sets of elements that affect trustworthiness in the general healthcare data visualization domain, the sets of factors that affect trustworthiness in a healthcare portal are unique. In order to ensure that interventions are trustworthy, it is necessary to carry out independent research on the topic of trustworthiness in healthcare interactive visualization tools as a separate topic.

A case study was conducted on a few different alternatives in order to enhance the performance of healthcare interactive visualization tools and rank the characteristics of healthcare interactive visualization tools in descending order of importance [8]. A consensus was reached among the authors regarding the characteristics to be used in the evaluation of healthcare interactive visualization tools, and these conclusions informed the decision-making process for identifying and selecting the criteria. For the purpose of this work, five characteristics of trustworthiness, four characteristics of visualization design, and three characteristics of interactive widgets were taken into consideration for the idealness assessment. The decision that experts in a particular field make collectively is what drives the process of alternative selection. Further, alternatives were chosen as per the popularity of interactive visualization tools among healthcare professionals. The authors of the study used fuzzy logic for this evaluation, so each healthcare data visualization was assigned a value between 0 and 1 for each characteristic.

Moreover, with regard to our specified characteristic set, each healthcare data visualization tool gained a value between 0 and 1 for each characteristic. In addition, the results of the evaluators' subjective cognition in linguistic words for each healthcare data visualization characteristic were based on the scale and the opinions of the experts, both of which are explained in the methodology portion of the paper. This work presents, on the basis of the identified characteristic set, the process of evaluating the six tools used for healthcare as well as the quantitative outcomes of that evaluation. The characteristics that were found and the alternatives are shown in Figure 2. The figure that follows discusses both the subsection description and the significance of the traits that were identified.

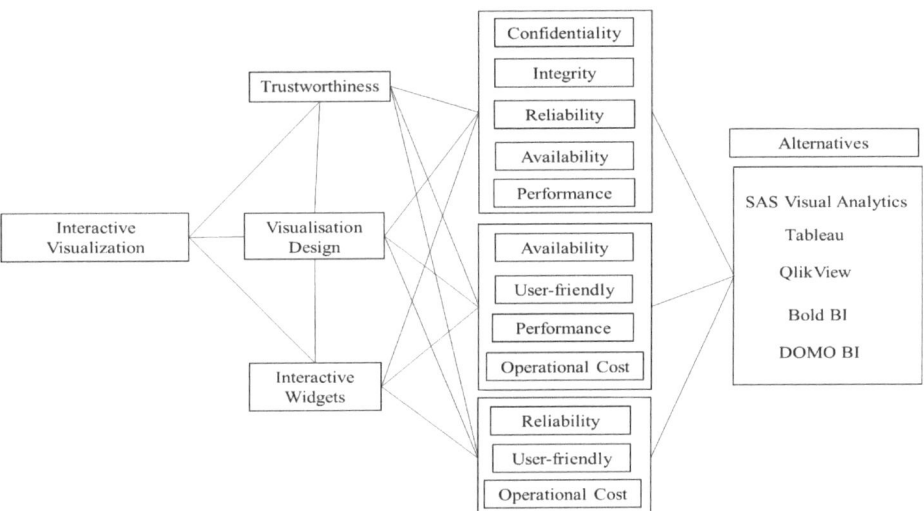

Figure 2. Assessment characteristics for interactive visualization of healthcare data.

Characteristics at the first level are further divided into sub-characteristics. Trustworthiness is affected by confidentiality, integrity, reliability, availability, and performance [19]. Visualization design is affected by availability, user friendliness, performance, and operational cost. Interactive widgets in a visualization tool depend on its characteristics, such as reliability, user friendliness, and operational cost. The first-level characteristics depend on each other for the best interactive visualization tool building. Hence, after creating its dependencies, it becomes a network-like structure problem. For such a multiple-criteria network-like structure problem, the Analytic Network Process (ANP) is a mathematical theory that was developed by Saaty [28] that is helpful for forecasting and presenting the influence of multiple decision criteria, their interactions, and their relative weights. ANP was named after the nature of its problem, which is a network-like structure of different criteria. To calculate the different weights of characteristics associated with this problem, we used ANP with fuzzy logic and TOPSIS for ranking the alternatives.

2.1.1. Trustworthiness

Interactive visualization tools are having an increasingly substantial impact on clinical decisions and diagnoses as a result of the significant increase in the number of healthcare solutions. On the other hand, there is scant evidence to support the notion that software can be trusted. An application or tool is said to have trustworthiness when it possesses the qualities that make it trustworthy for others, such as healthcare professionals. There are different characteristics of trustworthiness that contribute to building a trustworthy visualization tool. We identified five important characteristics, the details of which are as follows:

Confidentiality: To maintain healthcare data privacy, it must be protected from digital and physical intrusion. Confidentiality is closely tied to other aspects of information privacy, such as who can see, share, and use specific pieces of healthcare data. Information with a low level of confidentiality may be considered "public" or innocuous if disclosed to a larger audience. High-confidentiality information must be protected against disclosure for the sake of avoiding identity theft, account and system compromise, legal or reputational damage, and other undesirable outcomes. The importance of privacy in keeping healthcare data visualization trustworthy is thus demonstrated.

Integrity: Healthcare data integrity is vital because so much depends on it. A dataset error in healthcare data can impact a clinician's decision making. Healthcare data integrity means accuracy, completeness, and consistency. Healthcare data integrity includes security for regulatory compliance. It decreases consumer assurance and trustworthiness. There are several data integrity threats. Copy-transferred data should not be modified between updates. Error-checking and validation maintain data integrity when sent or reproduced without alteration.

Reliability: For a clinician or healthcare expert to use a visualization tool to ensure the accuracy of healthcare data, the data must be complete and correct. This is what is meant by "data reliability." One of the main goals of data integrity programs, which are also used to maintain data security, data quality, and regulatory compliance, is to make sure data is trustworthy. The term "data reliability" refers to how consistent information is between different databases, apps, or platforms. It also has to do with how trustworthy the source of information is. If the data are trustworthy enough, a trustworthy figure will always be right. Thus, it can be seen as a sign of honesty.

Availability: The frequency with which healthcare data can be used by a healthcare provider organization or a partner is a measure of data availability. A healthcare provider organization runs more smoothly when clinicians have access to data at all times. Important aspects of data availability include access to the data and a steady stream of data. Data that cannot be accessed are as good as useless. As a result, data availability is the only factor that can influence the trustworthiness of interactive data visualization. If workers were to have problems obtaining firm data, productivity would take a hit. Data accessibility is critical for most modern enterprises. The good news is that, by following data availability best practices, a forward-thinking firm may enjoy all the advantages of having sufficient data availability.

2.1.2. Visualization Design

User-Friendly: The goal of good visualization tool design is to ensure that a product is not only functional but also pleasurable and simple to use for healthcare experts. The interactive visualizations could be understood by every level of health expert, be it a researcher in healthcare or a doctor. The goal is to guarantee that every consumer of an interactive visualization tool is completely content with their experience using the product. An improved user experience is the result of a design that facilitates the user's goals and duties. The design must be simplified, the instructions must be clear and succinct, and the learning curve must be minimized.

Operational Cost: Visualization tool developers have never been in a position where they are not under pressure to cut expenses and maximize investment. This pressure has only risen as a result of COVID-19, as more and more hospitals and healthcare organizations have sped up their digitalization efforts in an effort to preserve a viable, virtual corporate presence. These operational cost optimizations have a direct impact on the design, trustworthiness, and interactive widgets of tools. Hence, operational cost is an important criterion for measuring a trustworthy and interactive visualization tool for healthcare professionals.

2.1.3. Interactive Widgets

The goal of interactive visualization is to improve the way in which people engage with information by using graphical representations of healthcare data. The term "interactive visuals" can also apply to the graphical displays that are employed by various technologies for analytics and business intelligence. The majority of the time, these representations are implemented in the form of interactive widgets. These widgets offer a simple method for comprehending insights that may be based on data that are constantly shifting. In order for healthcare data visualizations to be called interactive, they need to incorporate some sort of human input (such as the ability to click on a button or move a slider), and their response times need to be fast enough to demonstrate a genuine connection between the healthcare data input and the visual output.

Performance: Problems with performance are characterized by a reaction time for output that is significantly longer than the time that is anticipated for its execution in a healthcare interactive visualization tool. The performance could be caused by untrustworthy third-party healthcare data, such as databases or hardware, or it could be caused by the design of the visualization. Hence, performance issues can be affected by trustworthiness, visualization design, and interactive widgets as well.

All of the features that were covered earlier have some bearing on interactive visualization tools. In addition, each of the mentioned traits, by virtue of the implicit specifications that they carry, plays an important part in the ideality of interactive visualization for healthcare as a whole. The authors of the study began by compiling a list of the multiple characteristics that were pertinent to the investigation. Following that, a conversation was had with the team of healthcare and security tool development experts about finalizing the characteristics set. After having a group discussion about all of the detected features, the specialists deleted any characteristics that were deemed unnecessary or inconsistent. The individual disagreements that arose among the experts over the characteristic selection were brought to a minimum, and at the end of this expert group debate, a collection of trustworthy healthcare data visualization characteristics was decided upon. So, each of these characteristics was taken into consideration for this analysis.

2.2. Methodology

The Analytic Network Process (ANP) of MCDM can solve networked decision-making problems. T.L. Saaty invented the technique in 1965. The approach has changed and improved since then [28]. It estimates the relative relevance of criteria (characteristics). It helps specialists choose the judgement that best fits their goal and understanding of the situation. Fuzzy data improve this process and helps elicit more accurate healthcare data [29].

Fuzzy sets are crucial here. Fuzzy sets accurately reflect decision makers' foggy preferences. Fuzzy logic can eliminate doubts when defining an element's membership in a fixed set is challenging. This is very useful for categorizing elements. Fuzzy logic rarely addresses such issues [30]. TOPSIS also produces the highest alternate rating [8]. Its main draw is this ability. Thus, integrating fuzzy logic with the ANP-TOPSIS methodology makes this study more effective and allows it to be used to evaluate the efficacy of interactive visualization achieved through the software of a hybrid medical expert system.

This article evaluates each visualization tool's success using the ANP-TOPSIS main methods. The fuzzy TOPSIS approach first determines the weight of each characteristic for the fuzzy ANP method. To establish correct weights, correlations between attributes are examined. After determining these attributes' key weights, the fuzzy TOPSIS technique is used to assess decision makers' social and economic performance and risk. These methods require interactive visualization specialists and a hybrid medical expert system. The specialists must have at least three years of experience selecting, managing, and conceptualizing interactive visualizations utilizing a hybrid medical expert system. Figure 3 shows the integrated fuzzy ANP TOPSIS method:

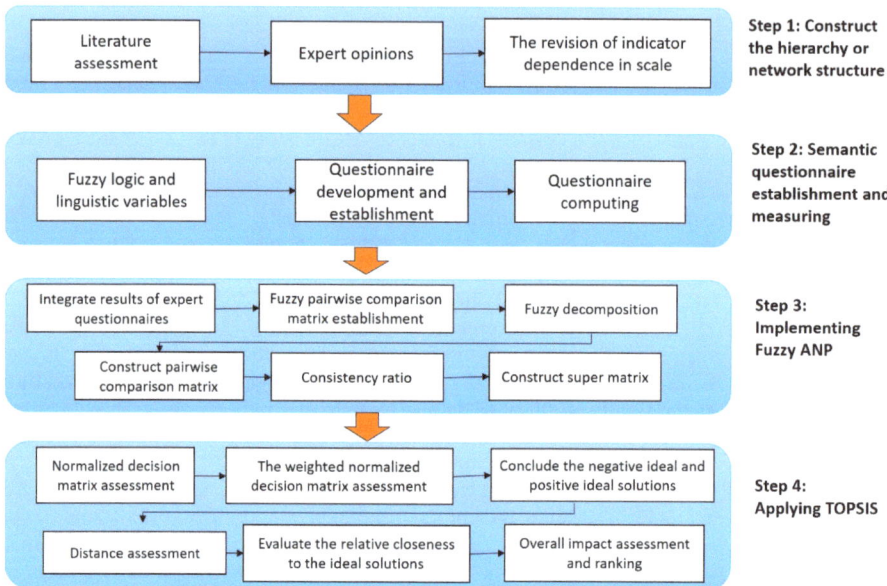

Figure 3. Flowchart of the proposed methodology.

2.2.1. Fuzzy Analytic Network Process

There is a significant potential for fuzzy-based ANP-TOPSIS to tackle MCDM challenges generated by imprecise and uncertain healthcare data [28,30]. When applied in a fuzzy environment, ANP yields characteristic weights that are more accurate, which in turn leads to outcomes that are more beneficial [28]. The TOPSIS method, when applied to problems involving MCDM, is one of the better-known techniques for ranking available solutions [28]. In this particular study, a total of 5 interactive visualization tools were used as alternatives and 12 characteristics of interactive visualization were used as criteria. When identifying and selecting the qualities, both the views of the specialists and well-known research works were taken into consideration.

Thomas Saaty [28] came up with the idea of incorporating the ANP, which is an extension of the AHP (Analytic Hierarchy Process). It enhances the capacity to handle interactions and dependencies between characteristics and sub-characteristics, which might alter the weights that are allocated to them. This can be a challenge when trying to build a model. Despite the many attempts to alter it so that it can account for erroneous human judgments, the ANP is severely constrained when it comes to evidentiary assessment fractions. The fundamental concept that underpins this is that the aggregation strategy utilized by the ANP is a reasonably straightforward one that can be applied to intervals as well as locally fuzzy priorities. However, in order to carry out the supermatrix priority derivation technique in the ANP, one must be familiar with complex real-number matrix operations. Nevertheless, none of the currently available methods for determining interval or fuzzy local priorities give results that can be incorporated into the calculation of the ANP matrix. This is the case despite the fact that these methods have been developed. In order to solve the unpredictability that surrounded the preferences of experts in a pairwise comparison matrix, the fuzzy ANP (PWCM) was developed. The following is a rundown of the various stages of the fuzzy ANP strategy that will be used in the calculation of the weights of the qualities:

Step 1: The process of constructing the network of the problem involves characterizing the relationships that exist among its numerous parts.

Step 2: In the following step of the procedure, triangular fuzzy numbers (TFNs) based on the scale proposed by Saaty [28] are used to compare various linked properties of the network pairwise and create comparison matrixes. The linguistic term "comparison" is used in this study, and the appropriate TFNs were assigned [30].

Step 3: Creating the Supermatrix.

In order to construct the supermatrix, it is necessary to ascertain the relative importance of each characteristic and sub-characteristic. As each comparison matrix's characteristics have a triangular fuzzy structure, the respective weights are calculated using Lotfi Zadeh's proposed extent analysis method [28]. This method consists of the following steps and is necessary because of the triangular, fuzzy membership structure.

Step 3.1: Finding the value of the fuzzy artificial degree for each of the following qualities is the first step in Zadeh's technique:

Let us assume that Pw is a pairwise comparison matrix in (Equations (1)–(5)):

$$Pw = [Q_{ij}]_{r \times s}, Q_{ij} = (l_{ij}, m_{ij}, u_{ij})$$

$$i = 1, 2, \ldots, r \quad j = 1, \ldots, s \tag{1}$$

$$S_i = \sum_{j=1}^{s} Q_{ij} \times \left[\sum_{i=1}^{r} \sum_{j=1}^{s} Q_{ij} \right]^{-1} \tag{2}$$

$$\text{where } \sum_{j=1}^{s} Q_{ij} = \left(\sum_{j=1}^{s} l_j, \sum_{j=1}^{s} r_j, \sum_{j=1}^{s} u_j \right) \forall i, \tag{3}$$

$$\sum_{i=1}^{r} \sum_{j=1}^{s} Q_{ij} = \left(\sum_{i=1}^{r} \sum_{j=1}^{s} l_{ij}, \sum_{i=1}^{r} \sum_{j=1}^{s} m_{ij}, \sum_{i=1}^{r} \sum_{j=1}^{s} u_{ij} \right), \text{ and} \tag{4}$$

$$\left[\sum_{i=1}^{r} \sum_{j=1}^{s} Q_{ij} \right]^{-1} = \left(\frac{1}{\sum_{i=1}^{r} \sum_{j=1}^{s} u_{ij}}, \frac{1}{\sum_{i=1}^{r} \sum_{j=1}^{s} m_{ij}}, \frac{1}{\sum_{i=1}^{r} \sum_{j=1}^{s} l_{ij}} \right) \tag{5}$$

Step 3.2: Calculating the relative likelihood of each Si over other characteristics (Equation (6)).

$$V(S_1 \geq S_2) = \begin{cases} 1 & \text{if } m_1 \geq m_2 \\ 0 & \text{if } l_1 \geq u_2 \\ \frac{l_2 - u_1}{(m_1 - u_1) - (m_2 - l_2)} & \text{otherwise} \end{cases} \tag{6}$$

Step 3.3: When using Equations (7) and (8), it can be difficult to determine how much weight each characteristic ought to be given in terms of the probability that a convex fuzzy number is greater than k other convex fuzzy numbers.

$$W'_i = V(S_k \geq S_1, S_2, \ldots \ldots S_r) = \min_{i=1,2,\ldots k,..r} (S_k \geq S_i) \quad (7)$$

$$w' = (W'_1, W'_2, \ldots, W'_r) \quad (8)$$

Step 3.4: Estimating the normalized weight vector using (Equation (9)).

$$w = (W_1, W_2, \ldots W_r) \quad (9)$$

Once the weights of each pairwise comparison matrix have been computed, the supermatrix can be created according to Equation (10):

$$W' = \begin{matrix} 1 = \text{Goal} \\ 2 = \text{Criteria} \\ 3 = \text{Sub} - \text{criteria} \end{matrix} \begin{bmatrix} 0 & 0 & 0 \\ W_{21} & W_{22} & 0 \\ 0 & W_{32} & W_{33} \end{bmatrix} \quad (10)$$

Step 4: Computing the actual weight vector of each sub-characteristic (Equation (11)).

$$W = \lim_{x \to \infty} W'^{2k+1} \quad (11)$$

2.2.2. Fuzzy Technique for Order of Preference by Similarity to Ideal Solutions

The fuzzy TOPSIS method was first put forth by M. M. D. Widianta et al. [31], and since then it has been widely used for evaluating alternatives in a range of contexts. This technique can be used to rank choices according to how similar or close they are to the ideal response. On this page [29], there is a lot of information about how to use fuzzy TOPSIS.

Step 1: Calculating the decision matrix that has been normalized.

Supposing that D_{nd} is the normalized fuzzy decision matrix (Equation (12)):

$$D_{nd} = [d_{ij}]_{r \times s} \; i = 1, \ldots \ldots r \; j = 1, \ldots \ldots, s \quad (12)$$

Every aspect of decision making, with the exception of the decision-making process itself, has been standardized according to the category that best fits each principle. The principle decides whether it is a benefit principle or a cost principle, which means that an increase in magnitude is advantageous in the first category; however, in the second category, a decrease in size is advantageous. To calculate each one, the following equations are used, which are classified by each component of the normalized decision-making process (Equation (13)):

$$d_{ij} = \left(\frac{l_{ij}}{u_j^+}, \frac{m_{ij}}{u_j^+}, \frac{u_{ij}}{u_j^+} \right) \quad (13)$$

where u_j^+ is the maximum u_{ij} for the benefit characteristic (Equation (14)).

$$d_{ij} = \left(\frac{l_j^-}{u_{ij}}, \frac{l_j^-}{m_{ij}}, \frac{l_j^-}{l_{ij}} \right) \quad (14)$$

where, l_j^- is the minimum l_{ij} for the cost characteristic.

Step 2: Calculating the weighted normalized decision matrix.

The weight of the characteristic is represented as wi, and the weighted normalized decision matrix is determined as follows (Equation (15)):

$$V = (v_{ij})_{r \times s} \text{ where } v_{ij} = r_{ij} \times w_{ij} \forall j = 1, \ldots \ldots, s, \text{ and } i = 1, \ldots \ldots, r \quad (15)$$

Step 3: The fuzzy positive ideal and the negative ideal as potential answers are suggested in this step.

$FPI = \left(v_{1j'}^+, \ldots v_{ij}^+\right)$ for the benefit characteristic; $FPI = \left(v_{1j'}^-, \ldots v_{ij}^-\right)$ for the cost characteristic.

Where v_i^+ is the maximum v_{ij}^-, v_{ij}^- is the minimum v_{ij}^+, and $i = 1, \ldots, r; j = 1, \ldots, s$.

Step 4: Calculating the distance of each alternative from positive ideal and negative ideal solutions (Equations (16) and (17)).

$$dia_j^+ = \sum_{j=1}^n dia_v\left(v_{ij}, v_j^+\right) i = 1, \ldots, r \tag{16}$$

$$dia_j^- = \sum_{j=1}^n dia_v\left(v_{ij}, v_j^-\right) i = 1, \ldots, r \tag{17}$$

The distance between two TFNs can be calculated (Equation (18)):

$$dia\left(\tilde{A}, \tilde{B}\right) = \sqrt{\frac{1}{3}\left((l_A - l_B)^2 + (m_A - m_B)^2 + (u_A - u_B)^2\right)} \tag{18}$$

Step 5: This step is performed to calculate the closeness coefficient factor (CCF) (Equation (19)).

$$CCF_j = \frac{dia_j^-}{\left(dia_j^+ + dia_j^-\right)} \tag{19}$$

Step 6: Prioritizing the alternatives.

The algorithm that is used to determine the closeness coefficient gives more weight to the choice that has the highest *CCFj* value; hence, the one that has the highest *CCFj* value is the one that comes out on top in the ranking list.

3. Results

Interactive visualization tools provide users with a number of alternatives for visualizing healthcare data for the purpose of medical diagnosis that go beyond the traditional options of pie, bar, and line charts. Some examples of these possibilities are 3D medical imaging and micro-CT, as well as X-rays, scatter plots, and other types of visualizations developed for particular diagnosis. Graphical representations of healthcare data are made available to healthcare experts with these tools, enabling them to conduct medical diagnoses by interacting with the representations. In the following, we shall examine the significance of a hybrid medical expert system in interactive visualization by utilizing procedures that consist of fuzzy networks. The numerical analysis of this attempt will provide a quantitative evaluation of the results it generates.

As a direct result of this, the purpose of this work is to conduct a case study on five alternatives of interactive visualization tools in order to investigate the qualities that characterize their appropriateness from the point of view of interactive visualization. The approach that was selected for this inquiry incorporates, as component elements, all of the possible identifiers that can be given, in addition to rating evaluations for each one. This was decided upon before the investigation began. In addition, these five interactive visualization tools were selected as alternatives for their comparative trustworthiness evaluation based on the decision that was arrived at by reaching a consensus amongst the owners of the relevant domains and the experts in these fields. This was done to ensure that the best possible results would be obtained from the evaluation. In order to make this study more productive and corroborative, an ANP-TOPSIS analysis was conducted under fuzzy settings. Under fuzzy settings, an evaluation of the ideality of a hybrid medical expert system was carried out with the support of ANP-TOPSIS. The evaluation focused on the context of interactive visualization. Following the equations indicated in the technique section (Equations (1)–(19)), the method was used to carry out this evaluation.

Following the conversion of the linguistic phrases to quantitative values (Steps 1–4 and Equations (1)–(11)), the values were then further refined into fuzzy-based, crisp numerical values (Step 5). Following this, numerical calculations were carried out in order to construct a pairwise comparison matrix, and the outcomes of these calculations, a summary of which can be found in Table 1, are shown below. The algorithm proceeded through the process of implementing fuzzy integer values and then subsequently transitioned into fuzzy-based crisp numeric values so that the final results could be written down in Table 1. Following this, numerical calculations were carried out in order to build a pairwise comparison matrix, and the results of these calculations, which are summarized in Table 1 and are shown below, may be found in the next paragraph.

Table 1. Pairwise comparisons matrixes of the groups.

Characteristic A/Characteristic B	Fuzzy Pairwise Comparisons Matrixes	Defuzzified Pairwise Comparisons Matrixes
Trustworthiness/Visualization Design	0.190, 0.170, 0.167	0.268
Trustworthiness/Interactive Widgets	0.364, 0.426, 0.44	0.277
Visualization Design/Interactive Widgets	0.319, 0.392, 0.401	0.370
Confidentiality/Integrity	0.148, 0.124, 0.118	0.015
Confidentiality/Reliability	0.348, 0.211, 0.106	0.390
Confidentiality/Availability	0.148, 0.113, 0.108	0.250
Confidentiality/Performance	0.192, 0.227, 0.222	0.390
Integrity/Reliability	0.152, 0.112, 0.108	0.350
Integrity/Availability	0.113, 0.075, 0.071	0.380
Integrity/Performance	0.226, 0.250, 0.253	0.450
Reliability/Availability	0.155, 0.122, 0.117	0.112
Reliability/Performance	0.192, 0.199, 0.196	0.248
Performance/Availability	0.306, 0.358, 0.373	0.390
Availability/User-Friendly	0.192, 0.199, 0.196	0.250
Availability/Performance	0.226, 0.250, 0.253	0.390
Availability/Operational Cost	0.155, 0.129, 0.124	0.233
User-Friendly/Performance	0.152, 0.112, 0.108	0.250
User-Friendly/Operational Cost	0.155, 0.093, 0.090	0.390
Performance/Operational Cost	0.113, 0.075, 0.071	0.350
Reliability/User-Friendly	0.192, 0.206, 0.203	0.380
Reliability/Operational Cost	0.148, 0.113, 0.108	0.450
User-Friendly/Operational Cost	0.192, 0.227, 0.222	0.112

In order to obtain the final results displayed in Table 1, the methodology was modified to include fuzzy wrappers (Equations (1)–(5)), estimation of triangular numbers, and degree of possibility. At long last, the specialists arrived at the pairwise comparison matrix by using Equations (7) and (8). Table 1 displays the defuzzified values of the group's characteristics. These values were computed using Equation (9), and the table was created. Table 2 displays the normalized weights of the group's characteristics after calculating the local priority vectors, the weighted supermatrix, and the supermatrix formation. The complete findings of this inquiry are summarized below for convenience. After this, certain numerical calculations were carried out with the intention of calculating the absolute weight vector for row values and the traits that are the most important, as demonstrated in Equations (10) and (11). When the fuzzy data from the judgment matrixes were put together, a pairwise contribution matrix was the result. Further, Table 2 shows the combined results through the network.

Table 2. Weights of Interactive Visualization.

Characteristic	Symbols	Independent Weight of the Groups	Overall Weights through Network	Percentage	Priority
Characteristics of Group 1 at Level 1					
Trustworthiness	C1	0.259	0.259	25.90%	3
Visualization Design	C2	0.416	0.416	41.60%	1
Interactive Widgets	C3	0.326	0.326	32.60%	2
Characteristics of Groups 1, 2, and 3 at Level 2					
Confidentiality	C11	0.115	0.030	2.977%	12
Integrity	C12	0.363	0.094	9.398%	4
Reliability	C13	0.255	0.066	6.602%	10
Availability	C14	0.268	0.069	6.939%	9
Performance	C15	0.277	0.072	7.172%	8
Availability	C21	0.156	0.065	6.482%	11
User-Friendly	C22	0.267	0.111	11.094%	2
Performance	C23	0.265	0.110	11.011%	3
Operational Cost	C24	0.212	0.088	8.809%	5
Reliability	C31	0.248	0.081	8.075%	6
User-Friendly	C32	0.341	0.111	11.103%	1
Operational Cost	C33	0.233	0.076	7.586%	7

The following part of the work provides a realistic assessment of the findings that were evaluated on particularly delicate interactive visualization software. The application of an ANP strategy while the conditions were fuzzy was used to obtain the combined weights of features; then, the software of TOPSIS, while the conditions were fuzzy, was used to obtain the global ranking of competing alternatives; this was carried out after the combined weights of features had been obtained. After this, we took the inputs on the technological data of five interactive visualization software systems and produced the summarized findings that are shown in Table 3 by including the standard scale that was defined in the technique. Passing the characteristic weights determined with the help of ANP to the TOPSIS technique when it is functioning in a fuzzy environment allows for the determination of the ranking order for the many options that can be chosen.

Table 3. Normalized decision matrix for alternatives with respect to criteria.

	SAS Visual Analytics	Tableau	QlikView	Bold BI	DOMO BI
Confidentiality	0.6578, 0.7570, 0.9190	0.6570, 0.7650, 0.9050	0.4560, 0.5330, 0.7330	0.8500, 0.9170, 0.9680	0.7720, 0.8560, 0.9450
Integrity	0.6490, 0.7640, 0.8800	0.6570, 0.7650, 0.9050	0.6578, 0.7570, 0.9190	0.8500, 0.9170, 0.9680	0.6578, 0.7570, 0.9190
Reliability	0.6570, 0.7650, 0.9050	0.6570, 0.7650, 0.9050	0.4560, 0.5330, 0.7330	0.8500, 0.9170, 0.9680	0.8500, 0.9170, 0.9680
Availability	0.6570, 0.7650, 0.9050	0.6570, 0.7650, 0.9050	0.6578, 0.7570, 0.9190	0.6570, 0.7650, 0.9050	0.4560, 0.5330, 0.7330
Performance	0.6578, 0.7570, 0.9190	0.8500, 0.9170, 0.9680	0.6578, 0.7570, 0.9190	0.6570, 0.7650, 0.9050	0.6578, 0.7570, 0.9190
Availability	0.4560, 0.5330, 0.7330	0.8500, 0.9170, 0.9680	0.8500, 0.9170, 0.9680	0.6570, 0.7650, 0.9050	0.6578, 0.7570, 0.9190
User-Friendly	0.6578, 0.7570, 0.9190	0.6570, 0.7650, 0.9050	0.4560, 0.5330, 0.7330	0.6570, 0.7650, 0.9050	0.4560, 0.5330, 0.7330
Performance	0.6578, 0.7570, 0.9190	0.6570, 0.7650, 0.9050	0.4560, 0.5330, 0.7330	0.8500, 0.9170, 0.9680	0.7720, 0.8560, 0.9450
Operational Cost	0.6490, 0.7640, 0.8800	0.6570, 0.7650, 0.9050	0.6578, 0.7570, 0.9190	0.8500, 0.9170, 0.9680	0.6578, 0.7570, 0.9190
Reliability	0.6570, 0.7650, 0.9050	0.6570, 0.7650, 0.9050	0.4560, 0.5330, 0.7330	0.8500, 0.9170, 0.9680	0.8500, 0.9170, 0.9680
User-Friendly	0.6570, 0.7650, 0.9050	0.6570, 0.7650, 0.9050	0.6578, 0.7570, 0.9190	0.6570, 0.7650, 0.9050	0.4560, 0.5330, 0.7330
Operational Cost	0.6578, 0.7570, 0.9190	0.8500, 0.9170, 0.9680	0.6578, 0.7570, 0.9190	0.6570, 0.7650, 0.9050	0.6578, 0.7570, 0.9190

Following the completion of a number of procedures that served as intermediaries, the normalized fuzzy decision matrix for five alternatives of interactive visualization tools (SAS Visual Analytics, Tableau, QlikView, Bold BI, and DOMO BI) was discovered. The findings of the analysis are contained within this matrix. Equations (12)–(15) can be used to help with the calculation of the normalized performance values of the fuzzy decision matrix. Table 4 displays the definitive findings, which were computed by combining Equations (16) and (17) to establish the positive and negative idealness of each alternative with reference to each characteristic (Tables 5 and 6). These equations were combined in order to ascertain the idealness of each alternative. The findings are arranged here according to the chronological order in which they were discovered. Equations (18) and (19) were used to compute the relative closeness score for each choice, which was then used to determine the degree of satisfaction; the results of this computation can also be found in Table 7. This was an after-thought calculation that was performed.

Table 4. Weighted normalized decision matrix.

	SAS Visual Analytics	Tableau	QlikView	Bold BI	DOMO BI
Confidentiality	0.0516, 0.0820, 0.0990	0.0516, 0.0990, 0.1220	0.0630, 0.1140, 0.1310	0.0630, 0.0979, 0.1310	0.0230, 0.0430, 0.0550
Integrity	0.0230, 0.0370, 0.0430	0.0230, 0.0370, 0.0430	0.0630, 0.0979, 0.1140	0.0516, 0.0820, 0.0990	0.0516, 0.0820, 0.0990
Reliability	0.0516, 0.0820, 0.0990	0.0516, 0.0990, 0.1220	0.0630, 0.1140, 0.1310	0.0630, 0.0979, 0.1310	0.0630, 0.0979, 0.1310
Availability	0.0230, 0.0370, 0.0430	0.0630, 0.0979, 0.1140	0.0516, 0.0820, 0.0990	0.0516, 0.0820, 0.0990	0.0516, 0.0820, 0.0990
Performance	0.0230, 0.0370, 0.0430	0.0230, 0.0370, 0.0430	0.0230, 0.0370, 0.0430	0.0230, 0.0370, 0.0430	0.0630, 0.0979, 0.1140
Availability	0.0630, 0.0979, 0.1140	0.0630, 0.0979, 0.1140	0.0516, 0.0820, 0.0990	0.0630, 0.0979, 0.1140	0.0516, 0.0820, 0.0990
User-Friendly	0.0516, 0.0990, 0.1220	0.0630, 0.1140, 0.1310	0.0630, 0.0979, 0.1310	0.0630, 0.1140, 0.1310	0.0630, 0.0979, 0.1310
Performance	0.0230, 0.0370, 0.0430	0.0630, 0.0979, 0.1140	0.0516, 0.0820, 0.0990	0.0630, 0.0979, 0.1140	0.0516, 0.0820, 0.0990
Operational Cost	0.0516, 0.0990, 0.1220	0.0630, 0.1140, 0.1310	0.0630, 0.0979, 0.1310	0.0630, 0.1140, 0.1310	0.0630, 0.0979, 0.1310
Reliability	0.0516, 0.0820, 0.0990	0.0230, 0.0370, 0.0430	0.0230, 0.0370, 0.0430	0.0630, 0.0979, 0.1140	0.0516, 0.0820, 0.0990
User-Friendly	0.0516, 0.0820, 0.0990	0.0516, 0.0990, 0.1220	0.0516, 0.0990, 0.1220	0.0630, 0.1140, 0.1310	0.0630, 0.0979, 0.1310
Operational Cost	0.0230, 0.0370, 0.0430	0.0630, 0.0979, 0.1140	0.0630, 0.0979, 0.1140	0.0630, 0.0979, 0.1140	0.0516, 0.0820, 0.0990

Table 5. Separation from positive solution.

	SAS Visual Analytics	Tableau	QlikView	Bold BI	DOMO BI
Confidentiality	0.9050	0.8990	0.9080	0.9360	0.9080
Integrity	0.9360	0.9360	0.9080	0.9280	0.9050
Reliability	0.9050	0.8990	0.9080	0.9280	0.9080
Availability	0.9360	0.9360	0.9080	0.9360	0.9080
Performance	0.9360	0.9080	0.9280	0.9360	0.9080
Availability	0.9280	0.9080	0.8990	0.9080	0.9280
User-Friendly	0.9360	0.9080	0.9360	0.9080	0.9360
Performance	0.8990	0.8990	0.9080	0.9280	0.9360
Operational Cost	0.9360	0.9360	0.9080	0.9280	0.9080
Reliability	0.9080	0.9080	0.9080	0.9360	0.9080
User-Friendly	0.9080	0.9080	0.9080	0.9360	0.9280
Operational Cost	0.9080	0.9080	0.9360	0.9080	0.9360

The study was carried out on five alternatives of interactive visualization tools, and the results showed that classification is more ideal and effective when it comes to dealing with interactive visualization. The evaluation was carried out on the basis of the criteria that were chosen. It is of the utmost importance to determine whether or not the results achieved are stable when one is attempting to demonstrate a framework for making decisions based on a number of different criteria. This can be achieved by determining whether or not the framework that is being demonstrated is stable. The sequence in which alternatives are presented is heavily influenced by the weights that are given to the various selection criteria. Alterations to the proportional weights of the various selection criteria have the potential to cause fluctuations in the ranks if they are not carried out carefully. In order to evaluate the dependability of the findings, the authors conducted a sensitivity analysis by following the technique provided in [5]. This allowed the authors to validate their findings. The sensitivity of the interactive visualization software to variations in performance can be investigated by incrementally adding a 5% penalty to the weights of each selection criterion while they are being implemented one at a time. The results of the sensitivity analysis are shown in graphical form in Figure 4, which are presented here for convenience. The outcomes unequivocally demonstrate that they maintain their constancy.

Table 6. Separation from negative solution.

	SAS Visual Analytics	Tableau	QlikView	Bold BI	DOMO BI
Confidentiality	0.0140	0.1420	0.0012	0.1730	0.0150
Integrity	0.1230	0.1420	0.0012	0.0012	0.0012
Reliability	0.0012	0.0150	0.1420	0.1420	0.0012
Availability	0.0140	0.1420	0.0120	0.0150	0.1420
Performance	0.0012	0.1420	0.1420	0.1420	0.0120
Availability	0.1420	0.0012	0.0012	0.1420	0.1230
User-Friendly	0.0150	0.1420	0.0012	0.0012	0.0012
Performance	0.1420	0.0150	0.1420	0.1420	0.0012
Operational Cost	0.1420	0.1420	0.0120	0.0150	0.1420
Reliability	0.0150	0.1420	0.1420	0.0012	0.0012
User-Friendly	0.1420	0.0120	0.0150	0.1420	0.0012
Operational Cost	0.2410	0.1230	0.2410	0.0150	0.1730

Table 7. Final ranking of alternatives.

S. No.	Visulization Applications	Closeness Coefficients
1	SAS Visual Analytics	0.52652
2	Tableau	0.53254
3	QlikView	0.48525
4	Bold BI	0.59547
5	DOMO BI	0.57635

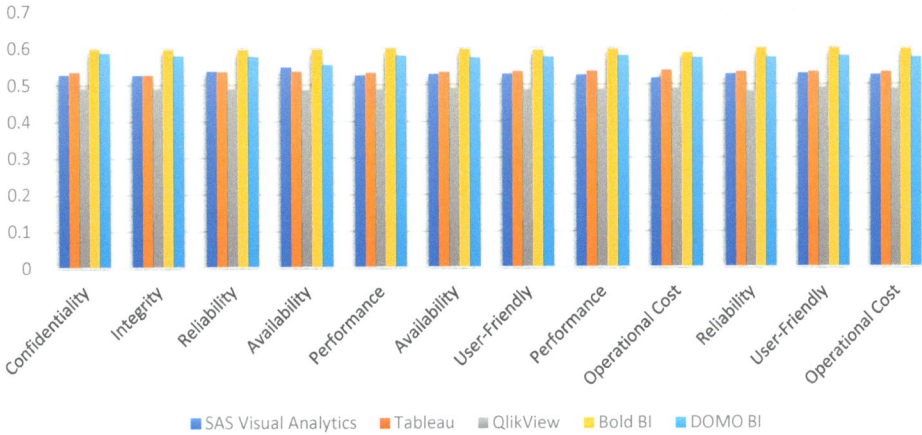

Figure 4. Sensitivity analysis in rankings when characteristics are varied from five percent.

4. Discussion

Our study proposed a novel approach to analyzing the trustworthiness of interactive visualization tools to assist healthcare experts in helping patients. After analyzing different tools for interactive visualization, we found the BoldBI visualization tool to fulfil the requirements of a trustworthy tool for patients as well as healthcare experts. To validate the results of this assessment, a comparative analysis was also performed with different methods of MCDM.

The use of a wide range of different methods of analysis can provide a conclusive means of determining whether or not the analyzed result and the projected method are superior. The author of this study has compared the results of the fuzzy ANP-COmplex PRoportional ASsessment (COPRAS) (Method 1), fuzzy ANP-VIekriterijumsko KOmpromisno Rangiranje (VIKOR) (Method 2), and fuzzy ANP-Elimination Et Choix Traduisant la Realité (ELECTRE) (Method 3) methodologies [2,6,9] with the results of the fuzzy ANP-TOPSIS technique to gauge the effectiveness of the proposed methodology. The results acquired through approaches such as fuzzy ANP-COPRAS, fuzzy ANP-VIKOR, and fuzzy ANP-ELECTRE are comparable to the results obtained through techniques such as fuzzy ANP-TOPSIS. The comparison is shown in a tabular representation in Table 8.

Table 8. Comparison with Other Methods.

S. No.	Visulization Applications	Method 0 (Proposed)	Method 1	Method 2	Method 3
1	SAS Visual Analytics	0.52652	0.52648	0.52365	0.52456
2	Tableau	0.53254	0.53025	0.53032	0.53789
3	QlikView	0.48525	0.48123	0.48456	0.48321
4	Bold BI	0.59547	0.59946	0.59778	0.59367
5	DOMO BI	0.57635	0.57526	0.57231	0.57149

It is clear, based on the information presented in Table 8, that the outcomes acquired by employing fuzzy ANP TOPSIS are more useful than the outcomes gained by employing any of the other methodologies. Therefore, using the hybrid method of fuzzy ANP-TOPSIS is more effective than using the other techniques to solve this particular problem. The trustworthiness of interactive visualization models was investigated and characterized by a number of different research projects. There has not been any quantitative research carried out on the impact of interactive visualization models' trustworthiness when used in fuzzy situations with a medical fuzzy expert system.

In addition, Spearman's correlation was tested using Equation (20) in order to determine whether or not there is a connection between the rankings that were produced utilizing the various approaches.

$$R = 1 - \frac{6 \sum d_i^2}{n(n^2 - 1)} \quad (20)$$

Here R denotes the Spearman's rank correlation coefficient, d is the difference between two ranks, and n denotes the total number of observations considered. The theoretical values of Spearman's ranking correlation coefficient run from +1 to 1. In this context, the sign indicates the nature of the link, whether it is positive or negative, and the value indicates the degree to which the association exists, as either strong, medium, or weak. The estimated values of the rank correlation coefficients calculated using Spearman's method, symbolized by the letter R, were 0.9736, 0.9845, and 0.9736 for Method 1, Method 2, and Method 3, respectively. It is possible to draw the conclusion that there is a significant positive link between the rankings produced by the two techniques (the suggested approach with Method 1, Method 2, and Method 3), since the value is extremely close to +1.

The visualization of medical data is no longer an option in the field of healthcare; rather, it is required for all contemporary medical institutions. It is anticipated that over the next six years, the global market for healthcare data analytics will expand by a factor of 3.5, growing from USD 11.5 billion in 2019 to USD 40.8 billion in 2025 [32]. The number of healthcare data that exist on the planet is staggering, and it will only continue to increase in the future. Not only has the collection and analysis of large numbers of healthcare data become crucial to diverse groups of experts working in fields such as economics, space research, and climate change, it has also become crucial to individuals and communities. This is because of the importance of the information that can be gleaned from healthcare data. Imaging as a visualization widget in medicine has the potential to identify and diagnose a wide variety of ailments, from cancer to heart issues, which has the potential to save the lives of millions of people. MRIs and CT scans are also quite effective, but the 2D images that are produced by these procedures require the examining physician to make certain assumptions in order to properly diagnose the patient's condition. Such types of visualization technology enable clinicians to build 3D images of MRI scans, which deliver crisper and higher-resolution photographs of blood vessels, organ tissues, and bones without the need for surgery. This results in significant savings in terms of both time and money.

5. Conclusions

Professionals and researchers have applied a wide range of techniques and strategies in order to build trustworthy and effective interactive visualizations. Their goal is to achieve this through the use of a variety of methods. A hybrid medical expert system is one of the best known of these technologies, and it plays an essential role. In this study, we investigated the trustworthiness of interactive visualization tools using the fuzzy ANP-TOPSIS method and ranked them accordingly. With the support of this methodology, researchers and developers will be able to design visualization tools that are more trustworthy. In spite of the results that we have obtained in this research work, there are other ways of making decisions that are based on a number of different methods (AHP, VIKOR, two-way fuzzy sets, etc.), and these other ways can be employed in order to achieve outcomes that are more productive. Further, the results of the empirical research that we conducted indicate that we have selected a method that is trustworthy for the purpose of this evaluation.

Funding: This research was supported by the Deanship of Scientific Research, Imam Mohammad Ibn Saud Islamic University, Saudi Arabia, grant no. 20-13-09-003.

Data Availability Statement: On reasonable request, the corresponding author will provide the information supporting the research study's conclusions.

Conflicts of Interest: The author declares no conflict of interest.

References

1. Javaid, M.; Haleem, A.; Vaishya, R.; Bahl, S.; Suman, R.; Vaish, A. Industry 4.0 technologies and their applications in fighting COVID-19 pandemic. *Diabetes Metab. Syndr. Clin. Res. Rev.* **2020**, *14*, 419–422. [CrossRef]
2. He, W.; Zhang, Z.; Li, W. Information technology solutions, challenges, and suggestions for tackling the COVID-19 pandemic. *Int. J. Inf. Manag.* **2021**, *57*, 102287. [CrossRef]
3. Adadi, A.; Berrada, M. Peeking Inside the Black-Box: A Survey on Explainable Artificial Intelligence (XAI). *IEEE Access* **2018**, *6*, 52138–52160. [CrossRef]
4. Murdoch, W.J.; Singh, C.; Kumbier, K.; Abbasi-Asl, R.; Yu, B. Interpretable machine learning: Definitions, methods, and applications. *Proc. Natl. Acad. Sci. USA* **2018**, *116*, 22071–22080. [CrossRef] [PubMed]
5. Ahuja, A.S. The impact of artificial intelligence in medicine on the future role of the physician. *PeerJ* **2019**, *7*, e7702. [CrossRef]
6. Stiglic, G.; Kocbek, P.; Fijacko, N.; Zitnik, M.; Verbert, K.; Cilar, L. Interpretability of machine learning-based prediction models in healthcare. *WIREs Data Min. Knowl. Discov.* **2020**, *10*, e1379. [CrossRef]
7. Available online: https://viso.ai/applications/computer-vision-in-healthcare/ (accessed on 12 April 2023).
8. Yamashita, R.; Nishio, M.; Do, R.K.G.; Togashi, K. Convolutional neural networks: An overview and application in radiology. *Insights Into Imaging* **2018**, *9*, 611–629. [CrossRef]
9. Mihajlovic, I. Everything you ever wanted to know about computer vision. *Preuzeto* **2019**, *31*, 2021.
10. Davenport, T.; Kalakota, R. The potential for artificial intelligence in healthcare. *Futur. Health J.* **2019**, *6*, 94. [CrossRef] [PubMed]
11. Seshadri, D.R.; Thom, M.L.; Harlow, E.R.; Gabbett, T.J.; Geletka, B.J.; Hsu, J.J.; Drummond, C.K.; Phelan, D.M.; Voos, J.E. Wearable Technology and Analytics as a Complementary Toolkit to Optimize Workload and to Reduce Injury Burden. *Front. Sports Act. Living* **2021**, *2*, 228. [CrossRef]
12. Vellido, A. The importance of interpretability and visualization in machine learning for applications in medicine and health care. *Neural Comput. Appl.* **2020**, *32*, 18069–18083. [CrossRef]
13. Dhillon, S.K.; Ganggayah, M.D.; Sinnadurai, S.; Lio, P.; Taib, N.A. Theory and Practice of Integrating Machine Learning and Conventional Statistics in Medical Data Analysis. *Diagnostics* **2022**, *12*, 2526. [CrossRef]
14. Zhang, G.; Atasoy, H.; Vasarhelyi, M.A. Continuous monitoring with machine learning and interactive data visuali-zation: An application to a healthcare payroll process. *Int. J. Account. Inf. Syst.* **2022**, *46*, 100570. [CrossRef]
15. Hoda, S.A.H.; Mondal, A.C. Studies on Multi-Criteria Decision-Making Based Healthcare Systems Using The Machine Learning. *J. Artif. Intell. Technol.* **2023**. [CrossRef]
16. Sacha, D.; Sedlmair, M.; Zhang, L.; Lee, J.A.; Weiskopf, D.; North, S.; Keim, D. Human-centered machine learning through interactive visualization. *Neurocomputing* **2017**, *268*, 164–175. [CrossRef]

17. Sarker, I.H. Machine Learning: Algorithms, Real-World Applications and Research Directions. *SN Comput. Sci.* **2021**, *2*, 160. [CrossRef] [PubMed]
18. Available online: https://www.tableau.com/en-gb/learn/articles/data-visualization (accessed on 5 April 2023).
19. Available online: https://www.b2binternational.com/2017/08/11/4-types-visualisations-role-play-market-research-process/ (accessed on 5 April 2023).
20. Mishra, P.; Pandey, C.; Singh, U.; Gupta, A. Scales of measurement and presentation of statistical data. *Ann. Card. Anaesth.* **2018**, *21*, 419. [CrossRef]
21. Dalati, S. Measurement and Measurement Scales. In *Modernizing the Academic Teaching and Research Environment: Methodologies and Cases in Business Research*; Springer: Berlin/Heidelberg, Germany, 2018; pp. 79–96.
22. Sharma, A.M. Data visualization. In *Data Science and Analytics*; Emerald Publishing Limited: Bingley, UK, 2020; pp. 1–22.
23. Grinstein, G.G.; Ward, M.O. Introduction to data visualization. In *Information Visualization in Data Mining and Knowledge Discovery*; Morgan Kaufmann: Burlington, MA, USA, 2002; Volume 1, pp. 21–45.
24. Thomas, J.; Harden, A. Methods for the thematic synthesis of qualitative research in systematic reviews. *BMC Med. Res. Methodol.* **2008**, *8*, 1–10. [CrossRef] [PubMed]
25. Sweet, S.A.; Grace-Martin, K.A. Modeling relationships of multiple variables with linear regression. In *Data Analysis with SPSS: A First Course in Applied Statistics*; Pearson: New York, NY, USA, 2012; pp. 161–188.
26. Xie, J.; Girshick, R.; Farhadi, A. Unsupervised deep embedding for clustering analysis. In Proceedings of the International Conference on Machine Learning, New York, NY, USA, 19–24 June 2016; pp. 478–487.
27. Ligthart, A.; Catal, C.; Tekinerdogan, B. Analyzing the effectiveness of semi-supervised learning approaches for opinion spam classification. *Appl. Soft Comput.* **2021**, *101*, 107023. [CrossRef]
28. Saaty, T.L. Decision making—The Analytic Hierarchy and Network Processes (AHP/ANP). *J. Syst. Sci. Syst. Eng.* **2004**, *13*, 1–35. [CrossRef]
29. Tavana, M.; Zandi, F.; Katehakis, M.N. A hybrid fuzzy group ANP–TOPSIS framework for assessment of e-government readiness from a CiRM perspective. *Inf. Manag.* **2013**, *50*, 383–397. [CrossRef]
30. Méndez-Durón, R. Do the allocation and quality of intellectual assets affect the reputation of open source software projects? *Inf. Manag.* **2013**, *50*, 357–368. [CrossRef]
31. Widianta, M.M.D.; Rizaldi, T.; Setyohadi, D.P.S.; Riskiawan, H.Y. Comparison of Multi-Criteria Decision Support Methods (AHP, TOPSIS, SAW & PROMENTHEE) for Employee Placement. *J. Phys. Conf. Ser.* **2018**, *953*, 012116. [CrossRef]
32. Available online: https://demigos.com/blog-post/healthcare-data-visualization/ (accessed on 4 April 2023).

Disclaimer/Publisher's Note: The statements, opinions and data contained in all publications are solely those of the individual author(s) and contributor(s) and not of MDPI and/or the editor(s). MDPI and/or the editor(s) disclaim responsibility for any injury to people or property resulting from any ideas, methods, instructions or products referred to in the content.

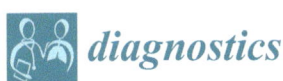

Article

Prediction of Acid-Base and Potassium Imbalances in Intensive Care Patients Using Machine Learning Techniques

Ratchakit Phetrittikun [1], Kerdkiat Suvirat [1], Kanakorn Horsiritham [2], Thammasin Ingviya [3,4] and Sitthichok Chaichulee [1,4,*]

[1] Department of Biomedical Sciences and Biomedical Engineering, Faculty of Medicine, Prince of Songkla University, Songkhla 90110, Thailand
[2] College of Digital Science, Prince of Songkla University, Songkhla 90110, Thailand
[3] Department of Family and Preventive Medicine, Faculty of Medicine, Prince of Songkla University, Songkhla 90110, Thailand
[4] Research Center for Medical Data Analytics, Faculty of Medicine, Prince of Songkla University, Songkhla 90110, Thailand
* Correspondence: sitthichok.c@psu.ac.th

Abstract: Acid–base disorders occur when the body's normal pH is out of balance. They can be caused by problems with kidney or respiratory function or by an excess of acids or bases that the body cannot properly eliminate. Acid–base and potassium imbalances are mechanistically linked because acid–base imbalances can alter the transport of potassium. Both acid–base and potassium imbalances are common in critically ill patients. This study investigated machine learning models for predicting the occurrence of acid–base and potassium imbalances in intensive care patients. We used an institutional dataset of 1089 patients with 87 variables, including vital signs, general appearance, and laboratory results. Gradient boosting (GB) was able to predict nine clinical conditions related to acid–base and potassium imbalances: mortality (AUROC = 0.9822), hypocapnia (AUROC = 0.7524), hypercapnia (AUROC = 0.8228), hypokalemia (AUROC = 0.9191), hyperkalemia (AUROC = 0.9565), respiratory acidosis (AUROC = 0.8125), respiratory alkalosis (AUROC = 0.7685), metabolic acidosis (AUROC = 0.8682), and metabolic alkalosis (AUROC = 0.8284). Some predictions remained relatively robust even when the prediction window was increased. Additionally, the decision-making process was made more interpretable and transparent through the use of SHAP analysis. Overall, the results suggest that machine learning could be a useful tool to gain insight into the condition of intensive care patients and assist in the management of acid–base and potassium imbalances.

Keywords: critical care; machine learning; acid–base balance; prediction; big data; health informatics

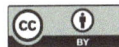

1. Introduction

Patients in intensive care units (ICUs) usually suffer from severe or life-threatening diseases and injuries [1]. Patients are provided with multiple life support systems to maintain their physiological functions. They are at high risk of clinical deterioration, which can occur frequently, abruptly, and without warning. Such problems need to be identified early and treated immediately. They require attentive and specific care with state-of-the-art diagnostic and curative technologies to ensure their normal body function.

Acid–base balance refers to the balance of acidity and alkalinity in the human body [2]. Carbon dioxide (CO_2) is crucial for acid–base balance in the body [3]. Patients may have a variety of conditions that can affect carbon dioxide balance, including respiratory disorders, renal dysfunction, and certain medications. Carbon dioxide balance is maintained by a delicate balance between the body's production of carbon dioxide and its removal by a respiratory and renal systems. The respiratory system removes carbon dioxide through breathing, while the kidneys regulate carbon dioxide levels by controlling the excretion of bicarbonate through the urine. Proper carbon dioxide balance is important. Excess carbon dioxide in the blood (hypercapnia) can lead to acidosis. On the other hand, a lack of carbon dioxide in the blood (hypocapnia) can lead to alkalosis. In the ICU, carbon dioxide balance is carefully monitored to ensure that patients are receiving the appropriate level of ventilation and that their kidneys are functioning properly. If an imbalance is detected, medical intervention may be needed to correct it. This may include administering oxygen or mechanical ventilation to assist breathing, or administering medications to regulate carbon dioxide levels.

Acid–base status is a key factor in understanding the physiological changes occurring in critically ill patients, as well as in making diagnoses, developing treatment plans, and monitoring progress [4]. Acid–base imbalance is a deviation from the usual balance of acids and bases in the body that causes the plasma pH to deviate from its normal range [2]. The balance of acids and bases in the body is tightly regulated because even tiny deviations from the normal range can have serious consequences for numerous organs, some of which are life-threatening. The body regulates the acid–base balance of the blood through various processes, such as the lungs (change in respiratory rate), the kidneys (excretion of excess acid or base), and buffer systems (use of bicarbonate, ammonia, proteins, and phosphate) [5]. An excess of acid is called acidosis, while an excess of base is called alkalosis. The process causing the imbalance is classified according to the source of the disturbance (respiration or metabolism) and the direction of the pH change. This results in the four main processes: respiratory acidosis, respiratory alkalosis, metabolic acidosis, and metabolic alkalosis. Metabolic acidosis and metabolic alkalosis can occur due to an imbalance in the production and excretion of acids and bases by the kidneys, while respiratory acidosis and respiratory alkalosis are caused by changes in carbon dioxide exhalation due to lung or respiratory disease. Patients may experience multiple acid–base disturbances. To determine a patient's acid–base balance, the physician needs to monitor the pH and the levels of carbon dioxide and bicarbonate in the blood. When an acid–base imbalance occurs, the body automatically attempts to compensate and restore the blood pH to normal through the respiratory and metabolic systems [2]. If the blood pH has changed significantly, this may indicate that the body's ability to adapt is failing and further investigation and treatment of the underlying cause of the acid–base disorder is needed.

Over half of the body's weight is made up of water. Electrolytes are minerals that carry an electric charge when they are dissolved in a liquid such as blood [6]. The kidneys help maintain electrolyte concentrations by filtering electrolytes and water from blood, returning some to the blood, and excreting any excess into the urine. Potassium is one of the electrolytes in the human body needed for the normal functioning of cells, neurons, and muscles. The body must maintain blood potassium levels within a certain range. High (hyperkalemia) or low (hypokalemia) levels of potassium in the blood can have disastrous consequences, such as cardiac arrhythmias or even cardiac arrest. The body can use the large reserves of potassium in the cells to keep blood potassium levels constant. Healthy kidneys can adjust potassium excretion to match fluctuations in potassium intake. Some medications and diseases can interfere with the transport of potassium, significantly affecting blood potassium levels. The interaction between acid–base and potassium balance involves transcellular cation exchange as well as changes in kidney function [7]. An imbalance in acid–base balance can lead to shifts in the transport of potassium into and out of cells [5]. This is particularly evident in metabolic acidosis, metabolic alkalosis, and, to a lesser extent, respiratory acid–base disorders. Hyperkalemia and hypokalemia can be detected during a routine blood test or when a physician detects certain abnormalities in an electrocardiogram. Physicians may assess the amount of potassium excreted in the urine or look for signs of diabetes, acidosis, or kidney disorders.

Generally, patients admitted to the ICU are evaluated based on clinical, pathological, and physiological data. They may experience worsening of symptoms or complications due to conditions such as heart failure. Often, the patient's worsening condition and dysfunction is not directly indicated, resulting in a delay in assessing the patient's risk and response to changes in the patient's condition. This can lead to more severe disease and loss of life. Timely treatment is therefore essential. Therefore, early detection can help patients have a better chance of survival. It can also reduce the use of medical resources.

Early detection of critical clinical conditions can lead to better health outcomes and lower healthcare costs [8]. Early warning scores (EWS) have been used to assess and determine a patient's severity based on clinical parameters routinely collected during an ICU stay [9]. Examples include Acute Physiology and Chronic Health Evaluation (APACHE) [10], Simplified Acute Physiology Score (SAPS) [11], Modified Early Warning Score (MEWS) [9], and National Early Warning Score (NEWS) [12]. These EWS scores employ pathological data, physiological data, and patient responses for calculation. They alert clinical staff when a patient's severity falls into the abnormality range, prompting them to immediately attend to the patient and plan treatment. However, most assessment tools were originally developed for manual bedside calculation. As electronic health records (EHRs) become ubiquitous, these tools are now closely integrated with modern EHRs. This allows scores to be calculated automatically based on patient data in EHRs. This makes patient care more convenient, faster, and more timely.

Machine learning has been shown to be able to find relationships in medical data that change over time with different patient conditions [13]. With patient data available in EHRs and real-time vital signs at the bedside, such as patient personal data (gender, age, and underlying disease), treatment history, physiological data, and laboratory results, it could be possible to develop an algorithm to determine the relationship between dynamic medical data and critical patient conditions by examining the relationships that occur around the patient at a critical time [14]. This could lead to modern data-driven EWS development that could be more accurate, specific, and real-time. It could also help physicians make informed decisions, making the process of patient care safer.

Many studies have shown that machine learning can predict or classify the clinical condition and clinical outcomes in intensive care patients [15–29]. For early prediction of sepsis, Kam et al. [15] developed a long short-term memory (LSTM) model, a deep learning model that incorporates past information, for early detection of systemic inflammatory response syndrome (SIRS) conditions that could lead to sepsis. Nemati et al. [16] developed a modified Weibull–Cox proportional hazards model for sepsis detection using data from EHR and high-resolution bedside monitoring. Zhang et al. [17] developed an LSTM model to predict sepsis using data (demographics, vital signs, laboratory values, and nutrition) from over 10,000 individual patients. Although these studies examined similar outcomes, the results cannot be compared because they used different datasets, and the definition of the outcomes was also different. Several studies investigated other critical clinical conditions. Kwon et al. [18] developed a deep learning algorithm for in-hospital cardiac arrest prediction. Tomasev et al. [19] developed a recurrent neural network model for continuous prediction of acute kidney injury. Wanyan et al. [20] developed a recurrent neural network model with contrastive loss to predict mortality, intubation, and ICU transfer in hospitalized COVID-19 patients. More recently, some studies employed more comprehensive clinical data and examined less critical clinical events. Lee et al. [21] used an autoregressive event time series model to predict the future occurrence of clinical events defined as drug administration, laboratory orders, medical procedures, and physiological measurements. Their model consists of three mechanisms with LSTM to process information from the distant past, a linear transformation model module to process recent information, and a probabilistic model to process periodicity. Their model can handle complex multivariate temporal time series of ICU data. Kaji et al. [22] trained LSTM to predict sepsis, myocardial infarction, and vancomycin antibiotic administration. Recently, some studies have begun to examine specific clinical conditions, such as hypocapnia [25], hypokalemia [27], hyperkalemia [28], and acid–base disturbances [29], but did not utilize time-series data. Many of the studies showed promising results with high performance measures, which can be further investigated in the clinic.

Although prediction by machine learning has the chance to improve the patient's health status, the problem with the reliability of the predictions is that they are not reliable for physicians because they are not interpretable. The problem can be addressed by applying an explanatory tool to the model so that it can provide the meaning of each predicted parameter (such as pulse, respiratory rate, and creatinine) for the prediction of critical illness (such as sepsis, acute kidney injury, acute lung injury). Current research trends address the use of interpretable machine learning models that can incorporate comprehensive and past information for early prediction of important clinical conditions, which could lead to early intervention, which in turn could lead to better patient outcomes.

Currently, machine learning development in the ICU is largely focused on predicting key outcomes, such as mortality, length of stay, and sepsis [15–17,22–24]. In other areas, such as acid–base disturbances and potassium imbalances, there are significant gaps that remain to be explored [25–29]. The acid–base and electrolyte balance is essential for the optimal functioning of physiological processes and cells, and an imbalance is often the result of an underlying disease and can have negative effects on clinical outcomes. Determining and, if possible, predicting the acid–base status of patients and using this information to control or regulate the balance can be beneficial in managing underlying diseases. The aim of this study is to investigate machine learning models to predict the occurrence of acid–base and potassium imbalances in intensive care patients. We used comprehensive patient data from Songklanagarind Hospital in Thailand. We employed 87 clinical predictors, including vital signs, general patient appearance, and laboratory measurements (chemistry labs, hematology labs, microscopy labs, and arterial blood gases).

2. Materials and Methods

2.1. Dataset

This study involved the de-identified data extracted from the EHR of Songklanagarind Hospital in Thailand. We used the vital signs, general appearance, and laboratory results of patients admitted to the hospital from August 2019 to April 2022 who spent at least 24 h in the medical intensive care unit (MICU). Our laboratory results involved blood chemistry tests, hematology tests, microbiology tests, and arterial blood gases. We included only the first MICU visit and excluded subsequent visits. We excluded patients in whom the duration of recorded vital signs and laboratory tests was less than 24 h and patients in whom all four laboratory tests were not examined during their ICU stay. Our dataset included 1089 patients with 1137 hospital admissions. Table 1 shows the characteristics of the patients in our dataset. Our study was approved by the Office of Human Research Ethics Committee, Faculty of Medicine, Prince of Songkla University (REC. 63-541-25-2).

Table 1. Dataset characteristics.

Characteristics	
Number of patients	1089
Number of admissions	1137
Age [1]	63.8 (18.1)
Gender	
Male [2]	602 (55.3%)
Female [2]	487 (44.7%)
Length of hospital stay [1]	27.2 (27.5)
Length of ICU stay [1]	7.0 (8.0)

[1] Values in Mean (S.D.); [2] Values in N (%).

2.2. Clinical Variables

In this study, we used vital signs, general appearance of the patient, and laboratory measurements as predictors. Vital signs and general appearance represent the important body functions of the patient. They are frequently monitored and carefully recorded in the EHR. Laboratory results are often used to predict the patient's current clinical condition.

We considered blood chemistry tests, hematology tests, microbiology tests, and blood gas tests. We selected only those variables for which there was an average of at least one measurement per day, calculated from the days patients spent in the MICU, for all patients. This resulted in a total of 87 variables. Figure 1 contains a list of all clinical variables considered in our study.

Vital signs (N=6)	Chemistry labs [Blood] (N=18)	Hematology labs [Blood] (N=32)	Microscopy labs [Urine] (N=13)	Arterial blood gases [Blood] (N=14)
Temperature (Temp)	Albumin (ALB)	Atypical lymphocyte (Atypl)	Bilirubin*	Respiratory mode*
Pulse rate (PR)	Alkaline phosphatase (ALP)	Band	Character*	pH
Respiratory rate (RR)	Alanine transaminase (ALT, SGPT)	Basophil (Baso)	Clarity*	Partial pressure of oxygen (pO2)
Oxygen saturation (SpO2)	Aspartate transaminase (AST, SGOT)	Complete blood count (CBC)	Color*	Partial pressure of carbon dioxide (pCO2)
Systolic blood pressure (SBP)	Blood urea nitrogen (BUN)	Eosinophil (Eos)	Hematuria*	Total concentration of carbon dioxide (ctCO2)
Diastolic blood pressure (DBP)	Calcium (CA)	Fibrinogen (Fib)	Glucose*	Actual base excess (ABE)
	Creatinine (CREAT)	Hemoglobin (Hb)	Ketone*	Standard base excess (SBE)
General appearance (N=4)	Chloride (Cl)	Hematocrit (Hct)	Leucocyte*	Oxygen saturation (sO2)
Pain value*	Globulin (GLOB)	Lymphocyte (Lymp)	Nitrite*	Bicarbonate concentration (cHCO3)
Sedation status*	Potassium (K)	Mean corpuscular hemoglobin (MCH)	Protein*	Potassium concentration (cK)
Oxygen supplement*	Sodium (Na)	Mean corpuscular hemoglobin concentration (MCHC)	Specific gravity (Sp. Gravi)	Sodium concentration (cNa)
Conciousness*	Phosphate (PHOS)	Mean corpuscular volume (MCV)	Urobilino*	Calcium concentration (cCa)
* Categorical variables	Total carbon dioxide (TCO2)	Mean platelet volume (MPV)	pH	Lactate concentration (cLac)
	Total protein (TP)	Erythrocyte distribution width (RDW)		Chloride concentration (cCl)
	Direct bilirubin (D-Bili)	Metamyelocytes (Meta)	Platelet blood smear (PLT smear)	Activated partial thromboplastin time (aPTT)
	Total bilirubin (T-Bili)	Monocyte (Mono)	Platelet count (PLT)	Activated partial thromboplastin time (aPTT) ratio
	eGFR by MDRD formula^ (eGFR-EP)	Myelocytes (Myelo)	Reticulocyte count (Retic)	Activated partial thromboplastin time (aPTT) control
	eGFR by CKD-EPI formula^ (eGFR-MD)	Nucleated red blood cells (NRBC)	Red blood cell (RBC) count	Prothrombin time (PT)
	^ eGFR: Estimated glomerular filtration rate	Polymorphonuclear (PMN)	White blood cell (WBC) count	Prothrombin time (PT) INR
		Toxic granulation	Corrected white blood cell (WBC) count	Prothrombin time (PT) control

Figure 1. Clinical variables in our dataset.

2.3. Clinical Conditions

Our study aims to predict clinical conditions that are common in intensive care patients so that early intervention can help improve patient outcomes. We identified 9 clinical conditions that occur in patients in our dataset: mortality, hypocapnia, hypercapnia, hypokalemia, hyperkalemia, metabolic acidosis, metabolic alkalosis, respiratory acidosis, and respiratory alkalosis. The criteria for hypocapnia and hypercapnia were defined according to Laserna et al. [30]. For hypokalemia and hyperkalemia, the European Resuscitation Council Guidelines for Resuscitation 2010 were used [31]. Regarding acid–base balance disorders, our study used the physiological approach according to Berend et al. [32] and Constable et al. [33]. Table 2 shows the criteria of each clinical condition.

Table 2. Criteria and statistics of clinical conditions.

Clinical Condition	Criteria	Admissions with Condition
Mortality	Death during ICU stay	213 (18.7%)
Hypocapnia	$pCO_2 < 35$ mmHg	360 (31.7%)
Hypercapnia	$pCO_2 > 45$ mmHg	296 (26.0%)
Hypokalemia	$K^+ < 3.5$ mmol/L	598 (52.6%)
Hyperkalemia	$K^+ > 5.5$ mmol/L	83 (7.3%)
Metabolic Acidosis	$pH < 7.35$, and $cHCO_3^- < 22$ mmol/L	202 (17.8%)
Metabolic Alkalosis	$pH > 7.45$, and $cHCO_3^- > 26$ mmol/L	430 (37.8%)
Respiratory Acidosis	$pH < 7.35$, and $pCO_2 > 45$ mmHg	258 (22.7%)
Respiratory Alkalosis	$pH > 7.45$, and $pCO_2 < 35$ mmHg	397 (34.9%)

2.3.1. Mortality

Mortality is defined as the patient's death while in the ICU. Mortality is a common prediction target and can serve as a benchmark for the algorithm. It is strongly associated with clinical variables in the EHR.

2.3.2. Hypocapnia and Hypercapnia

Hypocapnia is present when a pCO_2 level is less than 35 mmHg, while hypercapnia is present when a pCO_2 level is more than 45 mmHg [30]. They may lead to an acid–base imbalance. Low carbon dioxide levels lead to a decrease in the hydrogen ion concentration in the blood, making the pH more basic. On the other hand, high carbon dioxide levels lead to an increase in the hydrogen ion concentration in the blood, making the pH more acidic. Patients may complain of lethargy, mild headache, shortness of breath, nausea, hyperventilation or hypoventilation, or fatigue [34].

2.3.3. Hypokalemia and Hyperkalemia

More than 20 % of hospitalized patients were found to have hypokalemia, i.e., a K^+ of less than 3.5 mmol/L [31]. With lower serum potassium levels, there is a risk of muscle necrosis, which can develop into paralysis, with deterioration of respiratory function and an increase in cardiac arrhythmias [35].

Hyperkalemia can be life-threatening, especially in patients with chronic kidney disease (CKD), diabetes mellitus, or heart failure. Hyperkalemia is often caused by stress, illness, or dehydration. A K^+ of greater than 5.5 mmol/L is recommended as a threshold for treatment of hyperkalemia [31].

2.3.4. Metabolic Acidosis and Metabolic Alkalosis

Metabolic acidosis is present when there is a $cHCO_3^-$ of <22 mmol/L and a pH of <7.35 [32,33]. Patients with metabolic acidosis can have serious consequences for cellular function and an increased risk of disease and death.

Compensatory hypoventilation in critically ill patients may lead to hypoxia or pulmonary infection. Failure of the right compensatory ventilation results in an increase in pCO_2 that precipitates metabolic alkalosis, the criteria for which are a $cHCO_3^-$ of >26 mmol/L and a pH of >7.45 [36].

2.3.5. Respiratory Acidosis and Respiratory Alkalosis

Respiratory acidosis often occurs when the lungs are unable to remove all carbon dioxide produced by the body. It affects approximately 25% of patients with chronic respiratory failure. Patients with respiratory acidosis have a pH of <7.35 and a pCO_2 of >45 mmHg [32,33]. Respiratory acidosis is associated with a higher risk of mortality and a greater need for intubation [37].

Respiratory alkalosis is often caused by hyperventilation which most commonly occurs in response to hypoxia, metabolic acidosis, increased metabolic demands, and pain. The criteria for respiratory alkalosis are a pCO_2 of <35 mmHg and a pH of >7.45 [32,33].

2.3.6. Annotation of Clinical Conditions

We used laboratory measurements, i.e., blood chemistry and arterial blood gas values, to identify clinical conditions. We considered only the first occurrence of the same clinical condition for each admission. All clinical conditions were annotated using variable values in the EHR data without physician involvement. We considered the time of occurrence of a clinical condition to be the time when the associated laboratory values met the criteria. Table 2 shows the number of admissions with presence of each clinical condition identified in our dataset.

2.4. Data Preparation

This study used the vital signs and laboratory results around patients admitted into the ICU. These data were mixed between numerical and text values. We converted the numerical values of the same variable into the same scale. We encoded all discrete and text values into categories. For each patient and variable, a time series with a fixed 15 min interval was created and filled with measurements taken during the associated time interval. The 15 min interval was chosen as our sampling period based on the observation that vital signs and general appearance factors can be collected as frequently as every 15 min. If we had chosen a larger interval, our machine learning models may have lost the ability to learn about the temporal dynamics of clinical data. If we had chosen a smaller interval, the number of observations would have been too high. Missing values were filled using the fill-forward method, from the last observation to the next values, taking into account all vital signs and laboratory measurements obtained before admission to the MICU but during the same hospital stay. This was performed to avoid sparse time series that could lead to poor results. Figure 2 shows examples of time series for one patient, which illustrate the fluctuating character of data in intensive care patients.

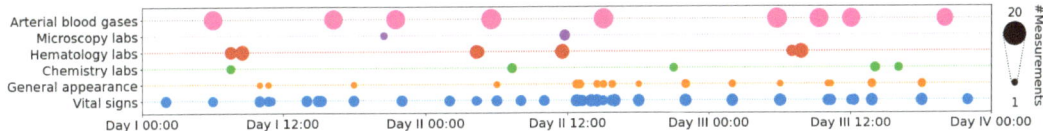

Figure 2. Illustration of our sequential clinical data randomly selected from a patient in the dataset during their 72 h stay in the ICU. The graph shows how often the clinical variables were measured, with more measurements during the day than at night.

2.5. Machine Learning Models

Our problem was cast as binary classification. We used a 12 h observation window. This was not a problem in patients who had recently been transferred to the ICU because the values of the clinical variables had been carried forward since the beginning of their stay when they were in other units. We investigated the performance of machine learning algorithms for predicting each clinical condition $T_P = \{1, 2, 4\}$ hours before its occurrence.

For each clinical condition, patients in whom the clinical condition occurred during their stay in the ICU were assigned to the positive group, whereas patients in whom the clinical condition did not occur were assigned to the negative group. For the positive group, we extracted the clinical signals in a 12 h observation window T_P hours before the onset of the clinical condition. For the negative groups, we extracted a 12 h observation window from the clinical signals at random for each patient (see Figure 3).

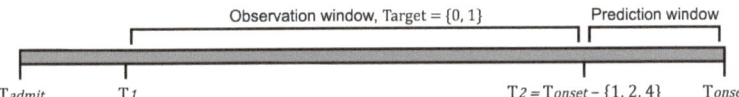

Figure 3. Diagram of our predictive tasks. The data in the observation window between T_1 and T_2 were used to predict the clinical condition occurring at time T_{onset}. For the positive sequences, the time of onset corresponded to the time of occurrence of the clinical condition. For the negative sequences, the time of onset was randomly chosen within the admission.

Regarding the evaluation procedures, our dataset included 1089 patients with 1137 admissions. A model received time-varying vital signs and laboratory results as inputs and generated the probability risk for each clinical condition between 0 and 1. We addressed data imbalance by performing sample weighting during the training of an algorithm.

We investigated four discriminative algorithms: *K* Nearest Neighbours (KNN), Support Vector Machine (SVM), Random Forest (RF), and Gradient Boosting (GB). Our goal was to explore simple but powerful classifiers that can be implemented at the edges. We conducted all experiments using the Python programming language and utilized SQL for retrieving all data from the database. We used the Scikit-learn (v.1.1.1), SHAP (v.0.41.0), Pandas (v.1.4.2), Numpy (v.1.21.6), and Matplotlib (v.3.5.2) frameworks.

2.5.1. K Nearest Neighbours

KNN is a versatile algorithm that works by finding the *K* closest data points to a given query point and uses the majority class of these data points as a prediction for the query point. With regards to hyperparameter optimization, we examined different numbers of neighbors ({3, 5, 7, 9}) and different weight functions (uniform and distance weights).

2.5.2. Random Forests

RF is a collection of decision trees, where each tree is trained on a randomly selected subset of the training data. The predictions of each tree are then combined to make a final prediction by considering the majority of votes. Random Forest can reduce overfitting, which is a common problem with decision trees, by training each tree on a different subset of the training data. RF can handle high-dimensional large data because it is inherently parallel. The weight associated with each leaf node reflects the importance of the variables. With regards to hyperparameter optimization, we examineddifferent numbers of trees in the forest (200, 400, 600) and maximum depth of the trees ({4, 8, 12, 16}).

2.5.3. Support Vector Machine

SVM is an algorithm that aims to find the hyperplane that maximally separates the different classes. SVM uses the kernel trick to transform the data into a higher dimensional space. The algorithm can effectively handle complex relationships in high-dimensional spaces between the features and the target with with high accuracy and reproducibility. For hyperparameter optimization, we examined different kernel types of trees in the forest (polynomial and radial basis function) and different regularization parameters (C parameter) ({1, 10, 100, 1000}).

2.5.4. Gradient Boosting

GB is an ensemble method in which a sequence of weak learners is trained, with each successive learner trained to correct the errors of the previous learner. The final prediction is produced by combining the predictions of all individual learners. GB is able to handle missing values, outliers, and a large number of features and is resistant to overfitting. Unlike SVM, GB can automatically learn nonlinear complex relationships in the data without explicit mapping. GB has achieved state-of-the-art results on many machine learning tasks. For hyperparameter optimization, we examined different numbers of boosting stages ({100, 200, 400}) and maximum depth of the tree ({4, 8, 12}).

2.6. Evaluation Metrics

A true positive (TP) is when a model correctly identifies a positive class; a true negative (TN) is when a model correctly identifies a negative class; a false positive (FP) is when the model incorrectly identifies a negative class, and a false negative (FN) is when the model incorrectly identifies a positive class. Sensitivity or recall represents the proportion of actual positives that are correctly predicted:

$$\text{Sensitivity or Recall} = \frac{TP}{TP + FN}. \qquad (1)$$

Specificity represents the proportion of actual negatives that are correctly predicted:

$$\text{Specificity} = \frac{TN}{TN + FP}. \qquad (2)$$

Precision represents the proportion of positive predictions that are actually correct:

$$\text{Precision} = \frac{TP}{TP + FP}. \qquad (3)$$

F1 score is a harmonic mean of precision and recall and represents a single metric that indicates how well a model finds relevant results:

$$F_1 \text{ Score} = \frac{2TP}{2TP + FP + FN}. \qquad (4)$$

A receiver operating characteristic (ROC) curve is a graphical representation that shows the trade-off between sensitivity and specificity by varying the classification threshold. A precision recall (PR) curve is similar to an ROC curve, but it shows the trade-off between precision and recall by varying the classification threshold. The PR curve is useful for evaluating the performance of a classifier when the class distribution is imbalanced (meaning that one class is significantly more prevalent than the other). Both the ROC curve and the PR curve are commonly used to evaluate the performance of binary classifiers. The area under the ROC curve (AUROC) and the area under the PR curve (AUPRC) are common metrics that can be used to evaluate the overall performance of a model.

Our study considers not only predictions but also understandable explanations. We used Shapley values [38] to determine how much each of the clinical features contributed to the prediction.

3. Results

The present study utilized clinical data from 1089 patients, encompassing 1137 admissions to the intensive care unit (ICU). A total of 87 clinical variables were considered, including vital signs, general appearance, chemical laboratories, hematology laboratories, microscopic labs, and arterial blood gases. The objective of the study was to predict nine clinical conditions: mortality, hypocapnia, hypercapnia, hypokalemia, hyperkalemia, metabolic acidosis, metabolic alkalosis, respiratory acidosis, and respiratory alkalosis. Although we used time series with a fixed 15 min interval as input, predictions can be made as the data come in, but the data must be formatted in time series with a fixed 15 min interval.

The results of the classification algorithms in predicting clinical conditions on the test set are presented in Table 3. The evaluation was conducted using a 12 h observation window and a 1 h prediction window, and the aim was to predict whether a clinical condition would occur within the subsequent hour. Precision, sensitivity (recall), specificity, and F1 score were calculated using the threshold that yielded the highest F1 score in the validation set.

We present both AUROC and AUPRC because the number of positive cases for each clinical condition varied. The former metric, AUROC, aims to minimize false negatives, while the latter metric, AUPRC, aims to minimize false positives. Based on the results presented in Table 3, the GB algorithm performed better than the other algorithms in 7 out of 9 clinical conditions: mortality (AUROC = 0.9822), hypocapnia (AUROC = 0.7524), hypokalemia (AUROC = 0.9191), hyperkalemia (AUROC = 0.9565), respiratory acidosis (AUROC = 0.8125), respiratory alkalosis (AUROC = 0.7685), and metabolic alkalosis (AUROC = 0.8284). The RF algorithm slightly outperformed GB in the remaining two clinical conditions: hypercapnia (AUROC = 0.8228) and metabolic acidosis (AUROC = 0.8682). The KNN algorithm was not effective in predicting any of the clinical conditions. The SVM algorithm performed competitively, but its performance did not surpass those of GB and RF. The clinical conditions that demonstrated the highest scores were mortality (AUROC = 0.9822 and AUPRC = 0.8557) and hypokalemia (AUROC = 0.9191 and AUPRC = 0.9455). In terms of predicting acid–base imbalances, the performance of the algorithms was similar, with AUROCs ranging between 0.7685 and 0.8699 and AUPRCs ranging between 0.5945 and 0.7150. Figure 4 shows the ROC curves compared for different classification algorithms for each clinical condition. Figure S1 shows the graphical comparison of F1 Score, AUROC, and AUPRC across different algorithms for each clinical condition.

Both precision and recall are important measurements because they provide different insights into the performance of a model. In some applications, a high recall rate may be more crucial in order to minimize the number of false-negative results, such as in screening tests. Conversely, a high precision rate may be more critical in applications where the cost of false-positive results is high, such as in diagnostic tests. The F1 score is a single metric that provides a balance between precision and recall and is less affected by imbalanced data. We used the decision threshold that gives the highest F1 score in the training set as the threshold for the test set to obtain precision, sensitivity, specificity, and F1 score. The clinical condition with the highest F1 score is hypokalemia (F1 = 0.8691), followed by mortality (F1 = 0.8101) and hypocapnia (F1 = 0.7115), respectively. Our F1 scores are in line with their AUROCs and AUPRC scores.

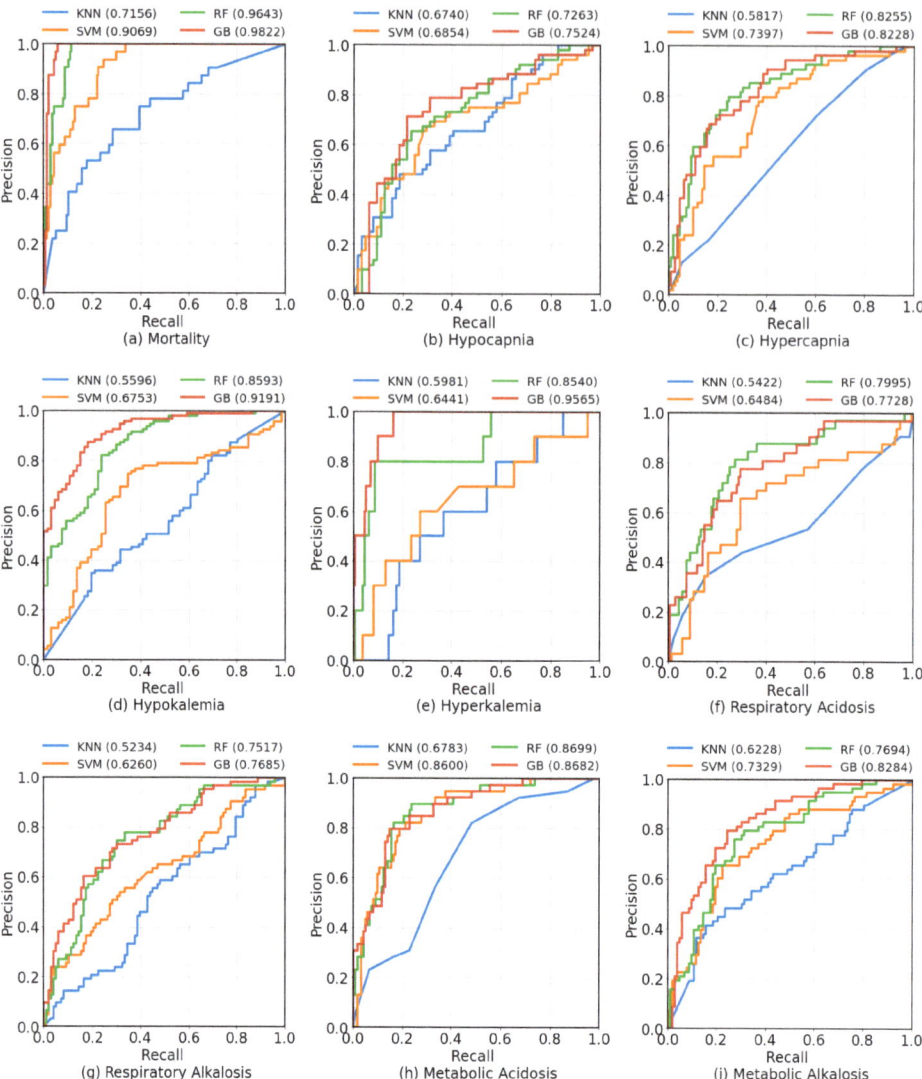

Figure 4. The ROC curves compare different algorithms for each target clinical condition. GB outperformed the other algorithms in most cases. There was a small number of positive cases for hyperkalemia.

Table 3. Performance for the next-hour prediction on each clinical condition on the test set.

Clinical Condition	N_1/N_0	Algorithm	Precision	Sensitivity	Specificity	F1 Score	AUROC	AUPRC
Mortality	213/924	K Nearest Neighbours	0.3333	0.5625	0.7410	0.4186	0.7156	0.4347
		Support Vector Machine	0.4746	0.8750	0.7770	0.6154	0.9069	0.6796
		Random Forests	0.6154	**1.000**	0.8561	0.7619	0.9643	0.8378
		Gradient Boosting	**0.6809**	**1.000**	**0.8921**	**0.8101**	**0.9822**	**0.8557**
Hypocapnia	360/777	K Nearest Neighbours	0.5484	0.6538	0.5625	0.5965	0.674	0.6353
		Support Vector Machine	0.6471	0.6346	0.7188	0.6408	0.6854	0.6282
		Random Forests	0.6429	0.6923	0.6875	0.6667	0.7263	0.615
		Gradient Boosting	**0.7115**	**0.7115**	**0.7656**	**0.7115**	**0.7524**	**0.6442**
Hypercapnia	296/841	K Nearest Neighbours	0.381	0.4444	0.6422	0.4103	0.5817	0.4107
		Support Vector Machine	0.5063	0.7407	0.6422	0.6015	0.7397	0.5382
		Random Forests	**0.6056**	**0.7963**	**0.7431**	**0.6880**	0.8255	**0.7036**
		Gradient Boosting	0.5909	0.7222	0.7523	0.6500	0.8228	0.6731
Hypokalemia	598/539	K Nearest Neighbours	0.6067	0.5684	0.4697	0.5870	0.5596	0.6779
		Support Vector Machine	0.75	0.7263	0.6515	0.738	0.6753	0.7359
		Random Forests	0.8061	0.8316	0.7121	0.8187	0.8593	0.8971
		Gradient Boosting	**0.8646**	**0.8737**	**0.8030**	**0.8691**	**0.9191**	**0.9455**
Hyperkalemia	83/1054	K Nearest Neighbours	0.0909	0.6000	0.6273	0.1579	0.5981	0.0714
		Support Vector Machine	0.0921	0.7000	0.5714	0.1628	0.6441	0.0981
		Random Forests	0.1600	0.8000	0.7391	0.2667	0.854	0.3053
		Gradient Boosting	**0.2083**	**1.0000**	**0.7640**	**0.3448**	**0.9565**	**0.6497**
Respiratory Acidosis	202/935	K Nearest Neighbours	0.2545	0.4375	0.6963	0.3218	0.5422	0.2938
		Support Vector Machine	0.3182	0.6562	0.6667	0.4286	0.6484	0.2797
		Random Forests	**0.4237**	**0.7812**	**0.7481**	**0.5495**	0.7995	0.5324
		Gradient Boosting	0.4068	0.7500	0.7407	0.5275	**0.8125**	**0.5945**
Respiratory Alkalosis	430/707	K Nearest Neighbours	0.4405	0.5873	0.5204	0.5034	0.5234	0.4175
		Support Vector Machine	0.4815	0.6190	0.5714	0.5417	0.6260	0.5335
		Random Forests	**0.6269**	0.6667	**0.7449**	0.6462	0.7517	0.6265
		Gradient Boosting	0.6081	**0.7143**	0.7041	**0.6569**	**0.7685**	**0.6924**
Metabolic Acidosis	258/879	K Nearest Neighbours	0.3492	0.5641	0.6639	0.4314	0.6783	0.4081
		Support Vector Machine	0.4648	0.8462	0.6885	0.6000	0.8600	0.5921
		Random Forests	**0.5385**	**0.8974**	0.7541	**0.6731**	**0.8699**	0.6870
		Gradient Boosting	0.5333	0.8205	**0.7705**	0.6465	0.8682	**0.7150**
Metabolic Alkalosis	397/740	K Nearest Neighbours	0.4583	0.5690	0.6176	0.5077	0.6228	0.5258
		Support Vector Machine	0.5846	0.6552	0.7353	0.6179	0.7329	0.6153
		Random Forests	0.5946	0.7586	0.7059	0.6667	0.7694	0.6143
		Gradient Boosting	**0.6389**	**0.7931**	**0.7451**	**0.7077**	**0.8284**	**0.6719**

Bold texts highlight the highest scores in each metric for each clinical condition. N_1 represents the number of samples with positive outcomes. N_0 represents the number of samples with positive outcomes. (Total = 1137).

Table 4 shows the predictive performance of GB at different prediction windows ($T_P = \{1,2,4,8\}$) on the test set. The performance of the prediction algorithm decreased as the gap between the prediction and the onset increased. This was expected and due to the fact that the further into the future the prediction was made, the more uncertainty there was about the outcome. Figure S2 shows the graphical comparison of F1 Score, AUROC, and AUPRC across different early prediction periods for each clinical condition.

Figure 5 presents ROC curves at different early prediction periods ($T_P = \{1,2,4,8\}$ h before onset). These ROC curves illustrate how the performance of the GB classifier changes as the prediction window increases. It appears that some clinical conditions were more robust towards early prediction than others as the performance of the classifier was relatively stable as the prediction window increased. Based on the results presented in Table 4, small decreases in AUROC and AUPRC (less than 0.05) were observed in the clinical conditions of mortality, hypocapnia, metabolic acidosis, and metabolic alkalosis when the prediction window was extended from 1 to 8 h. However, large decreases were observed in the clinical conditions of hypercapnia, hypokalemia, hyperkalemia, respiratory acidosis, and respiratory alkalosis.

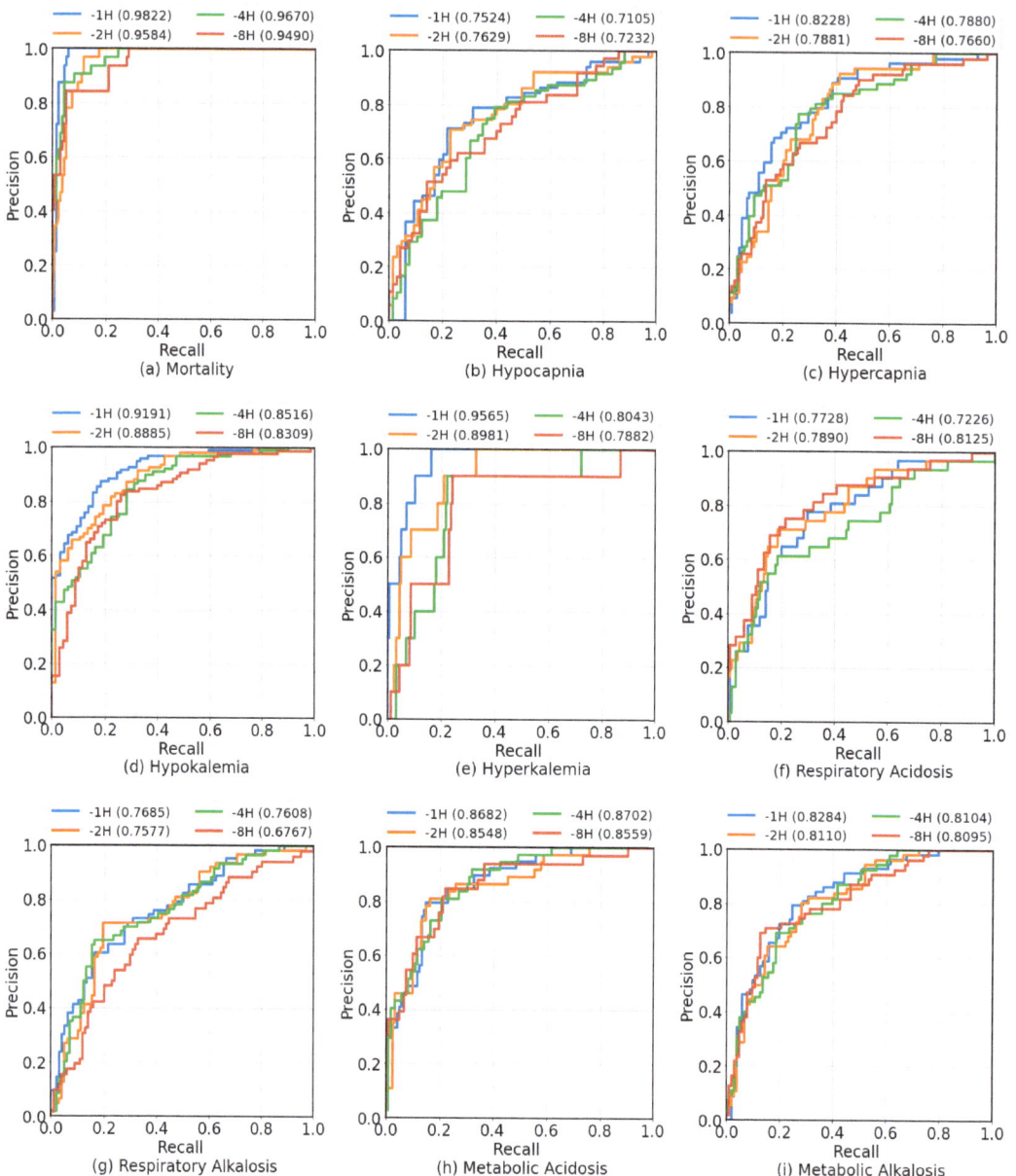

Figure 5. The ROC curves compare different early prediction periods (1, 2, 4, and 8 h before onset) using GB for each target clinical condition.

Table 4. Predictive performance of the GB classifier at different prediction windows ($T_P = \{1,2,4,8\}$).

Clinical Condition	N_1/N_0	Before Onset	Precision	Sensitivity	Specificity	F1 Score	AUROC	AUPRC
Mortality	213/924	1 h	0.6809	1.000	0.8921	0.8101	0.9822	0.8557
		2 h	0.6078	0.9688	0.8561	0.7470	0.9584	0.8148
		4 h	0.5769	0.9375	0.8417	0.7143	0.9670	0.8820
		8 h	0.5400	0.8438	0.8345	0.6585	0.9490	0.8462
Hypocapnia	360/777	1 h	0.7115	0.7115	0.7656	0.7115	0.7524	0.6442
		2 h	0.6491	0.7255	0.6923	0.6852	0.7629	0.7207
		4 h	0.6034	0.7292	0.6515	0.6604	0.7105	0.5997
		8 h	0.4808	0.6757	0.6143	0.5618	0.7232	0.6099
Hypercapnia	296/841	1 h	0.5909	0.7222	0.7523	0.6500	0.8228	0.6731
		2 h	0.5217	0.6792	0.6972	0.5902	0.7881	0.6081
		4 h	0.5600	0.7925	0.6972	0.6562	0.7880	0.6496
		8 h	0.4857	0.6667	0.6727	0.5620	0.7660	0.6142
Hypokalemia	598/539	1 h	0.8646	0.8737	0.8030	0.8691	0.9191	0.9455
		2 h	0.8191	0.828	0.7500	0.8235	0.8885	0.9127
		4 h	0.7895	0.8427	0.7059	0.8152	0.8516	0.8866
		8 h	0.7907	0.8000	0.7429	0.7953	0.8309	0.8475
Hyperkalemia	83/1054	1 h	0.2083	1.0000	0.7640	0.3448	0.9565	0.6497
		2 h	0.1579	0.9000	0.7019	0.2687	0.8981	0.2761
		4 h	0.1636	0.9000	0.7143	0.2769	0.8043	0.1573
		8 h	0.1667	0.9000	0.7205	0.2812	0.7882	0.1628
Respiratory Acidosis	202/935	1 h	0.4068	0.7500	0.7407	0.5275	0.8125	0.5945
		2 h	0.3382	0.7419	0.6667	0.4646	0.7890	0.5339
		4 h	0.3607	0.7097	0.7111	0.4783	0.7728	0.4539
		8 h	0.3333	0.6129	0.7185	0.4318	0.7226	0.3975
Respiratory Alkalosis	430/707	1 h	0.6081	0.7143	0.7041	0.6569	0.7685	0.6924
		2 h	0.6618	0.7143	0.7653	0.6870	0.7577	0.6250
		4 h	0.5733	0.7167	0.6768	0.6370	0.7608	0.6250
		8 h	0.5082	0.5962	0.7030	0.5487	0.6767	0.5167
Metabolic Acidosis	258/879	1 h	0.5333	0.8205	0.7705	0.6465	0.8682	0.7150
		2 h	0.5000	0.8378	0.7480	0.6263	0.8548	0.6490
		4 h	0.4918	0.8108	0.7459	0.6122	0.8702	0.6686
		8 h	0.4375	0.8485	0.7073	0.5773	0.8559	0.6923
Metabolic Alkalosis	397/740	1 h	0.6389	0.7931	0.7451	0.7077	0.8284	0.6719
		2 h	0.5970	0.7143	0.7404	0.6504	0.8110	0.6571
		4 h	0.5455	0.7636	0.6602	0.6364	0.8104	0.6775
		8 h	0.5513	0.7818	0.6602	0.6466	0.8095	0.6799

N_1 represents the number of samples with positive outcomes. N_0 represents the number of samples with positive outcomes. (Total = 1137).

Figure 6 shows the importance of each clinical variable on the GB classifier on each clinical condition. The feature importance was calculated using the impurity-based Gini importance. This method quantifies the importance of each feature by measuring the decrease in node impurity that results from splitting on that feature. The total decrease in node impurity was normalized by the proportion of samples reaching that node and was averaged across all trees in the ensemble model. The resulting value reflect the influence of that feature on the model's predictions.

According to Figure 6, patient consciousness was a significant factor in predicting mortality. The features related to carbon dioxide in the blood would be ranked highly for predicting hypocapnia and hypercapnia, as these clinical conditions are characterized by abnormal levels of carbon dioxide in the blood. Similarly, the features related to potassium would be ranked highly for predicting hypokalemia and hyperkalemia, as these clinical conditions are characterized by abnormal levels of potassium in the body. For acid–base imbalances, features related to acid, base, bicarbonate, and carbon dioxide would be ranked highly, as these factors play a key role in regulating acid–base balance in the body.

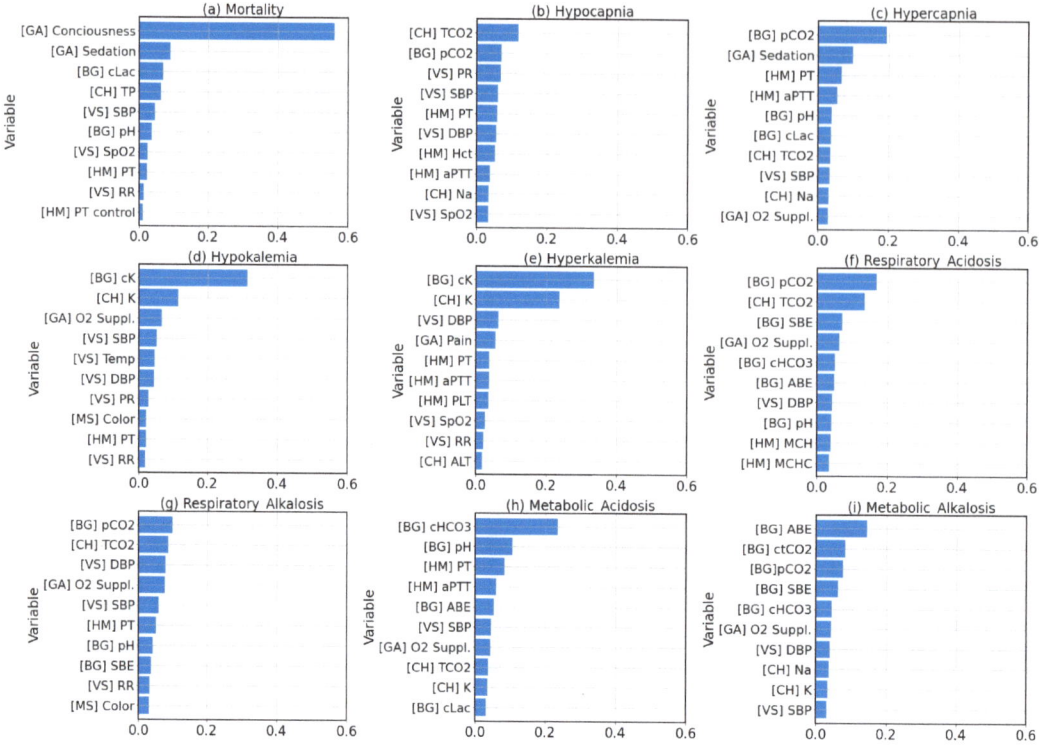

Figure 6. Feature importances calculated from the GB classifer for each clinical condition.

4. Discussion

Machine learning can be a tool to provide timely decision support, simplify the vast amount of information commonly available in the ICU, and highlight the most important elements for each patient. This study focused on the prediction of acid–base and potassium imbalances in intensive care patients. We also looked into predicting mortality, which was used as a baseline to demonstrate the effectiveness of our data embedding strategy and the prediction algorithm in a typical scenario. Our mortality prediction results were in line with other studies [20,23,24] despite ours employing our institutional dataset. Table 3 and Figure 4 indicate that tree-based algorithms, i.e., RF and GB, outperformed the other algorithms for the early prediction of one hour. In general, all of the algorithms used in the study performed better than a random guess. Based on the results, mortality and hypokalemia were the two clinical conditions with the highest F1 Scores, AUROCs, and AUPRCs. Hypocapnia, hypercapnia, respiratory alkalosis, and metabolic alkalosis all had AUROCs of more than 0.65, indicating that they have potential for further study as clinical conditions that can be accurately predicted using machine learning.

When optimizing the hyperparameters, we observed that for KNN, a larger number of neighbors tended to lead to better performance, as this increases the probability that similar data points are present in the neighborhood. For SVM, the regularization parameter C controls the trade-off between maximizing the margin and minimizing the misclassification error. Larger values of C tended to lead to better results, as an attempt was made to increase the margin while attempting to correctly classify all training points. For RF, a larger number of trees tended to lead to better performance because the probability of overfitting was reduced, while the criteria used for data partitioning tended not to have a large effect on performance. For GB, the number of decision trees and the maximum depth of each decision tree were important parameters. We found that a larger number of trees and a lower maximum depth tended to lead to better performance. We observed slightly different sets of hyperparameters for each clinical condition for each model.

With regards to algorithms, GB and RF differ in how the trees are built and how their predictions are combined. GB builds a sequence of weak learners. GB adjusts the weights of data points misclassified by the previous tree to give more weight to difficult cases. RF independently trains many fully grown decision trees and then votes on classifying new data. RF is generally good when there are many features or when the data are high-dimensional. RF can effectively decorrelate the trees and reduce overfitting. RF also handles missing data and categorical variables well. GB is more prone to overfitting than RF, but it can find nonlinear interactions between variables. GB is also sensitive to the scale of the feature; few features may dominate the model. Both RF and GB can work well in different situations. and the choice depends on the dataset and specific problem. For hypercapnia, respiratory acidosis, and metabolic acidosis, it happens that RF scored higher than GB. We suspect that GB may have difficulty handling the complexity and may overfit in these problems.

From the results in Table 4 and Figure 5, the scores for respiratory acidosis and respiratory alkalosis decreased significantly as the prediction window increased. The scores for mortality, hypokalemia, and metabolic alkalosis remained relatively robust, even as the prediction window increased, allowing predictions for these clinical conditions to be made several hours in advance. The scores for hypokalemia decreased as the prediction window increased, eventually making early prediction more difficult. This may be due to the small number of positive samples for hyperkalemia. It is generally more difficult to make accurate predictions with a small number of positive samples, as there is less data available to train the prediction algorithm. This suggests that, due to their intrinsic characteristics, certain clinical conditions may be more difficult to predict than others, even with the use of machine learning techniques. With regards to the four cardinal acid–base disorders, the results suggest that the machine learning models seemed to learn about the physiological regulation of the HCO_3^-/CO_2 buffering system and were able to predict the acid–base disorders. These models may be effective in providing decision support for nurses and clinicians in the ICU setting.

4.1. Comparison to Other Studies

Many studies have demonstrated the ability of machine learning to predict clinical outcomes and clinical conditions in intensive care patients. The performance of a model may vary depending on the specific dataset and prediction task. Most studies have been conducted in a domain-specific context, such as predicting clinical events that may occur during surgery. For hypocapnia, Chen et al. [25] developed machine learning models to predict six different outcomes, including hypocapnia, using GB with physiological signals. The authors obtained an AUROC of 0.8551 and an AUPRC of 0.4451. Their results with GB outperformed those of the LSTM. Our study achieved AUPRCs of 0.6099–0.6442, which were higher than those of the authors. For hypercapnia, Fan et al. [26] developed an RF model to predict hypercapnia during one-lung ventilation using RF. They obtained an AUROC of 0.7450, which is comparable to our study, which obtained AUROCs of 0.7660–0.8228. Regarding hypokalemia and hyperkalemia, Zhou et al. [27] developed a GB model for predicting severe hypokalemia with an AUROC of 0.73. Our study obtained higher AUROCs of 0.8309–0.9191 for hypokalemia. Similarly, Kwak et al. [28] investigated the prediction of hyperkalemia with an AUROC of 0.85 for both RF and GB. Ours achieved AUROCs of 0.7882–0.9565. For the four acid–base disorders, Cherif et al. [29] developed a mathematical model for predicting acid–base disorders that takes into account the physiological regulation of the buffer system. The model can predict the primary disturbances and provides pathophysiological insights. This study supports our hypothesis that the acid–base disorders can be predicted using machine learning algorithms.

4.2. Calibration Curves

Figure 7 shows calibration curves that plot the mean predicted probability against the frequency of the event on the test set. A perfect model would have a calibration curve that is a straight line with a slope of one and an intercept of zero. If the curve is above the straight line, it means the model is overconfident, while a curve below the line means the model is underconfident. Calibration curves can be used to evaluate how well a model is able to predict events within different probability ranges. Compared with other algorithms, the GB models were better calibrated. The GB model of hypokalemia appears to be well-calibrated. The GB models seem to provide a risk score in the range between 0–1 better than other algorithms.

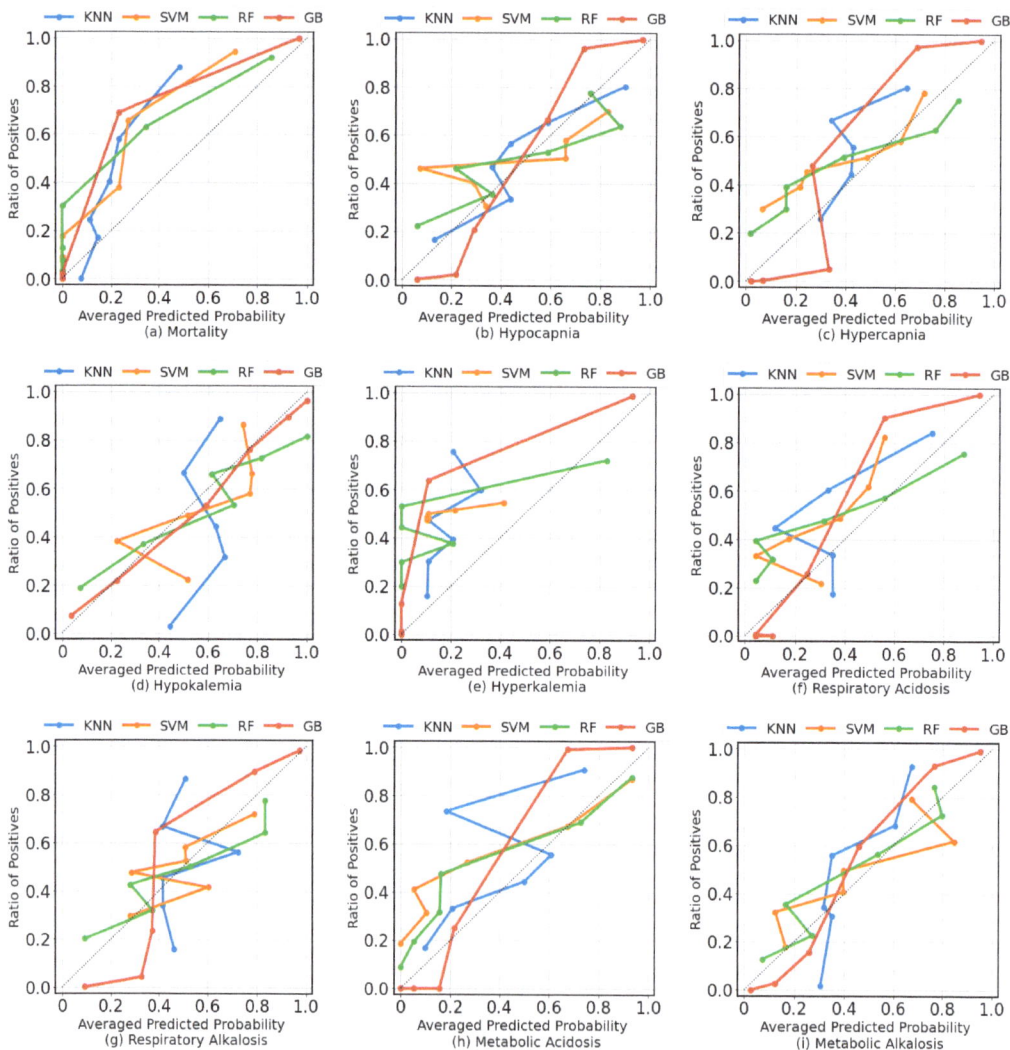

Figure 7. Calibration curves demonstrate the degree of calibration of each classifier for every clinical condition in the test set. Most of the calibration curves indicate that the classifiers are well-calibrated.

4.3. Feature Importance

Overall, the feature importance results in Figure 6 provide insight into the factors that the model is considering important when making predictions, which can help to increase understanding of the model's decision-making process and inform further development or refinement of the model. Our results of feature importance indicate that the model had a strong understanding of the context surrounding the clinical conditions it was predicting. For mortality, the top features identified by the model (such as consciousness, SBP, SpO_2, and RR) are included in commonly used ICU bedside scoring indexes, such as APACHE [10] and MEWS [9]. The models for predicting mortality were effective due, in part, to the inclusion of patient consciousness as input features. For hypocapnia and hypercapnia, pCO_2 and TCO_2, which are direct predictors of hypocapnia and hypercapnia, came up on top of the lists of feature importance. For hypokalemia and hyperkalemia, both types of potassium measurements from both chemistry labs and arterial blood gases were the most important variables. For acid–base imbalances, the variables indicating acid–base balance, electrolytes, and gasses in blood (such as SBE, ABE, pCO_2, TCO_2, $cHCO_3$, K^+, and Na^+) are strong predictors. It is likely that the model, although not specifically designed to process temporal data, learned the temporal dynamics of the changes as well as the relationship between the different predictors to make predictions about the occurrence of these clinical conditions.

In Figure 8, the temporal importance of each clinical variable was averaged across all clinical conditions in the test set. Hence, the model's predictions were based on multiple time points, with the most recent and earlier measurements being weighted more heavily. This means that the model takes into account the temporal dynamics of the data when making predictions.

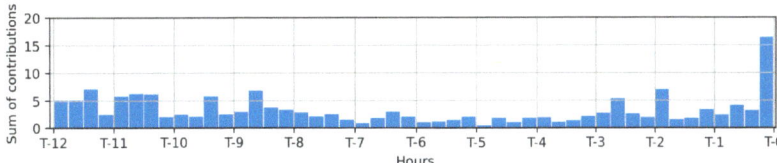

Figure 8. Temporal importance was calculated by averaging across all clinical variables and all clinical conditions in the test set. This measure reflects the degree of influence of each time point on the prediction. We observed that greater weight was given to the most recent and earlier measurements. This may indicate that the algorithms are able to capture changes in clinical variables over time.

4.4. Feature Explanations

The explainability of models is critical in healthcare because healthcare providers are responsible for the actions taken. It is important that the decisions made by machine learning models are understandable to the user. Figure 9 presents a visualization of a sample patient in the test set over a period of 30 h, as well as the model outputs and the visualization of the contributions of each feature at each time step to the output of the model. The top 40 important clinical variables were selected for this visualization. The contributions were calculated using SHAP values from the SHAP framework [38], which were summed over different time steps of the same values and again summed over different clinical conditions. Some clinical variables, i.e., vital signs and arterial blood gases, were measured more frequent than the others. The models can identify variables that are outside of their normal ranges, e.g., the periods with low blood pressure and high respiratory rate, that may need attention of medical doctors.

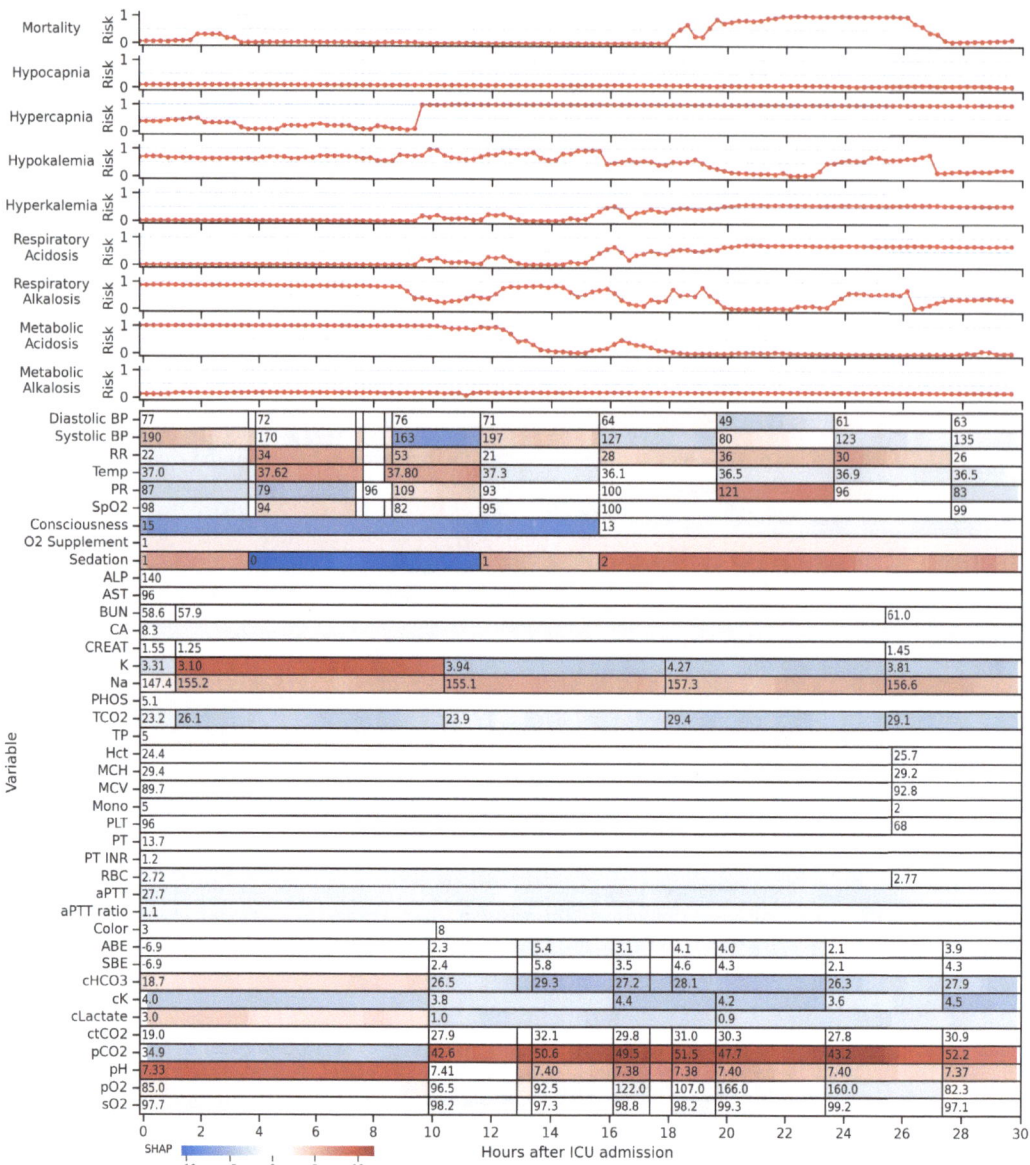

Figure 9. Feature visualization of one sample patient in the test set with model outputs provides valuable insights into how the models are making predictions based on the clinical data. By transforming the raw data into time series with a fixed 15 min interval and fill forward imputation, the models can analyze patterns over time and predict the patient's score for the clinical condition. The models can also flag variables outside their normal range, indicating areas requiring attention from clinicians. It is worth noting that only the top 40 most important clinical variables are shown, and some measurements are skipped due to space limitations. Overall, the feature visualization with model outputs is a powerful tool for understanding how the models are making predictions and identifying areas where clinicians can take action to improve patient outcomes.

4.5. Limitations

There are several limitations to this study. First, the dataset used was relatively small compared to larger datasets, such as MIMIC [39] and eICU [40], but the results do demonstrate that it is possible to develop algorithms using data from a single local institution. Second, our study defined acid–base disturbances using the simple thresholding technique, not from the point of view of the carbonic-acid–bicarbonate buffer system. Future studies may take into account the dynamics of the physiological regulation and buffer system. Third, the study did not consider other factors, such as medications or diagnoses made by physicians, which may have an impact on the results. The reason is that these data are too fine-grained, and it might be difficult for machine learning algorithms to learn from them effectively with a small dataset. If we take these factors into account, we could study the impact of chronic conditions on critically ill patients, which in turn can improve the performance of the algorithms. Expanding the dataset to include data from other ICUs within the same institution could help address this limitation. Fourth, balancing a dataset using methods, such as SMOTE (Synthetic Minority Over-sampling Technique) [41], can improve the performance of a machine learning model in minority class prediction by creating synthetic samples by interpolating between existing minority class samples and then increasing the number of minority class samples in the training dataset. Fifth, the study did not use more complex modeling techniques, such as recurrent neural networks or transformers, which have built-in temporal dynamics functionality, due to the desire to use smaller computational units and maintain interpretability of features. Additionally, marginal performance improvements of these complex modeling techniques were observed in other studies compared to ensemble tree algorithms. Finally, the study was conducted using data from a single institution, and the results may not be generalizable to other hospitals or healthcare settings.

4.6. Future Work

Future work involves examining the generalizability of the algorithms across different datasets, such as MIMIC and eICU, or with different cohorts. This can provide insight into how well the model would perform on a broader population. To achieve this, it is important to ensure that the variables used in the algorithm are also present in the target dataset. As suggested by the study by Desautels et al. [42], the performance and robustness of the algorithm can be improved through the use of transfer learning on a target dataset, such that knowledge learned from one dataset can be applied to improve the performance on a different but related dataset. Next, the performance of the model could potentially be improved when a model is trained with data from bedside monitoring systems, such as continuous vital signs. This is because bedside monitoring data provide a more detailed and granular view of a patient's physiology and disease progression over time. With this type of data, the model is able to detect subtle changes in a patient's condition that may not be apparent with less frequent measurements, such as those taken during routine care. The use of data from bedside monitoring systems would also allow the model to account for the dynamic nature of critical illness, which is characterized by rapid physiologic changes. Finally, it would be interesting to investigate whether the factors from bedside monitoring tools, such as APACHE II or SAPS, which are currently utilized in the clinic, can be used to predict acid–base and potassium imbalances. If these factors are found to be useful, they could be incorporated into clinical decision-making tools and treatment protocols without requiring additional data to be collected.

5. Conclusions

Acid–base disorders occur when there is an imbalance in the normal pH of the body. This can be caused by problems with kidney or respiratory function or by an excess of acids or bases that the body cannot properly eliminate. Acid–base disorders can also affect potassium levels in the body by altering the transport of potassium. It is important to monitor and regulate both acid–base balance and potassium levels to maintain proper physiological and cellular function of the body. This study used machine learning to predict acid–base and potassium imbalances in intensive care patients, which could be useful in controlling or regulating the balance and thus beneficial to the management of the underlying disease. We were interested in nine clinical conditions related to the acid–base and potassium imbalances: mortality, hypocapnia, hypercapnia, hypokalemia, hyperkalemia, metabolic acidosis, metabolic alkalosis, respiratory acidosis, and respiratory alkalosis. The study used an institutional dataset of 1089 patients with 87 clinical variables, including vital signs, patient appearance, and laboratory measurements. The results showed that GB generally had the best performance, with AUROCs ranging from 0.6767 to 0.9822 and AUPRCs ranging from 0.5945 to 0.9455 for the different clinical conditions and different prediction windows. The highest performances were seen in the prediction of mortality and hypokalemia, and the predictions for mortality, hypokalemia, and metabolic alkalosis remained relatively robust even when the prediction window was increased, indicating the potential for early prediction. We used the SHAP framework to make the decision-making process of our machine learning models interpretable and transparent. The results were promising and could be useful for clinicians to gain insights into the underlying clinical condition.

Supplementary Materials: The following supporting information can be downloaded at: https://www.mdpi.com/article/10.3390/diagnostics13061171/s1, Table S1: Summary of the functions in the scikit-learn library and the hyperparameters that are optimized during the training of an algorithm; Figure S1: Visualization of F1 score, AUROC, and AUPRC for each algorithm and for each clinical condition; Figure S2: Visualization of F1 score, AUROC, and AUPRC for each early prediction window and for each clinical condition; Figure S3: PR curves compare different algorithms for each clinical condition; Figure S4: PR curves compare different early prediction windows for each clinical condition; Figure S5: Confusion matrices of GB classifiers on the test set for a one hour early prediction window for each clinical condition.

Author Contributions: Conceptualization, T.I. and S.C.; methodology, R.P.; software, R.P. and K.S.; validation, R.P., S.C. and K.H.; formal analysis, R.P.; investigation, R.P.; resources, S.C.; data curation, R.P. and T.I.; writing—original draft preparation, R.P. and S.C.; writing—review and editing, R.P. and S.C.; visualization, R.P. and S.C.; supervision, S.C.; project administration, S.C.; funding acquisition, S.C. All authors have read and agreed to the published version of the manuscript.

Funding: R.P. and K.S. gratefully acknowledge their graduate scholarships from the Faculty of Medicine, Prince of Songkla University under grant number 02/2563 and 01/2564, respectively. R.P. also received a thesis research grant from the graduate school, Prince of Songkla University. This work was supported by the Health Systems Research Institute (HSRI) under grant number HSRI 63-147. The APC was jointly funded jointly by Research and Development Office (RDO) and Faculty of Medicine, Prince of Songkla University.

Institutional Review Board Statement: The study was conducted in accordance with the Declaration of Helsinki, and approved by the Office of Human Research Ethic Committee, Faculty of Medicine, Prince of Songkla University under Approval No. REC. 63-541-25-2 (Date: 13 January 2021).

Informed Consent Statement: Patient consent was waived due to the retrospective nature of the study. The study analyzed de-identified clinical data of the patients.

Data Availability Statement: The de-identified clinical data presented in this study are available on request from the corresponding author, subject to approval by the Office of Human Research Ethic Committee. The data are not publicly available due to institutional policies.

Conflicts of Interest: The authors declare no conflict of interest.

Abbreviations

The following abbreviations are used in this manuscript:

ABE	Actual Base Excess
ALB	Albumin
ALP	Alkaline Phosphatase

ALT	Alanine Transaminase
APACHE	Acute Physiology And Chronic Health Evaluation
aPTT	Activated Partial Thromboplastin Time
AST	Aspartate Transaminase
AUPRC	Area Under The Precision Recall Curve
AUROC	Area Under The Receiver Operating Characteristic Curve
BUN	Blood Urea Nitrogen
CA	Calcium
cCa_2^+	Calcium Concentration
cCl^-	Chloride Concentration
$cHCO_3^-$	Bicarbonate Concentration
cK^+	Potassium Concentration
CKD	Chronic Kidney Disease
Cl^-	Chloride
cLac	Lactate Concentration
cNa^+	Sodium Concentration
CO_2	Carbon Dioxide
CREAT	Creatinine
$ctCO_2$	Total Concentration Of Carbon Dioxide
DBP	Diastolic Blood Pressure
EHR	Electronic Health Record
EWS	Early Warning Score
GB	Gradient Boosting
GLOB	Globulin
ICU	Intensive Dare Unit
K^+	Potassium
KNN	K Nearest Neighbours
LSTM	Long Short-Term Memory
MCH	Mean Corpuscular Hemoglobin
MCHC	Mean Corpuscular Hemoglobin Concentration
MCV	Mean Corpuscular Volume
MEWS	Modified Early Warning Score
MICU	Medical Intensive Care Unit
Mono	Monocyte
Na^+	Sodium
NEWS	National Early Warning Score
pCO_2	Partial Pressure Of Carbon Dioxide
PHOS	Phosphate
PLT	Platelet
pO_2	Partial Pressure Of Oxygen
PR	Pulse Rate
PT	Prothrombin Time
RBC	Red Blood Cell
RF	Random Forest
ROC	Receiver Operating Characteristic
RR	Respiratory Rate
SAPS	Simplified Acute Physiology Score
SBE	Standard Base Excess
SBP	Systolic Blood Pressure
SHAP	Shapley Additive Explanations
SIRS	Systemic Inflammatory Response Syndrome
sO_2	Oxygen Saturation
SpO_2	Oxygen Saturation
SQL	Structured Query Language
SVM	Support Vector Machine
TCO_2	Total Carbon Dioxide
TP	Total Protein

References

1. Adhikari, N.K.; Fowler, R.A.; Bhagwanjee, S.; Rubenfeld, G.D. Critical care and the global burden of critical illness in adults. *Lancet* **2010**, *376*, 1339–1346. [CrossRef] [PubMed]
2. Bhagavan, N.; Ha, C.E. Water, Electrolytes, and Acid–Base Balance. In *Essentials of Medical Biochemistry*; Elsevier: Amsterdam, The Netherlands, 2015; pp. 701–713. [CrossRef]
3. Quinteros, L.M.; Roque, J.B.; Kaufman, D.; Raventós, A.A. Importance of carbon dioxide in the critical patient: Implications at the cellular and clinical levels. *Med. Intensiv. (Engl. Ed.)* **2019**, *43*, 234–242. [CrossRef]
4. Forsal, I.; Bodelsson, M.; Wieslander, A.; Nilsson, A.; Pouchoulin, D.; Broman, M. Analysis of acid–base disorders in an ICU cohort using a computer script. *Intensive Care Med. Exp.* **2022**, *10*. [CrossRef] [PubMed]
5. Hamm, L.L.; Hering-Smith, K.S.; Nakhoul, N.L. Acid-Base and Potassium Homeostasis. *Semin. Nephrol.* **2013**, *33*, 257–264. [CrossRef] [PubMed]
6. Kazda, A.; Jabor, A.; Zámečník, M.; Mašek, K. Monitoring Acid-Base and Electrolyte Disturbances in Intensive Care. In *Advances in Clinical Chemistry*; Elsevier: Amsterdam, The Netherlands, 1989; Volume 27, pp. 201–268. [CrossRef]
7. Adrogué, H.J.; Madias, N.E. Changes in plasma potassium concentration during acute acid–base disturbances. *Am. J. Med.* **1981**, *71*, 456–467. [CrossRef]
8. Charlton, P.H.; Pimentel, M.; Lokhandwala, S. Data Fusion Techniques for Early Warning of Clinical Deterioration. In *Secondary Analysis of Electronic Health Records*; Springer International Publishing: Berlin/Heidelberg, Germany, 2016; pp. 325–338. [CrossRef]
9. Subbe, C. Validation of a modified Early Warning Score in medical admissions. *QJM* **2001**, *94*, 521–526. [CrossRef]
10. Knaus, W.A.; Draper, E.A.; Wagner, D.P.; Zimmerman, J.E. APACHE II: A Severity of Disease Classification System. *Crit. Care Med.* **1985**, *13*, 818–829. [CrossRef] [PubMed]
11. Moreno, R.P.; Metnitz, P.G.H.; Almeida, E.; Jordan, B.; Bauer, P.; Campos, R.A.; Iapichino, G.; Edbrooke, D.; Capuzzo, M.; Le Gall, J.-R. SAPS 3—From evaluation of the patient to evaluation of the intensive care unit. Part 2: Development of a prognostic model for hospital mortality at ICU admission. *Intensive Care Med.* **2005**, *31*, 1345–1355. [CrossRef] [PubMed]
12. Jones, M. NEWSDIG: The National Early Warning Score Development and Implementation Group. *Clin. Med.* **2012**, *12*, 501–503. [CrossRef]
13. Cosgriff, C.V.; Celi, L.A.; Stone, D.J. Critical Care, Critical Data. *Biomed. Eng. Comput. Biol.* **2019**, *10*, 117959721985656. [CrossRef] [PubMed]
14. Johnson, A.E.W.; Ghassemi, M.M.; Nemati, S.; Niehaus, K.E.; Clifton, D.; Clifford, G.D. Machine Learning and Decision Support in Critical Care. *Proc. IEEE* **2016**, *104*, 444–466. [CrossRef] [PubMed]
15. Kam, H.J.; Kim, H.Y. Learning representations for the early detection of sepsis with deep neural networks. *Comput. Biol. Med.* **2017**, *89*, 248–255. [CrossRef] [PubMed]
16. Nemati, S.; Holder, A.; Razmi, F.; Stanley, M.D.; Clifford, G.D.; Buchman, T.G. An Interpretable Machine Learning Model for Accurate Prediction of Sepsis in the ICU. *Crit. Care Med.* **2018**, *46*, 547–553. [CrossRef] [PubMed]
17. Zhang, D.; Yin, C.; Hunold, K.M.; Jiang, X.; Caterino, J.M.; Zhang, P. An interpretable deep-learning model for early prediction of sepsis in the emergency department. *Patterns* **2021**, *2*, 100196. [CrossRef] [PubMed]
18. Kwon, J.; Lee, Y.; Lee, Y.; Lee, S.; Park, J. An Algorithm Based on Deep Learning for Predicting In-Hospital Cardiac Arrest. *J. Am. Heart Assoc.* **2018**, *7*, e008678. [CrossRef] [PubMed]
19. Tomašev, N.; Glorot, X.; Rae, J.W.; Zielinski, M.; Askham, H.; Saraiva, A.; Mottram, A.; Meyer, C.; Ravuri, S.; Protsyuk, I.; et al. A clinically applicable approach to continuous prediction of future acute kidney injury. *Nature* **2019**, *572*, 116–119. [CrossRef] [PubMed]
20. Wanyan, T.; Honarvar, H.; Jaladanki, S.K.; Zang, C.; Naik, N.; Somani, S.; Freitas, J.K.D.; Paranjpe, I.; Vaid, A.; Zhang, J.; et al. Contrastive learning improves critical event prediction in COVID-19 patients. *Patterns* **2021**, *2*, 100389. [CrossRef]
21. Lee, J.M.; Hauskrecht, M. Modeling multivariate clinical event time-series with recurrent temporal mechanisms. *Artif. Intell. Med.* **2021**, *112*, 102021. [CrossRef]
22. Kaji, D.A.; Zech, J.R.; Kim, J.S.; Cho, S.K.; Dangayach, N.S.; Costa, A.B.; Oermann, E.K. An attention based deep learning model of clinical events in the intensive care unit. *PLoS ONE* **2019**, *14*, e0211057. [CrossRef]
23. Na Pattalung, T.; Chaichulee, S. Comparison of machine learning algorithms for mortality prediction in intensive care patients on multi-center critical care databases. *IOP Conf. Ser. Mater. Sci. Eng.* **2021**, *1163*, 012027. [CrossRef]
24. Na Pattalung, T.; Ingviya, T.; Chaichulee, S. Feature Explanations in Recurrent Neural Networks for Predicting Risk of Mortality in Intensive Care Patients. *J. Pers. Med.* **2021**, *11*, 934. [CrossRef] [PubMed]
25. Chen, H.; Lundberg, S.M.; Erion, G.; Kim, J.H.; Lee, S.I. Forecasting adverse surgical events using self-supervised transfer learning for physiological signals. *NPJ Digit. Med.* **2021**, *4*, 167. [CrossRef] [PubMed]
26. Fan, Y.; Ye, T.; Huang, T.; Xiao, H. Machine learning-based construction of a clinical prediction model for hypercapnia during one-lung ventilation for lung surgery. *Res. Sq.* **2022**. [CrossRef]
27. Zhou, Z.; Huang, C.; Fu, P.; Huang, H.; Zhang, Q.; Wu, X.; Yu, Q.; Sun, Y. Prediction of in-hospital hypokalemia using machine learning and first hospitalization day records in patients with traumatic brain injury. *CNS Neurosci. Ther.* **2022**, *29*, 181–191. [CrossRef] [PubMed]
28. Kwak, G.H.; Chen, C.; Ling, L.; Ghosh, E.; Celi, L.A.; Hui, P. Predicting Hyperkalemia in the ICU and Evaluation of Generalizability and Interpretability. *arXiv* **2021**, arXiv:2101.06443.

29. Cherif, A.; Maheshwari, V.; Fuertinger, D.; Schappacher-Tilp, G.; Preciado, P.; Bushinsky, D.; Thijssen, S.; Kotanko, P.; et al. A mathematical model of the four cardinal acid–base disorders. *Math. Biosci. Eng.* **2020**, *17*, 4457–4476. [CrossRef] [PubMed]
30. Laserna, E.; Sibila, O.; Aguilar, P.R.; Mortensen, E.M.; Anzueto, A.; Blanquer, J.M.; Sanz, F.; Rello, J.; Marcos, P.J.; Velez, M.I.; et al. Hypocapnia and Hypercapnia Are Predictors for ICU Admission and Mortality in Hospitalized Patients With Community-Acquired Pneumonia. *Chest* **2012**, *142*, 1193–1199. [CrossRef]
31. Soar, J.; Perkins, G.D.; Abbas, G.; Alfonzo, A.; Barelli, A.; Bierens, J.J.; Brugger, H.; Deakin, C.D.; Dunning, J.; Georgiou, M.; et al. European Resuscitation Council Guidelines for Resuscitation 2010 Section 8. Cardiac arrest in special circumstances: Electrolyte abnormalities, poisoning, drowning, accidental hypothermia, hyperthermia, asthma, anaphylaxis, cardiac surgery, trauma, pregnancy, electrocution. *Resuscitation* **2010**, *81*, 1400–1433. [CrossRef]
32. Berend, K.; de Vries, A.P.; Gans, R.O. Physiological Approach to Assessment of Acid–Base Disturbances. *N. Engl. J. Med.* **2014**, *371*, 1434–1445. [CrossRef]
33. Constable, P.D. Clinical Assessment of Acid-Base Status: Comparison of the Henderson-Hasselbalch and Strong Ion Approaches. *Vet. Clin. Pathol.* **2000**, *29*, 115–128. [CrossRef]
34. Rawat, D.; Modi, P.; Sharma, S. *Hypercapnea*; StatPearls Publishing: St. Petersburg, FL, USA, 2022.
35. Gennari, F.J. Hypokalemia. *N. Engl. J. Med.* **1998**, *339*, 451–458. [CrossRef] [PubMed]
36. GALLA, J.H. Metabolic Alkalosis. *J. Am. Soc. Nephrol.* **2000**, *11*, 369–375. [CrossRef] [PubMed]
37. Plant, P.K. One year period prevalence study of respiratory acidosis in acute exacerbations of COPD: Implications for the provision of non-invasive ventilation and oxygen administration. *Thorax* **2000**, *55*, 550–554. [CrossRef]
38. Lundberg, S.M.; Erion, G.; Chen, H.; DeGrave, A.; Prutkin, J.M.; Nair, B.; Katz, R.; Himmelfarb, J.; Bansal, N.; Lee, S.I. From local explanations to global understanding with explainable AI for trees. *Nat. Mach. Intell.* **2020**, *2*, 56–67. [CrossRef]
39. Johnson, A.; Bulgarelli, L.; Pollard, T.; Horng, S.; Celi, L.A.; Mark, R. MIMIC-IV. *Phys. Net.* **2022**. [CrossRef]
40. Pollard, T.J.; Johnson, A.E.W.; Raffa, J.D.; Celi, L.A.; Mark, R.G.; Badawi, O. The eICU Collaborative Research Database, a freely available multi-center database for critical care research. *Sci. Data* **2018**, *5*, 180178. [CrossRef] [PubMed]
41. Cihan, P.; Ozger, Z.B. A new approach for determining SARS-CoV-2 epitopes using machine learning-based in silico methods. *Comput. Biol. Chem.* **2022**, *98*, 107688. [CrossRef]
42. Desautels, T.; Calvert, J.; Hoffman, J.; Mao, Q.; Jay, M.; Fletcher, G.; Barton, C.; Chettipally, U.; Kerem, Y.; Das, R. Using Transfer Learning for Improved Mortality Prediction in a Data-Scarce Hospital Setting. *Biomed. Inform. Insights* **2017**, *9*, 117822261771299. [CrossRef] [PubMed]

Disclaimer/Publisher's Note: The statements, opinions and data contained in all publications are solely those of the individual author(s) and contributor(s) and not of MDPI and/or the editor(s). MDPI and/or the editor(s) disclaim responsibility for any injury to people or property resulting from any ideas, methods, instructions or products referred to in the content.

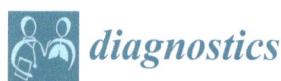

Review

Emerging Technology-Driven Hybrid Models for Preventing and Monitoring Infectious Diseases: A Comprehensive Review and Conceptual Framework

Bader M. Albahlal

College of Computer and Information Sciences, Imam Mohammad Ibn Saud Islamic University, Riyadh 13318, Saudi Arabia; bmalbahlal@imamu.edu.sa

Abstract: The emergence of the infectious diseases, such as the novel coronavirus, as a significant global health threat has emphasized the urgent need for effective treatments and vaccines. As infectious diseases become more common around the world, it is important to have strategies in place to prevent and monitor them. This study reviews hybrid models that incorporate emerging technologies for preventing and monitoring infectious diseases. It also presents a comprehensive review of the hybrid models employed for preventing and monitoring infectious diseases since the outbreak of COVID-19. The review encompasses models that integrate emerging and innovative technologies, such as blockchain, Internet of Things (IoT), big data, and artificial intelligence (AI). By harnessing these technologies, the hybrid system enables secure contact tracing and source isolation. Based on the review, a hybrid conceptual framework model proposes a hybrid model that incorporates emerging technologies. The proposed hybrid model enables effective contact tracing, secure source isolation using blockchain technology, IoT sensors, and big data collection. A hybrid model that incorporates emerging technologies is proposed as a comprehensive approach to preventing and monitoring infectious diseases. With continued research on and the development of the proposed model, the global efforts to effectively combat infectious diseases and safeguard public health will continue.

Keywords: blockchain; IoT devices; AI algorithms; big data analytics; deep learning

Citation: Albahlal, B.M. Emerging Technology-Driven Hybrid Models for Preventing and Monitoring Infectious Diseases: A Comprehensive Review and Conceptual Framework. *Diagnostics* **2023**, *13*, 3047. https://doi.org/10.3390/diagnostics13193047

Academic Editors: Wan Azani Mustafa and Hiam Alquran

Received: 30 June 2023
Revised: 11 September 2023
Accepted: 11 September 2023
Published: 25 September 2023

Correction Statement: This article has been republished with a minor change. The change does not affect the scientific content of the article and further details are available within the backmatter of the website version of this article.

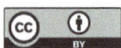

Copyright: © 2023 by the author. Licensee MDPI, Basel, Switzerland. This article is an open access article distributed under the terms and conditions of the Creative Commons Attribution (CC BY) license (https://creativecommons.org/licenses/by/4.0/).

1. Introduction

The coronavirus pandemic has had a devastating impact on the world, spreading to 188 countries and causing more than 1 million deaths. Governments have reacted by executing arrangement bundles, such as closing schools and limiting individuals to their homes, which have been effective in abating the development of the infection. Figure 1 shows the COVID-19 statistics for the most affected countries in the world [1]. The COVID-19 pandemic led to the cancellation of numerous imperative world occasions, including the Tokyo Olympics and Dubai Expo [1–3]. The arrangement of approach bundles has brought about expansive, useful, and quantifiable well-being results [4]. To restrain the spread of the infection, governments have executed measures such as police watches, CCTV, rambles, and geo-fences [4], which require a critical number of social assets. In reaction to the COVID-19 widespread, researchers and government authorities around the world have been working tirelessly to create a remedy and foresee the potential development direction of the infection since its introductory location by the World Health Organization (WHO). To tackle this difficult challenge, scholars have explored the integration of emerging technologies in hybrid models for preventing and monitoring infectious diseases. This manuscript presents a comprehensive overview of such hybrid models, emphasizing the assimilation of innovative technologies, such as blockchain, Internet of Things (IoT), big data, and artificial intelligence (AI) [5]. Blockchain technology has garnered significant attention as a potential solution, offering secure and transparent mechanisms for tracking and tracing the transmission of infections [6]. By leveraging blockchain, hybrid systems enable contact tracing while upholding data confidentiality and security. Moreover, the integration of IoT sensors and big data compilation has demonstrated promising potential in disease surveillance [1]. These technologies facilitate the collection and analysis of massive datasets, enabling the real-time monitoring of infectious diseases [4]. This data-centric approach amplifies our knowledge of disease dynamics, enabling effective response strategies and timely interventions. AI plays a pivotal role in symptom identification and bolstering drug manufacturing [7]. By harnessing AI algorithms, researchers can scrutinize symptoms and patterns associated with the virus, enabling early detection and swift response [8]. Additionally, AI-driven drug manufacturing processes expedite the development and production of efficacious treatments. Considering the present challenges and existing research, this investigation proposed a hybrid conceptual framework model that integrates blockchain, IoT, big data, and AI technologies. The hybrid conceptual framework model aims to offer comprehensive and proactive solutions for disease prevention and monitoring [9]. By leveraging these emerging technologies, this model possesses the potential to transform disease control strategies, with a focus on preventive measures to tackle the ongoing pandemic.

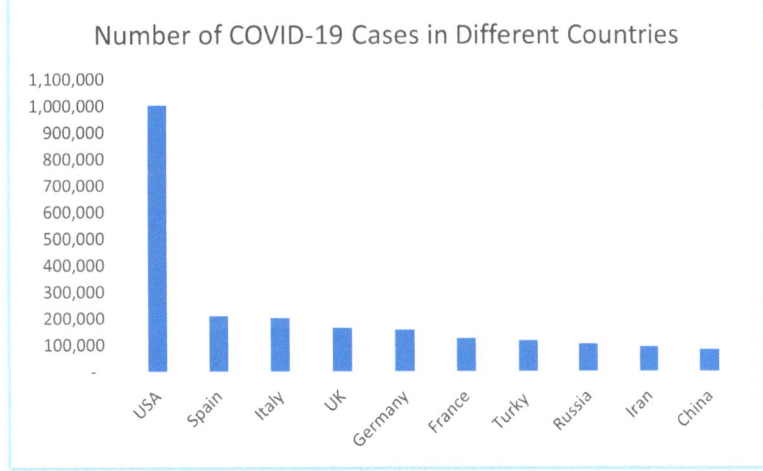

Figure 1. The effect of COVID-19 in the world [1].

In the subsequent sections, a detailed review of the hybrid models utilized for disease prevention and monitoring, analyzing their effectiveness by incorporating blockchain, IoT, big data, and AI, is presented. Furthermore, the proposed hybrid conceptual framework model, highlighting its potential to tackle the current pandemic through proactive and preventative measures, is discussed.

2. Literature Review

The advent of the novel COVID-19 virus has prompted a substantial amount of research into the creation of useful methodologies for the prevention and monitoring of diseases. The primary objective of this literature review is to provide a comprehensive overview of the hybrid models utilized to tackle the issues presented by infectious illnesses, with an explicit emphasis on the emerging technologies, such as blockchain, IoT, big data, and AI.

2.1. Emerging Technologies

By combining these technologies, this model seeks to revolutionize the way we respond to public health crises, opening new possibilities for the future. Most importantly, the hybrid conceptual framework model advocates for a preventive strategy to reduce the spread of the virus and its impact on society. This paper seeks to explore the potential of this innovative framework and its ability to revolutionize our response to the pandemic.

2.1.1. Blockchain

Blockchain innovation can be utilized to guarantee the secure and tamper-resistant capacity and sharing of sensitive well-being information. It provides a decentralized and straightforward stage where information can be safely stored and controlled through cryptography. Within the setting of irresistible illnesses, records, tests, inoculation information, and other pertinent data can be stored in the blockchain, guaranteeing the security and authenticity of the information [10]. Individuals from all over the world are working hard to discover the best arrangements to anticipate the spread of contamination and rapidly recognize viral carriers since coronavirus is exceedingly infectious. The potential utilization cases of blockchain in healthcare are various, extending from information sharing and security to obtaining information. Examples include blockchain stages planned for clinical trials or accuracy of prescribed medication. Within the current setting of widespread administration, blockchain is rising as a significant innovation arrangement, providing a straightforward, solid, and cost-effective arrangement to encourage fruitful decision-making, which may viably contribute to speedier mediation amid this emergency. The blockchain phase is composed of three primary components: information, disseminated records, and agreement calculation. These components can be utilized for clinical trial administration, therapeutic supply chain, client security assurance, information conglomeration, contact tracing, and episode follow-up [11].

2.1.2. Internet of Things

Internet of Things (IoT) devices, including wearable sensors, environmental sensors, and medical equipment, can gather information about infectious diseases in real time. IoT devices, for instance, can track vital signs, such as respiratory rate, heart rate, and body temperature, to identify early signs of infections. Environmental sensors can track the air quality and look for pathogens nearby. The collected data can be securely transmitted by these IoT devices to the blockchain for additional analysis. Big data analytic techniques can be used to process and analyze the enormous amount of data gathered from IoT devices as well as other pertinent data sources, such as social media, electronic health records, and public health databases. Infectious-disease-related patterns, correlations, and trends can be found using this analysis. Using cutting-edge analytic algorithms, machine learning and data mining make it possible to detect disease events, forecast the spread of infections, and evaluate the effectiveness of prevention measures [12]. IoT collects data through sensors and provides intelligent perception, recognition, and management. IoT is monitored, connected, and interacts in real time. It transmits data through the network, creating a pervasive connection between IoT and people. IoT digitizes the real world, and its application is wide-ranging, including smart environments (homes, offices, and factories) and personal and social domains [8]. The three main characteristics of IoT development are connectivity, perception, and intelligence. The integration and convergence of network communications, big data analysis, edge computing, deep learning, artificial intelligence, and blockchain enable IoT to achieve an all-around perception. When the system connects to the internet, it connects via the hub (or gateway). For example, smart security devices (access control, smart locks, and cameras) can connect to internet big-data services and cloud services to gain a better understanding of COVID-19 monitoring and tracing [6].

2.1.3. Artificial Intelligence

Artificial intelligence (AI) algorithms can be employed to provide decision support in various aspects of infectious disease prevention and monitoring. For instance, machine learning models can predict the likelihood of an individual contracting a specific disease based on their health records and environmental data. AI can also help in contact tracing by analyzing data from multiple sources and identifying potential infection hotspots. Natural language processing (NLP) techniques can be used to extract relevant information from the medical literature and assist in drug discovery or treatment recommendations [5]. AI techniques have recently been used as a powerful tool for coronavirus data analytics, prediction, and drug/vaccine discovery. Studies show that AI has mostly been employed for solving coronavirus-related issues through two key approaches: machine learning (ML) and deep learning (DL). ML is a subfield of AI, and its objective is to understand the structure of data and match them to models that can be expressed and utilized by people. ML algorithms allow computers to perform training on data inputs and use statistical analysis solutions to output values that fall within a specified range. Thus, ML can be used to build models from sample data to automate decision-making processes using data inputs. In the fight against coronavirus, ML can be used for services such as facial recognition to detect infected people or temperature detection on the human body for possible virus infection [10]. For instance, an AI company in the US has recently utilized ML-powered interactive graphs to track the virus migration across China [9] and to create an alert system through which users can receive information about whether an infected individual has travelled within their vicinity. This solution helps to find infected individuals and provide them with medical resources. DL methodologies have also been exploited to implement intelligent coronavirus fighting solutions. Conceptually, DL uses multiple neural network layers in a deep architecture [13].

2.1.4. Big Data

Big data offers an effective way to map and combine various data sources to gain insight into the tracking of the COVID-19 outbreak. Furthermore, it enables us to comprehend virus structure and treatment, as big data platforms can be equipped with sophisticated modelling tools that enable the construction of complex simulation models using the COVID-19 data stream. Therefore, text mining algorithms are essential. Nevertheless, the sheer amount of data and the speed at which it must be processed necessitates the use of AI-based intervention [14].

3. Review and Comparison of the Existing Techniques

A comprehensive review and comparison of existing techniques is presented in this section regarding the prevention and monitoring of infectious diseases. The objective is to provide a thorough assessment of the strengths, weaknesses, and effectiveness of various approaches employed in detecting and monitoring infectious diseases, particularly in the context of the COVID-19 pandemic. The review encompasses a wide range of techniques, including big data analytics, artificial intelligence, nature-inspired computing, blockchain, Internet of Things, and other emerging technologies. By systematically analyzing and comparing these techniques, the article aims to identify the most promising and effective strategies for disease prevention, contact tracing, and data management. Through this review and comparison, valuable insights and recommendations can be derived to guide future research and development efforts in the field of infectious disease surveillance and control.

3.1. Descriptive Analysis

Agbehadji et al. [14] discussed the use of computing models, such as big data, AI, and nature-inspired computing (NIC), in detecting and predicting COVID-19 cases and contact tracing. It also emphasizes the potential of nature-inspired computing to enhance detection accuracy [14]. Another study provided an overview of the potential applications of big data and AI in managing the COVID-19 pandemic [5]. Nguyen et al. [6] presented a conceptual architecture that integrates blockchain and AI for fighting against coronavirus. The architecture consists of four layers: coronavirus data sources, blockchain functions, AI functions, and stakeholders. Data from various sources, including clinical labs, hospitals, and social media, were consolidated to create raw data, which were then developed into big data [6]. A previous study explored the use of technologies, such as the Internet of Things (IoT), unmanned aerial vehicles (UAVs), blockchain, AI, and 5G, to mitigate the impact of the COVID-19 outbreak [1]. A blockchain-based infrastructure for contact tracing, ensuring user privacy, was proposed in [4]. Simulations using different values in the blockchain network supported the proposed framework.

The study in [7] reviewed the role of IoT in healthcare and its significance in dealing with pandemics. The use of biomedical sensors, gateways, and cloud for collecting and analyzing patients' physiological parameters was discussed in [7]. A literature review methodology was used to identify the challenges faced by healthcare sectors in dealing with the COVID-19 epidemic outbreak [8]. The challenges were categorized into physical, operational, resource-based, organizational, technological, and external healthcare challenges. Potential solutions using AI and IoT were proposed in [8]. A blockchain-based system using Ethereum smart contracts and oracles was proposed, implemented, and evaluated to track reported COVID-19 cases [9]. The system tracks the number of new cases, deaths, and recovered cases obtained from trusted sources. Ramallo-González et al. [15] proposed an IoT platform for a contact information sharing and risk notification system, named CIoTVID, to trace and isolate the source of COVID-19 infection. The system is comprised of four layers: data acquisition, data aggregation, machine intelligence, and services. Services are developed on the blockchain platform, and the data generated from these services are stored in distributed blockchain databases [15]. Another framework was proposed for a contact information sharing and risk notification system using blockchain, smart contract, and Bluetooth technologies [10]. The system aims to trace and isolate the source of COVID-19 infection. It also includes four layers: user interaction, mobile service, smart contract service, and data storage [10].

A theoretical model called virus epidemic prediction system (VEPS) was proposed for predicting infectious diseases [11]. The model incorporates technologies such as IoT sensors, FoT (Fog of Things), cloud, and blockchain, each with their own advantages. IoT sensors and Fog node devices process and store health datasets over a blockchain network [11]. Tan et al. utilized a decentralized blockchain-based vehicle-recording mechanism, performed cooperatively by vehicular cloud and edge units, for infection tracking on specific vehicles and individuals [12]. A hybrid medical data acquisition module was attached to the integrated cloud-assisted vehicular ad hoc network (VANET) infrastructure for the non-contact measurement of passengers' physical status, remotely facilitated by the vehicular cloud [12]. To address the privacy concerns of existing contact tracing solutions, a contact tracing scheme called BeepTrace allows worldwide collaborations to integrate existing tracing and positioning solutions with the help of blockchain technology [16]. In another study Zhang et al. [13] proposed a blockchain-based system to provide the secure management of home quarantine, which can help in outbreak control. The system uses advanced cryptographic primitives to ensure privacy and security attributes for various events. To demonstrate the application of the system, they used an IoT system with a desktop computer, laptop, Raspberry Pi single-board computer, and the Ethereum smart contract platform [13]. Ferreti et al. [17] utilized a mathematical model to estimate the basic reproductive number (R0) and quantify the contribution of different transmission routes of SARS-CoV-2, also discussing the use of digital contact tracing through mobile phone applications to avoid delays in traditional manual contact-tracing procedures.

Topol [18] highlighted the potential of AI, particularly deep neural networks (DNNs), in various medical applications, such as interpreting medical scans, improving diagnostic accuracy, and reducing misinterpretation. However, the paper also acknowledged the limitations and challenges in the use of AI in medicine, including the need for validation in real-world clinical environments and addressing biases and inequities. In cardiology, DNNs have been used for the diagnosis of heart attacks and arrhythmia and the classification of echocardiograms with comparable or better accuracy than cardiologists. The FDA has approved several proprietary AI algorithms for image interpretation, and the use of AI in medical imaging is expanding rapidly [18].

Deebak and Al-Turjman [19] proposed an intelligent Edge–IoT framework (IE-IoT) to detect potential threats in the early stage of COVID-19. The learning models used in the analysis were ANN, CNN, and RNN. The proposed IE-IoT can utilize the communication technologies of IoT, such as BLE, Zigbee, and 6LoWPAN, to examine the factor of power consumption. Hamid et al. [20] presented a systematic review of IoMT-based systems for COVID-19 prevention and detection. They also proposed a framework named 'COV-AID' that remotely monitors and diagnoses the disease. The framework encompasses the benefits of IoMT sensors and extensive data analysis and prediction [20]. Sanida et al. [21] proposed an approach that uses a robust hybrid deep convolutional neural network (DCNN) consisting of a combination of VGG blocks (visual geometry group) and an inception module for prompt and accurate identification [21]. In a recent study by Dubey et al. [22], ensemble deep learning (EDL) was superior to deep transfer learning (TL) in both non-augmented and augmented frameworks for the classification of COVID-19 patients based on hybrid deep-learning-based lung segmentation.

3.2. Tabular Analysis for the Emerging Techniques for Pandemic Management

Table 1 presents an analysis of the emerging technologies used in various research studies related to the management and monitoring of infectious diseases, particularly in the context of the COVID-19 pandemic. Furthermore, Table 1 provides a comprehensive overview of the tools utilized in each study and the corresponding results and summary.

Table 1. Analysis of the emerging technologies used in the following research studies.

Article	Tool Used	Results and Summary
A1	IoT, Drones, AI, Blockchain, and 5G	Managing disease impact
A4	Blockchain	Privacy of contact tracing and risk assessment
A5	Big data and AI	Management of the ongoing outbreak
A6	Blockchain and AI	Outbreak tracking, user privacy protection, and safe day-to-day operations
A7	IoT	Smart hospital and health worker management
A8	AI-IoT and cloud-based system	Management and monitoring of healthcare workers
A9	Blockchain	Blockchain-based solution for trust, transparency, and traceability and streamlines the communication
A10	Blockchain	contact information sharing and risk notification system
A11	Blockchain, IoT, and FoT (Fog of Things)	Location-specific information about the person with a health record
A12	Cloud-based, VANETs, and Blockchain	Vehicular ad hoc networks for medical surveillance and infection tracking of suspected passengers
A13	IoT and Blockchain	A home-quarantine management system.
A14	Big data, AI, and NIC	Accurate detection and optimized contact tracing
A15	IoT	CIoTVID open application for the propagation of the pandemic
A16	Blockchain	Application BeepTrace for collaboration and positioning solutions
A17	Mathematical mode reproductive number (R0)	Digital contact tracing through mobile phone apps
A18	AI and Deep neural networks (DNNs)	Pattern recognition
A19	Intelligent Edge-IoT framework (IE-IoT)	Detect potential threats in their early stages

Table 1. Cont.

Article	Tool Used	Results and Summary
A20	IoMT-based systems	Extensive data analysis and prediction
A21	Hybrid DCNN consisting of a combination of VGG blocks	Prompt and accurate identification
A22	Hybrid deep learning	Reduce the spread of the disease

Each study in the table demonstrates the utilization of emerging technologies to tackle different aspects of the pandemic. By summarizing the tools used and the outcomes achieved, the table provides a comprehensive overview of the research landscape in the field of infectious disease management. It showcases the diversity of approaches and the potential of these emerging technologies in combating the spread of infectious diseases and improving public health outcomes.

3.3. Evaluation Matrix of the Emerging Techniques for Pandemic Management

Tables 2 and 3 serve as a visual representation of the technology usage in the selected research articles, enabling researchers and readers to identify the most adopted technologies in the field. Table 2 provides a summary of the emerging technologies used in various research studies. It presents a comparison of different technologies, such as big data, AI, blockchain, IoT-FoT (Internet of Things-Fog of Things), cloud-based solutions, NIC, and 5G. Each row represents a specific research article, while the columns represent the different emerging technologies. It also indicates the presence of a technology in each research article, e.g., in Article 1, in which big data and AI are both utilized, while blockchain, IoT-FoT, and NIC are not utilized in this study. Out of the total research articles considered, two articles employed big data, four articles incorporated artificial intelligence, nine articles utilized blockchain, and so on.

Table 2. Matrix of the emerging technologies used in the following research studies.

Article	Emerging Technologies							
	Big Data	Artificial Intelligence	Blockchain	IoT-FoT	Cloud-Based	NIC	5G	Others
A1		✓	✓	✓			✓	✓
A4			✓					
A5	✓	✓						
A6		✓		✓				
A7				✓				
A8				✓	✓			
A9			✓					
A10			✓					
A11			✓	✓				
A12			✓		✓			✓
A13			✓	✓				
A14	✓	✓				✓		
A15				✓				
A16			✓					
Σ	2	4	9	6	2	1	1	2

Table 3. A concise overview of the capabilities of different emerging techniques in managing and monitoring the pandemic spread.

Techniques	Hybrid System Features				
	Tracking	Data Privacy	Communication	Contact Tracing	Medication
Big Data	✓		✓		
IoT-FoT	✓		✓	✓	
AI	✓			✓	✓
Blockchain		✓	✓	✓	✓
Cloud-based			✓		
NIC		✓		✓	
5G		✓	✓		
∑	3	3	5	4	2

Table 3 provides a concise summary of the technologies' presence, allowing for comparisons and observations regarding the trends and patterns in their application. This summary also allows for a quick overview of the prevalence and distribution of the emerging technologies among the reviewed studies.

The purpose of this matrix is to assess and compare different techniques in terms of their capabilities for managing and monitoring the spread of a pandemic. Tables 1 and 2 illustrate the emerging techniques that provide features for managing and monitoring the spread of the pandemic. Table 3 evaluates various techniques, including big data, IoT-FoT, AI, and blockchain, based on their capabilities in different aspects of a hybrid system for pandemic management. The evaluated features of the hybrid system, including big data, IoT-FoT, and AI, are capable of tracking. For data privacy techniques, such as blockchain, NIC, and 5G, these features are identified. The communication feature is facilitated by using the techniques of big data, IoT-FoT, blockchain, cloud-based solutions. The techniques that enable contact tracing, a critical aspect of pandemic management, are IoT-FoT, AI, blockchain, and NIC.

This quick comparison of these techniques based on their specific features aids researchers and practitioners in understanding the strengths and limitations of each technique within the context of a hybrid system for pandemic management.

3.4. Graphical Representation

Figure 2 provides a comparison and evaluation of the technologies based on their performance across the different functions. It also presents a comprehensive overview of how the emerging technologies align with the desired features of the evaluated systems, highlighting areas of strength and potential areas for improvement or further exploration. Overall, Figure 2 serves as a visual summary of the relationship between emerging technologies and the functions of the evaluated systems, facilitating a better understanding of the strengths and weaknesses of each technology in the context of specific research.

Figure 3 represents different emerging technologies and represents the number of research papers that have employed each technology. Each technology is represented by a colored bar, and the height of the bar indicates the frequency or number of research papers that have utilized that technology. In Figure 3, the taller the bar, the greater the number of technologies employed in that article, such as in Article 1. The summary of the graph includes insights such as which technologies have been widely adopted in the analyzed research studies, indicating their relevance and potential impact in the context of the studied area. It also highlights the technologies that are less prevalent or have been underutilized, suggesting potential opportunities for further research and exploration.

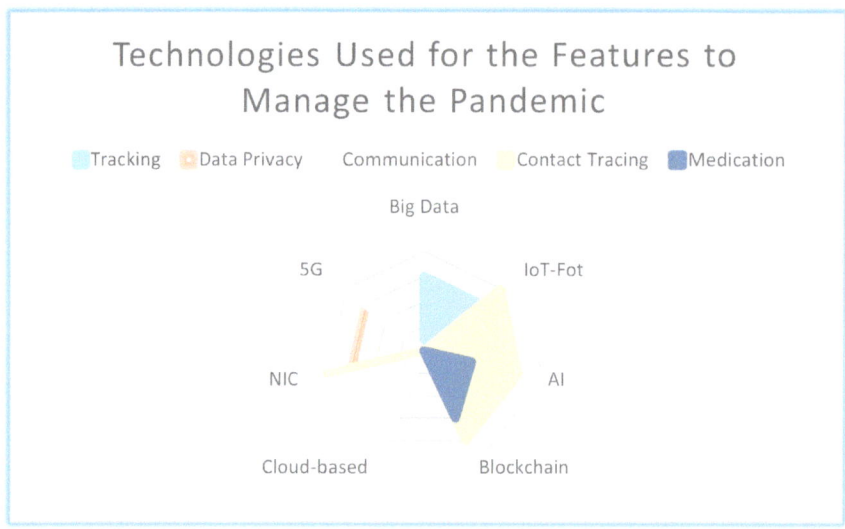

Figure 2. Illustrates a comparison of the emerging technologies used for the features to manage the pandemic.

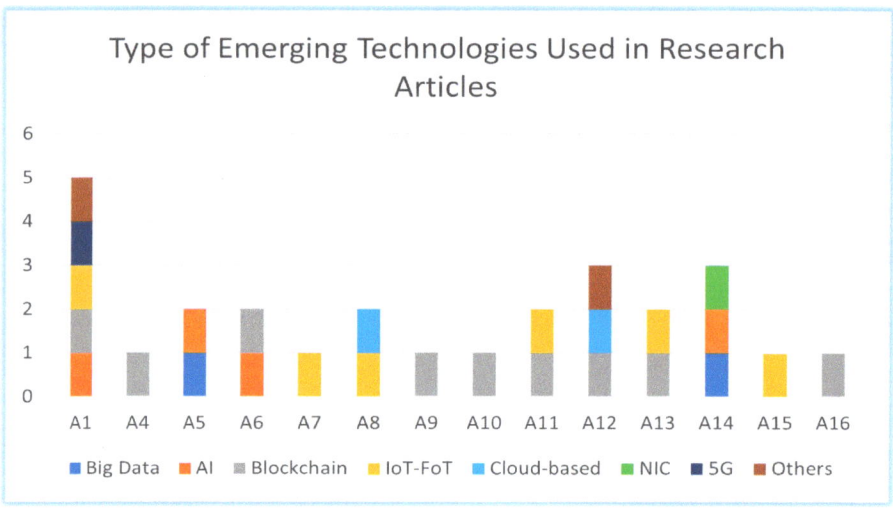

Figure 3. Illustrates the type of emerging technologies used in each research article.

4. Proposed Model

The proposed hybrid system is called hybrid disease prevention, monitoring, and management system (HDPMMS). This hybrid system, which combines emerging technologies, including blockchain, IoT, big data, and AI, provides a comprehensive solution for disease prevention, monitoring, and management (see Figure 4). The HDPMMS aims to address the challenges posed by infectious diseases by leveraging the capabilities of these technologies.

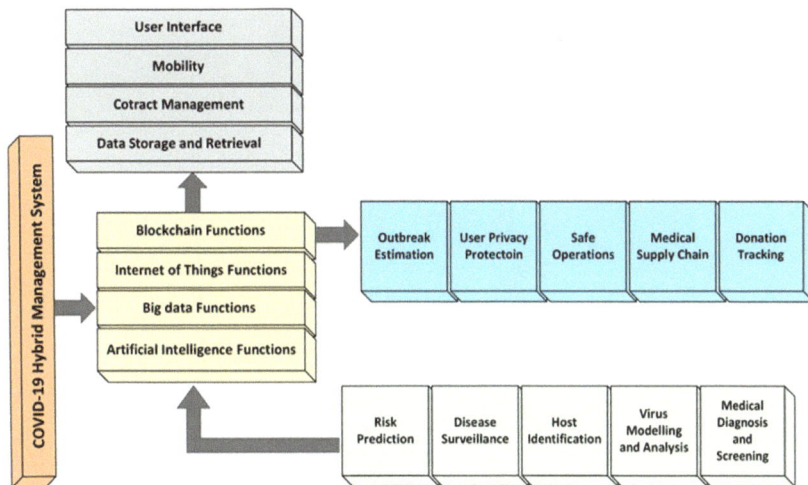

Figure 4. Proposed model based on blockchain, IoT, big data, and AI to provide the most comprehensive solution to infectious diseases.

4.1. The Key Components of the HDPMMS

Blockchain-based secure contact tracing and source isolation: The HDPMMS utilizes blockchain technology to enable secure and transparent contact tracing. It ensures that the transmission of infections can be effectively tracked, and source isolation can be implemented securely. By leveraging the decentralized nature of blockchain, the system enhances data privacy and security, reducing the risk of unauthorized access and tampering.

Integration of IoT sensors for real-time data collection: IoT sensors are integrated into the HDPMMS to collect real-time data on vital health parameters. These sensors can monitor various physiological indicators, such as body temperature, heart rate, and respiratory rate. The continuous data collection allows for the early detection of potential outbreaks and enables proactive interventions.

Big data analytics for data-driven insights: The HDPMMS incorporates big data analytic techniques to analyze the collected data from IoT sensors and other sources. Through data preprocessing, cleaning, and analysis, the system can derive meaningful insights and identify patterns related to disease dynamics. This enables researchers and healthcare professionals to make informed decisions and develop data-driven strategies for disease prevention and control.

AI for symptom identification and drug manufacturing support: The HDPMMS employs AI algorithms to support symptom identification and drug manufacturing. AI algorithms can analyze vast amounts of patient data and medical records, identifying patterns and symptoms associated with specific diseases. This aids in early detection, accurate diagnosis, and timely interventions. AI can also assist in drug-manufacturing processes, such as predicting the efficacy of potential therapeutics and optimizing drug development.

The HDPMMS represents a proactive approach to disease prevention and monitoring by integrating the power of blockchain, IoT, big data, and AI technologies. By combining these technologies, the system aims to provide real-time insights, secure contact tracing, early detection of outbreaks, and support for effective drug development. The HDPMMS has the potential to revolutionize disease control strategies, enabling timely interventions and proactive measures to combat the ongoing pandemic and future global health threats.

4.2. The Key Functions of the HDPMMS

The hybrid disease prevention, monitoring, and management system incorporates various functions to effectively address disease prevention and monitoring. Secure contact tracing: The HDPMMS utilizes blockchain technology to enable secure contact tracing. It allows for the recording and tracking of individuals' interactions, ensuring that the transmission of infectious diseases can be effectively monitored and traced. The decentralized and tamper-resistant nature of the blockchain ensures data integrity and privacy.

Source isolation: The HDPMMS facilitates source isolation by identifying and isolating the origin of the infection. By leveraging blockchain technology, the system can securely track the source of infection and prevent further spreading. This function is crucial in containing outbreaks and minimizing the impact of infectious diseases.

Real-time data collection: The HDPMMS integrates IoT sensors to collect real-time data on vital health parameters. These sensors monitor individuals' physiological indicators, such as body temperature, heart rate, and respiratory rate. Continuous data collection enables the early detection of potential outbreaks and provides real-time insights into individuals' health conditions.

Data analytics and insights: The HDPMMS incorporates big data analytic techniques to analyze the collected data. Through data preprocessing, cleaning, and analysis, the system derives meaningful insights and identifies patterns related to disease dynamics. This function enables healthcare professionals and researchers to make informed decisions, develop data-driven strategies, and allocate resources effectively for disease prevention and control.

Symptom identification: The HDPMMS employs AI algorithms to identify symptoms associated with infectious diseases. By analyzing vast amounts of patient data and medical records, AI algorithms can detect patterns and identify specific symptoms indicative of diseases. This function aids in early detection, accurate diagnosis, and timely interventions.

Drug-manufacturing support: The HDPMMS utilizes AI to support drug-manufacturing processes. AI algorithms can analyze molecular structures, predict the efficacy of potential therapeutics, and optimize drug development. This function enables researchers and pharmaceutical companies to expedite the drug discovery and development process, thus leading to more effective treatments for infectious diseases.

Overall, the HDPMMS combines secure contact tracing, source isolation, real-time data collection, data analytics, symptom identification, and drug-manufacturing support to provide a comprehensive approach to disease prevention and monitoring. By leveraging the emerging technologies, the HDPMMS aims to enhance early detection, proactive interventions, and effective response strategies, ultimately mitigating the impact of infectious diseases on a global scale.

5. Results

Implementing the HDPMMS framework can enhance disease surveillance capabilities by enabling real-time data collection and analysis. The integration of IoT sensors and the utilization of big data analytics allow for the early detection of outbreaks, prompt response to emerging threats, and accurate monitoring of disease trends. This leads to more effective disease surveillance and better-informed decision-making.

Improved contact tracing and source isolation: The HDPMMS's secure contact-tracing function through blockchain technology enables the efficient and transparent tracking of individuals' interactions. By accurately identifying and isolating the source of the infection, the system helps to contain the spread of infectious diseases more effectively. This capability minimizes the risk of further transmission and contributes to the overall control of outbreaks.

Timely symptom identification and diagnosis: The integration of AI algorithms in the HDPMMS enables timely and accurate symptom identification. By analyzing patients' data and medical records, the system can detect specific symptoms associated with infectious diseases, allowing for early diagnosis and appropriate treatment. This leads to improved patient outcomes and facilitates the implementation of targeted interventions.

Facilitated drug-manufacturing and development process: The HDPMMS's AI-driven drug-manufacturing support function streamlines the drug discovery and development process. By leveraging AI algorithms to analyze molecular structures and predict drug efficacy, researchers and pharmaceutical companies can expedite the development of effective therapeutics. This accelerates the availability of treatments and improves the overall management of infectious diseases.

Proactive and data-driven decision-making process: The HDPMMS provides decision-makers with data-driven insights and actionable information. By utilizing big data analytics, the system generates meaningful insights and patterns related to disease dynamics. This empowers healthcare professionals, policymakers, and researchers to make proactive decisions, allocate resources efficiently, and implement targeted interventions to prevent and control the spread of infectious diseases.

The implementation of the HDPMMS results in improved disease surveillance, efficient contact tracing and source isolation, timely symptom identification, facilitated drug manufacturing, and proactive decision-making. These outcomes contribute to the overall effectiveness of disease prevention and monitoring efforts, helping to mitigate the impact of infectious diseases and safeguard public health.

6. Conclusions

In conclusion, the HDPMMS presents a comprehensive and innovative approach to address the challenges posed by infectious diseases. By integrating blockchain, IoT, big data analytics, and AI, the HDPMMS offers a holistic solution for disease prevention and monitoring. Through the implementation of the HDPMMS, several key benefits can be achieved. The system enables secure contact tracing and source isolation, ensuring the effective control of disease transmission. Real-time data collection from IoT sensors facilitates the early detection of outbreaks and provides valuable insights into individuals' health conditions. The application of big data analytics allows for data-driven decision-making, enhancing disease surveillance and response strategies. Additionally, AI supports symptom identification and drug manufacturing, improving diagnosis and facilitating the development of effective therapeutics.

The HDPMMS emphasizes proactive measures and preventive solutions, rather than over-reliance on treatments and cures. By leveraging emerging technologies, the system empowers healthcare professionals, researchers, and policymakers to take prompt actions, allocate resources efficiently, and implement targeted interventions to mitigate the impact of infectious diseases.

The HDPMMS has the potential to revolutionize disease prevention and monitoring strategies, leading to improved public health outcomes. However, it is important to acknowledge that the implementation of such a hybrid system requires the careful consideration of ethical, legal, and privacy implications. Collaboration among various stakeholders, including healthcare organizations, technology providers, and regulatory bodies, is crucial to ensure the responsible and effective deployment of the HDPMMS.

Henceforth, further research and development are needed to refine the HDPMMS and optimize its performance. Continued advancements in technology, data management, and algorithmic capabilities will contribute to the ongoing evolution of this hybrid system. By harnessing the power of emerging technologies, the HDPMMS offers promising prospects for addressing the ongoing pandemic and future global health threats, ultimately improving the health and well-being of populations worldwide.

Funding: This research received no external funding.

Institutional Review Board Statement: Not applicable.

Informed Consent Statement: Not applicable.

Data Availability Statement: Not applicable.

Conflicts of Interest: The author declares no conflict of interest.

Abbreviations

The following abbreviations are used in this manuscript:

AI	Artificial Intelligence
DCNN	Deep Convolutional Neural Network
DNNs	Deep Neural Networks
FDA	Food and Drug Administration
DL	Deep Learning
ML	Machine Learning
VGG	Visual Geometry Group
COVID-19	Coronavirus Disease 2019
IoT	Internet of Things
WHO	World Health Organization
NLP	Natural Language Processing
NIC	Network and Information Center
5G	Fifth Generation (Wireless Technology)
FOT	Fog of Things
VANETs	Vehicular Ad Hoc Networks
HDPMMS	Hybrid Disease Prevention, Monitoring, and Management System

References

1. Chamola, V.; Hassija, V.; Gupta, V.; Guizani, M. A Comprehensive Review of the COVID-19 Pandemic and the Role of IoT, Drones, AI, Blockchain, and 5G in Managing Its Impact. *IEEE Access* **2020**, *8*, 90225–90265. [CrossRef]
2. Wong, A.Y.; Ling, S.K.; Louie, L.H.; Law, G.Y.; So, R.C.; Lee, D.C.; Yau, F.C.; Yung, P.S. Impact of the COVID-19 Pandemic on Sports and Exercise. *Asia Pac. J. Sports Med. Arthrosc. Rehabil. Technol.* **2020**, *22*, 39–44. [CrossRef]
3. Shrestha, N.; Shad, M.Y.; Ulvi, O.; Khan, M.H.; Karamehic-Muratovic, A.; Nguyen, U.S.D.; Baghbanzadeh, M.; Wardrup, R.; Aghamohammadi, N.; Cervantes, D.; et al. The Impact of COVID-19 on Globalization. *One Health* **2020**, *11*, 100180. [CrossRef]
4. Klaine, P.V.; Zhang, L.; Zhou, B.; Sun, Y.; Xu, H.; Imran, M. Privacy-Preserving Contact Tracing and Public Risk Assessment Using Blockchain for COVID-19 Pandemic. *IEEE Internet Things Mag.* **2020**, *3*, 58–63. [CrossRef]
5. Bragazzi, N.L.; Dai, H.; Damiani, G.; Behzadifar, M.; Martini, M.; Wu, J. How Big Data and Artificial Intelligence Can Help Better Manage the COVID-19 Pandemic. *Int. J. Environ. Res. Public Health* **2020**, *17*, 3176. [CrossRef] [PubMed]
6. Nguyen, D.; Ding, M.; Pathirana, P.N.; Seneviratne, A. Blockchain and AI-Based Solutions to Combat Coronavirus (COVID-19)-Like Epidemics: A survey. *IEEE Access* **2021**, *9*, 95730–95753. [CrossRef]
7. Kumar, M.; Nayar, N.; Mehta, G.; Sharma, A. Application of IoT in Current Pandemic of COVID-19. *IOP Conf. Ser. Mater. Sci. Eng.* **2021**, *1022*, 012063. [CrossRef]
8. Kumar, S.; Raut, R.D.; Narkhede, B.E. A Proposed Collaborative Framework by Using Artificial Intelligence-Internet of Things (AI-IoT) in COVID-19 Pandemic Situation for Healthcare Workers. *Int. J. Healthc. Manag.* **2020**, *13*, 337–345. [CrossRef]
9. Marbouh, D.; Abbasi, T.; Maasmi, F.; Omar, I.; Debe, M.; Salah, K.; Jayaraman, R.; Ellahham, S. Blockchain for COVID-19: Review, Opportunities, and a Trusted Tracking System. *Arab. J. Sci. Eng.* **2020**, *45*, 49–50. [CrossRef] [PubMed]
10. Song, J.; Gu, T.; Fang, Z.; Feng, X.; Ge, Y.; Fu, H.; Hu, P.; Mohapatra, P. Blockchain Meets COVID-19: A Framework for Contact Information Sharing and Risk Notification System. In Proceedings of the 2021 IEEE 18th International Conference on Mobile Ad Hoc and Smart Systems (MASS), Denver, CO, USA, 4–7 October 2021; pp. 269–277. [CrossRef]
11. Tewari, N.; Kumar, R.; Joshi, M.; Budhani, S. A Blockchain and FOT (Fog of Things) Based Framework and Technique for Anticipating an Infectious Illness Sent by a Harmful Respiratory Infection. In Proceedings of the 2021 10th International Conference on System Modeling & Advancement in Research Trends (SMART), Moradabad, India, 10–11 December 2021; pp. 368–372. [CrossRef]
12. Tan, H.; Kim, P.; Chung, I. Practical Homomorphic Authentication in Cloud-Assisted VANETs with Blockchain-Based Healthcare Monitoring for Pandemic Control. *Electronics* **2020**, *9*, 1683. [CrossRef]
13. Zhang, J.; Wu, M. Blockchain Use in IoT for Privacy-Preserving Anti-Pandemic Home Quarantine. *Electronics* **2020**, *9*, 1746. [CrossRef]
14. Agbehadji, I.E.; Awuzie, B.O.; Ngowi, A.B.; Millham, R.C. Review of Big Data Analytics, Artificial Intelligence and Nature-Inspired Computing Models towards Accurate Detection of COVID-19 Pandemic Cases and Contact Tracing. *Int. J. Environ. Res. Public Health* **2020**, *17*, 5330. [CrossRef] [PubMed]
15. Ramallo-González, A.P.; González-Vidal, A.; Skarmeta, A.F. CIoTVID: Towards an Open IoT-Platform for Infective Pandemic Diseases such as COVID-19. *Sensors* **2021**, *21*, 484. [CrossRef] [PubMed]

16. Xu, H.; Zhang, L.; Onireti, O.; Fang, Y.; Buchanan, W.J.; Imran, M.A. BeepTrace: Blockchain-Enabled Privacy-Preserving Contact Tracing for COVID-19 Pandemic and Beyond. *IEEE Internet Things J.* **2021**, *8*, 3915–3929. [CrossRef]
17. Ferreti, L.; Wymant, C.; Kendall, M.; Zhao, L.; Nurtay, A.; Abeler-Dörner, L.; Parker, M.; Bonsall, D.; Fraser, C. Quantifying SARS-CoV-2 Transmission Suggests Epidemic Control with Digital Contact Tracing. *Science* **2020**, *368*, eabb6936. [CrossRef] [PubMed]
18. Topol, E.J. High-performance medicine: The convergence of human and artificial intelligence. *Nat. Med.* **2019**, *25*, 44–56. [CrossRef] [PubMed]
19. Deebak, B.D.; Al-Turjman, F. EEI-IoT: Edge-Enabled Intelligent IoT Framework for Early Detection of COVID-19 Threats. *Sensors* **2023**, *23*, 2995. [CrossRef] [PubMed]
20. Hamid, S.; Bawany, N.Z.; Sodhro, A.H.; Lakhan, A.; Ahmed, S. A Systematic Review and IoMT Based Big Data Framework for COVID-19 Prevention and Detection. *Electronics* **2022**, *11*, 2777. [CrossRef]
21. Sanida, T.; Tabakis, I.M.; Sanida, M.V.; Sideris, A.; Dasygenis, M. A Robust Hybrid Deep Convolutional Neural Network for COVID-19 Disease Identification from Chest X-ray Images. *Information* **2023**, *14*, 310. [CrossRef]
22. Dubey, A.K.; Chabert, G.L.; Carriero, A.; Pasche, A.; Danna, P.S.; Agarwal, S.; Mohanty, L.; Nillmani Sharma, N.; Yadav, S.; Jain, A. Ensemble Deep Learning Derived from Transfer Learning for Classification of COVID-19 Patients on Hybrid Deep-Learning-Based Lung Segmentation: A Data Augmentation and Balancing Framework. *Diagnostics* **2023**, *13*, 1954. [CrossRef] [PubMed]

Disclaimer/Publisher's Note: The statements, opinions and data contained in all publications are solely those of the individual author(s) and contributor(s) and not of MDPI and/or the editor(s). MDPI and/or the editor(s) disclaim responsibility for any injury to people or property resulting from any ideas, methods, instructions or products referred to in the content.

MDPI AG
Grosspeteranlage 5
4052 Basel
Switzerland
Tel.: +41 61 683 77 34

Diagnostics Editorial Office
E-mail: diagnostics@mdpi.com
www.mdpi.com/journal/diagnostics

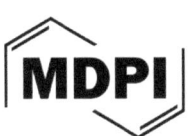

Disclaimer/Publisher's Note: The title and front matter of this reprint are at the discretion of the Guest Editors. The publisher is not responsible for their content or any associated concerns. The statements, opinions and data contained in all individual articles are solely those of the individual Editors and contributors and not of MDPI. MDPI disclaims responsibility for any injury to people or property resulting from any ideas, methods, instructions or products referred to in the content.

www.ingramcontent.com/pod-product-compliance
Lightning Source LLC
LaVergne TN
LVHW072319090526
838202LV00019B/2312